Menopause is one of the most loaded words in a woman's vocabulary, conjuring up, as it does, visions of a neurotic, dried-up, rapidly ageing woman struggling with uncontrollable hot flushes, a spreading waistline, mood swings, brittle bones, a softening mind and the threat of a host of dread diseases waiting to take over an increasingly fragile body.

In this meticulously researched, reader-friendly book, approved by a number of medical experts, Nicole Jaff gives short shrift to the traditional image of the menopausal woman, dispels many of the myths surrounding this stage of a woman's life, tackles the controversial issue of hormone replacement therapy sensibly and tactfully offers valuable advice for getting through an often trying time.

Her theme is 'knowledge is power' and she aims to provide her readers with enough practical information to enable them to work with the professionals; to participate sensibly in decisions about treatment; and to look on menopause not as the beginning of the end of a useful life but as the start of a new phase in which women can take charge of themselves as women and spend the rest of their lives 'living authentically with humour, vitality, wisdom and wit'.

When an unnecessary hysterectomy plunged **Nicole Jaff** into premature menopause, she was prompted to research the subject of menopause in depth. This set her on the path to menopause consultancy, helping women to avoid the same mistakes by arming them with the information they need to make informed decisions about their health. She lives with her husband Nicholas and has two daughters, Sophie and Elizabeth.

Praise for *Menopause Today*:

'Nicole Jaff has braved the highways of conflicting information about hormone replacement therapies to bring us a new updated edition of *Menopause Today*. Jaff, who is not a medical doctor, has read widely, carefully and analytically on her subject. She has also consulted with specialists in the medical profession. Her book goes a long way to cutting through the mumbo jumbo of myth and fear that has accumulated around the 'change'. She does not claim to have all the answers and she asks her readers to ask questions of their doctors. Most importantly, Jaff lays the responsibility of women's bodies squarely at the feet of women themselves. She inspires readers to approach their health with diligence and intelligence. She knows that this is not always easy; her understanding is both psychological and physical. Women who are at this stage of their lives owe it to themselves to read this book.'

– Maureen Isaacson, *Sunday Independent* Books Editor

'My computer tells me that this is the 100th book that I have reviewed over the past years. It is the best written with the most clear English of any that I have received.'

– John McGarry, *Journal of the British Menopause Society*

'*Menopause Today* is essential reading not only for those women approaching the menopause but also for those who have experienced the menopause and who want clarity of the changes that occurred during this inevitable period in their lives. A must read.'

– Professor Derick Raal, Head of Endocrinology, University of the Witwatersrand

'Menopause is a natural process for a woman and not an illness, yet so many women dread its onset, fearing it to be a time fraught with anxiety and emotion. Nicole Jaff's knowledge of the processes of peri- and postmenopause, coupled with her innate understanding of a woman's psyche, make her ideal to address this commonly misunderstood female health issue. Nicole has tremendous empathy for helping women understand what is happening to them during menopause and her empowering approach to wellness means women walk away from her talks knowing and believing menopause can be a positive time of vibrant health and happiness.'

– Frith Thomas, editor of *Women&Home* magazine SA

'Jaff's research is thorough and the book is cleverly put together ... *Menopause Today* will enable you to understand this phase of your life as a middle-aged woman and to prepare for it.'

– *Die Burger*

'The author takes the reader on a brief – and riveting – history of Hormone Replacement Therapy and how the whole topic has turned on its head in recent years ... Her key message in the book, which strives to be non-judgemental about the unique choices which women make during their menopausal years, is that every woman is different.'

– *The Witness*

'Nicole Jaff supports the view that knowledge is power and she's assembled a practical, well-researched book that hones in on this significant period in a woman's life. Figuring out the ins-and-outs of hormone fluctuations is mostly a daunting challenge for the layperson, and she tackles the topics in a very accessible, down-to-earth way.'

– *Cape Times*

'Nicole Jaff, the menopause consultant, really was amazing. All of a sudden, I realised that this gorgeous vibrant woman was in the same stage of her life as myself and looked great despite the cursed menopause. Not only was her talk inspiring and amusing, but it helped one realise that the symptoms are varied and instead of thinking one is crazy, we don't have to suffer unnecessarily. Individuals are all different and we need different remedies to get back on track.'

– Colleen Theakstone, after a *Women&Home* Menopause Workshop

---

'I cannot describe the wonderful feeling I left with KNOWING finally that I was not alone in feeling all the strange feelings and experiencing the debilitating and confusing stage of life – menopause!'

– Beverley Flis, *FairLady* reader

'Nicole Jaff's talk was informative and most interesting and many of the women present left feeling so much happier that they were not alone. [She] opened our eyes to the true facts of menopause and left us feeling more equipped to deal with the years ahead.'

– Linda Nathan, chairman, Durban Branch UJW

'Thanks for such a WONDERFUL book. What an absolute relief to find a source containing the plain truth ... After reading your book, I certainly feel more empowered to deal with this phase in my life! I keep your book handy and refer to it often.'

– Andrea Matthewson

'Nicole Jaff's book is a user-friendly, comprehensive guide that covers the issues that concern women during the peri and postmenopausal years and shows them how to live healthy, and fulfilled lives after menopause. *Menopause Today* provides readers with practical information which will help them to work with their healthcare professionals and to participate knowledgeably and sensibly in decisions about their own treatment and health ... I heartily recommend Nicole Jaff's presentation on *Menopause Today*. It is a must for every woman and for men as well.'

– Hazel Cohen, director, RCHCC

'I heartily endorse Nicole's presentation and material and hope that she may impact many, many more women's lives.'

Yvonne Wilson

'This book is recommended by the South African Menopause Society (SAMS). It is a comprehensive, thoroughly researched and user-friendly guide that will empower menopausal women to make informed decisions about managing menopause in conjunction with their healthcare provider.'

Menopause

The **Complete** Guide

REVISED EDITION

NICOLE JAFF

PENGUIN BOOKS

Published by the Penguin Group
Penguin Books (South Africa) (Pty) Ltd, 24 Sturdee Avenue, Rosebank,
Johannesburg 2196, South Africa
Penguin Group (USA) Inc, 375 Hudson Street, New York, New York 10014,
USA
Penguin Group (Canada), 90 Eglinton Avenue East, Suite 700, Toronto,
Ontario, Canada M4P 2Y3 (a division of Pearson Penguin Canada Inc)
Penguin Books Ltd, 80 Strand, London WC2R 0RL, England
Penguin Ireland, 25 St Stephen's Green, Dublin 2, Ireland (a division of
Penguin Books Ltd)
Penguin Group (Australia), 250 Camberwell Road, Camberwell, Victoria 3124,
Australia (a division of Pearson Australia Group Pty Ltd)
Penguin Books India Pvt Ltd, 11 Community Centre, Panchsheel Park, New
Delhi – 110 017, India
Penguin Group (NZ), 67 Apollo Drive, Mairangi Bay, Auckland 1310, New
Zealand (a division of Pearson New Zealand Ltd)

Penguin Books (South Africa) (Pty) Ltd, Registered Offices:
24 Sturdee Avenue, Rosebank, Johannesburg 2196, South Africa

www.penguinbooks.co.za

First published by Penguin Books (South Africa) (Pty) Ltd 2008

Text copyright © Nicole Jaff 2008

ISBN 978 0 143 02575 7

Typeset by Compleat
Cover photograph: Patrick Toselli
Cover design: Mr Design
Printed and bound by Pinetown Printers, KwaZulu-Natal

For my family, Nicholas, Sophie and Elizabeth, for their unwavering love and support. And to my mother, Joan Bernitz, who showed me a wider world.

CONTENTS

Acknowledgements

Both editions of this book could not have come into being without the help and dedication of a host of medical experts. With humour and endless patience, Dr Merwyn Jacobson, medical director of Vitalab, Centre for Assisted Conception, gave huge amounts of his time to helping and encouraging me; teaching me about the intricacies of the female reproductive system and guiding me around the many pitfalls of trying to explain the complex process of menopause. He forced me to pay minute attention to detail and curbed my tendency to make sweeping statements. To him I owe the title of Chapter 5: 'If I shake you, will you rattle?'

Professor Derrick Raal, the director of the Carbohydrate & Lipid Metabolism Research Unit and professor and head of the Division of Endocrinology and Metabolism at the University of the Witwatersrand, took time out of his very busy life to explain to me, using wonderful metaphors, the medical mechanics of the endocrine system, cardiovascular disease and diabetes. Consistently helpful and considerate, he never failed to return my calls and answer my queries, even late at night.

Other professionals who gave me the benefit of their expertise and offered invaluable help and advice were: Dr Carol-Ann Benn, senior consultant at Chris Hani Baragwanath Hospital, lecturer in the department of surgery at the Faculty of Health Sciences, University of the Witwatersrand, and national director of Netcare Breast Care, Centre of Excellence; Ria Buys, registered dietician; Dr Susan Brown, Faculty of Health Sciences at the University of the Witwatersrand; Prof Linda Cardozo, King's College Hospital in London, professor of urogynaecology and consultant gynaecologist; Dr Dimitri Constantinou, the director of the Centre for Exercise and Sports Management, Faculty of Health Sciences at the University of the Witwatersrand; Dr Paul Dalmeyer, reproductive specialist; Dr Michael Davey, gynaecologist, founder member and president of the South African Meno-pause Society; Dr Jenny Edge, surgeon at the Christiaan Bar-nard Memorial Hospital in Cape Town; Dr Gereth Edwards, plastic and reconstructive surgeon; Dr Gillian Keast, friend and general practitioner; Dr Gary Levy, dermatologist; Dr Stanley Lipschitz, specialist physician and specialist geri-atrician; Dr Joanne Miller, ophthalmologist; Ms Shira Moch, part-time lecturer in the department of pharamacology at the Faculty of Health Sciences, University of the Witwatersrand; Dr Naomi Rapeport, specialist physician; Dr Kogie Reddi, pathologist, Lancet Laboratories; Dr Russell Seider, director of screening and diagnostic mammography at the Oxford Road Institute for Mammography and Bone Densitometry; Dr Trudy Smith, principal specialist and senior lecturer in the department of obstetrics and gynaecology, Johannesburg Hospital and University of the Witwatersrand; Dr Michael Suzman, clinical assistant in surgery at the Weill Medical College of Cornell University and director of plastic surgery at Westchester Medical Group, White Plains, New York; Dr Susan Tager, clinical head of neurology at the Wits Univer-sity Donald Gordon Medical Centre; Anne Till, registered dietician and director of Anne Till & Associates; Professor Lizette van Rensburg, professor of human genetics and cancer genetics at the University of Pretoria.

Any errors are mine alone.

Introduction to the revised edition

In the introduction to the first edition of *Menopause Today* I wrote that 'knowledge is power', believing then, as I do now, that once a woman is armed with the correct information, the visit to the doctor's office will be less traumatic and she won't be 'bullied' into making a decision which might prove to be wrong for her.

I wrote the book so that women would not suffer as I did when I experienced an abrupt surgical menopause without adequate knowledge or understanding the consequences of the procedure. This book is intended for all women battling through the perimenopause as well as those who have finally reached menopause, and are overwhelmed by the huge amounts of information with which they are bombarded by the media and the Internet. My intention is to help them understand the way their body works during this very important time of their lives so they can approach menopause without fear, in the knowledge that it is not a disease, but the start of a time of life that can be lived energetically and happily.

It is vital for women to work in partnership with their healthcare practitioners and not leave their doctor's office feeling confused and anxious. I address their fears that on the one hand, they face a future of crumbling bones, disease and dementia; that they will live out their lives, sexless and worthless unless they start a regimen of hormone therapy (HT), and on the other, that they are placing themselves at risk for cancers, stroke and heart disease if they do decide to use HT to alleviate the symptoms of menopause, like night sweats and hot flushes, that are affecting their quality of life. I believe that menopause is a time of balance, and if we take responsibility for our health we will be just fine.

The response to the first edition of this book was both humbling and heartening – women read it carefully, discussed it with their doctors, shared it with their friends, kept it next to their beds, and gave it to their mothers. They consulted it to answer the numerous questions that arose in their daily lives in relation to peri- and postmenopause.

Equally gratifying were the doctors' responses. Far from objecting to a non-medical person writing about this subject, they were enormously receptive. Many of them congratulated me, reviewed the book with insight and generosity, and kept it in their consulting rooms, where they recommended it to their patients. Now I frequently find myself sharing a platform or conducting workshops with these doctors. I am invited to address their congresses, which I do with some trepidation, but always with a sense that in discussing the troublesome issues surrounding the contentious subject of menopause, I may be helping other women.

I am very grateful to have been given this forum; to be able to assure women that there is someone in their corner who will ask the questions and attempt to find the answers that will help them. But as I wrote originally, menopause is a vast subject, the research is constantly changing, and opinions surrounding it are forceful and diverse.

In the three years since the first edition of *Menopause Today* was published, new research has emerged which has made it imperative to update the book. There have been exciting developments in diagnosing and treating breast cancer and new research on genetic testing. Treatments have become available for osteoporosis which are more sophisticated and easier to use. Problematic areas have emerged which should be addressed and women must be made of aware of the new choices available to them.

What has not changed is that menopause comes at a complicated time of life for many women, their bodies are aging, their lives are changing, and they are bombarded with conflicting advice because they live in a world which has identified and targeted them as a lucrative market. The information derived from the Women's Health Initiative (WHI), which acted as a huge catalyst in the pharmaceutical industry because it turned so much conventional wisdom about hormone therapy upside down, has not convinced many doctors that they should practice evidence-based medicine. They are still sceptical about the results of the WHI and some continue to prescribe HT to all women instead of assessing each individual case.

I am also concerned about a new trend that is emerging which mirrors the attitude of Dr Robert Wilson, whom I write about in Chapter 3. This movement suggests that menopausal women, with few exceptions, should be on HT at all costs; that they need HT to live happy productive lives even if they don't have symptoms. This is in spite of the fact that the position of the most prominent menopause societies is that women should only take HT for severe menopause symptoms that compromise their quality of life or for prevention of bone loss in women with premature menopause.

In addition, many doctors do not fully explain the risks and benefits of HT to their patients, despite the research, nor do they regard their patients as individuals who should be carefully informed before they use HT. Equally worrying is the increase in the number of doctors using bioidentical hormones that have not been approved by the various medical regulatory bodies in different countries. There is a disquieting tendency for these healthcare practitioners to prescribe HT as 'anti-ageing' medicine, so that many women find themselves spending large amounts of money on a cocktail of hormones that they have been told will keep them young, sexy and disease free; claims that are not based on rigorous research. Middle-aged women still fear ageing and our society continues to value youth and beauty above age and experience, which feeds into the promises of many unscrupulous people who sell these so-called anti-ageing hormones to menopausal women as magic bullets.

This book should be a tool for peri- and postmenopausal women who are not afraid of ageing and accept that we are genetically programmed to age; women who want to age as healthily as possible in the final third of their lives, so that their menopausal years are good ones. It is a book for women who want to take responsibility for their health and who are wary of being sold treatments which may benefit the seller more than the buyer. It is for women who believe they have the right to current information which will inform their choices and the decisions they will make about their health in menopause. It is for women who believe they are in partnership with their doctors. It is for all women who believe that menopause is not an ending but the beginning of some of the best years of their lives.

Introduction to the first edition

It was very disconcerting. There I was at an international menopause conference, surrounded by experts from the United States, Europe, the United Kingdom and South Africa, all of them in conflict about the benefits and risks of hormone replacement therapy (HRT). The divergent views assailing me from all sides left me bewildered and anxious.

Each expert had a different perspective on the absolute and relative risks of HRT and, at times, the debate grew acrimonious as the attitudes of the different menopause societies became apparent. There was endless and heated discussion, examination of the data and arguments about whether or not menopausal women should use HRT. Even more scary and confusing were the comments from the audience of doctors and gynaecologists, who appeared to listen only to the parts of the debate they wanted to hear. After hours of lectures on the subject I couldn't imagine how an average woman with no access to medical resources, little or no experience in the field and who could only rely on her own doctor for information, must feel.

By the end of the first day of the conference my level of anxiety was intense. The more I heard, the less I understood. I couldn't clarify my thoughts and decide what would suit me, let alone all the women who were constantly asking me for advice on HRT. On reflection, it is extraordinary that we women are so dependent on the bias of those who are our caregivers, so many of whom are men. I found myself equally confused by the conservatives who overwhelmed me with significant statistics on the benefits of HRT and the alternative medicine practitioners and advocates of women's rights who told me to trust my inner guidance. In the first case, I find it very difficult to extrapolate from the statistics and make them apply to my own personal situation and in the latter I am not sure I want to depend on my inner guidance, which might be great when choosing a partner or friend, but isn't knowledgeable enough to tell me why something that has so many risks and benefits should be good or bad for my body in the long run. It seems a terrible risk to take.

I thought of all the headlines that have bombarded women over the past few years: `HRT use plunges as debate goes on', `Women urged to avoid HRT', `Facts haven't borne out concerns over HRT risks', `Cancer society advises against HRT', `HRT debate puts women in quandary', `Hormones might lower Alzheimer's risk', `Time to replace HRT says expert', `Breast cancer risks drop after hormones', `Stroke risk ends large HRT study', `HRT a big mistake says health body', `Firm busts may hide breast cancer'. Then, just as women decide that it's too risky to use HRT, they see an item on Sky TV stating: `107,000 women have stopped HRT unnecessarily'. They go to their doctors bearing this information. Instead of clarifying the situation the doctors spew out dozens of statistics aimed at showing women just how good it is for them to use HRT. There is also insidious advertising from the pharmaceutical companies, which seems to promise eternal youth; ardent testimonials from their friends and the suggestion from many caregivers that using HRT benefits hair and skin, making it appear more youthful. In addition, some practitioners suggest that estrogen may prevent memory loss and dementia. Are we then being irresponsible by refusing to take HRT? Will we feel `old' and `dried out' if we don't? Since we will spend at least a third of our lives in menopause will we be compromising the quality of those lives in the next 20 to 30 years if we aren't `compliant' and don't take HRT?

I realised that much of the confusion about menopause arises because women haven't time to sift through the huge volume of information available. If it is difficult for a busy gynaecologist with medical training to make sense of all the data, it is probably even more difficult for ordinary women to do so. I have at least 60 books on menopause, each with a different perspective. Among them are two books with the same title, *The Estrogen Alternative*, but they give totally contradictory advice. The subtitle of one is 'What every Woman Needs to Know about Hormone Replacement Therapy and SERMs, the New Estrogen Substitutes', while the other is subtitled 'Natural Hormone Therapy with Botanical Progesterone'. Which one should we believe?

The books in my library range from *The Good News about Women's Hormones* by Geoffrey Redmond MD to the bible on menopause, *The Wisdom of Menopause* by Dr Christiane Northrup. The former contains some 500 pages of impenetrable information. A paragraph on page 375, for instance, dealing with high cholesterol levels, enlightens readers with the following: `There is a dangerous interaction of these [cholesterol lowering] drugs with certain other medications, including antibiotic erythromycin, immunosuppressants such as cyclosporin, and two other drugs, nicotinic acid and gemfibrozil. All of these can cause a situation known as rhabdomyolisis …' The book by Northrup, who is a woman doctor who has spent many years actively caring for women in a concerned, knowledgeable and sympathetic fashion, is user-friendly and practical but densely written.

Many women coping with the stresses and angst of mid-life don't have the time to work through that amount of information to find out, once again, that they need to depend on that elusive inner guidance. `When it comes to hormone replacement therapy, the science we look to for answers is inconsistent … The blessing is that this dilemma forces us to tune in more fully to our inner wisdom, and to make our choices in full partnerships with our intuition and intellect,' writes Northrup. There are, of course, feminist-oriented books, like Leslie Kenton's *Passage to Power*, but these often leave women feeling guilty and inadequate, with a sense that they are somehow failing to create an exhaustingly healthy and spiritually aware life.

The Internet, with literally hundreds of thousands of sites of menopause information, can be very useful, but it takes hours to sift through these sites and without a sound knowledge base it is extremely difficult to know an expert opinion from a charlatan one, or to decipher medical writing, which is often obscure and ambiguous.

Menopause comes at a complicated time of life for women. While women's rights activists are quite correct when they say that menopause is not a disease, it happens when there are tremendous changes taking place in a woman's life and in her psyche. She is also acutely aware that her body is ageing and, depending on the society in which she finds herself, she often feels adrift, less useful and certainly less attractive than she used to be. I have talked to many women who are grappling with exhausting physical symptoms like hot flushes, mood swings, palpitations and memory loss at the same time as they are struggling with questions about their life choices. They feel less well, more tired, their weight seems to be skyrocketing and they are uncertain about their future.

Menopause is a field of research that is rapidly changing. We live in an environment where middle-aged women are an extremely important market element. Information directed at women is often biased and self-interested; busy doctors don't have time to read the latest research and are often bitterly divided among themselves and arrogant in their approach to women. These traits are not confined to male doctors; some of the most inflexible practitioners I have met are women.

Because there is so much complex, conflicting information about menopause and it is expressed in medical terminology that is difficult to understand, women are unable to ask pertinent questions or to decipher the answers so that they can make important decisions about their health. They often have a built-in conviction that in spite of the fact that they are paying for the consultation and have an inalienable right to understand their condition and make decisions which feel right for them, they are not really entitled to information. Even the most confident women are strangely diffident when questioning their doctors' opinions or asking them to clarify explanations and recommendations.

If women want to know more about menopause, they should be able to read about it in user-friendly language, which is informative and simple to understand. They should be comfortable discussing the latest research with their medical practitioners and they should be able to grasp the different options that are available to them, so that they are clear about their choices. They should feel empowered to make sensible decisions for themselves.

There are hundreds of books about menopause. Women have to wade through endless chapters on self-expression and power surges, and long explanations of why menopause is or is not a disease, before they can actually understand what is happening to their bodies. There seems to be so much mystery surrounding the process and terminology of menopause. I believe this is a hangover from the bad old days when women weren't 'allowed' to think for themselves and found it easier to submit to the dictates of their doctors, not understanding the workings of their own bodies or the consequences of the medicines prescribed. Many doctors say that they are careful to explain the process of menopause but if you ask most women whether they found these explanations helpful it turns out that they often felt patronised and found the brief, formulaic descriptions of the process, couched in unfamiliar and confusing terms, inadequate.

As I write this, sitting in front of my computer, surrounded by my library of books on the subject, I understand how women feel. I have read all the books but because each expert has such a different way of using the terminology and describing the process of menopause and such different convictions about the subject, I'm not surprised that women feel anxious and helpless about making an informed decision.

I know that when I understand something clearly I can deal with it properly, so in writing this book I have tried to simplify the wide body of information in a user-friendly way that is accessible to women. The menopause is a very complicated process, so if you can, take time to read the explanations carefully, even if it all seems very confusing. I hope that when you have read the book you will be able to visit your doctor with a basic understanding of menopause and ask relevant questions without being afraid of sounding like an idiot.

Knowledge is power. When we understand something we can deal with our fears and all the implications; we can make sensible choices and we can feel empowered. The visit to the doctor's office becomes less traumatic and we can read about menopause or discuss it with our friends logically and calmly. Armed with knowledge, we can't be bullied, either by those who have a passionate belief in HRT or those who have a passionate conviction that alternative therapies are the only way. With knowledge we can make the best choices for our bodies, our lifestyles and our psyches. We can live well with menopause.

How to make the most of the book

I have tried to use as few technical terms as possible. The medical terms are usually in italics next to the more down-to-earth word or phrase. There is a full glossary of these words at the end of the book. So next time the doctor talks about *hyperplasia* you'll know he means that the lining of your womb is thickened. Some sections of the book are drier and more technical than others but I have included them so that you will understand how your body works and can make responsible health choices. You can use the book as a reference, dipping into it when you need a particular piece of information, or you can read it right through. It is written in such a way that by the time you reach the end all the pieces of the puzzle will have fallen into place and most of the mysteries of menopause will have been unveiled. Each chapter ends with a series of empowerment points, which are later collated in one section and which you can glance at before you visit your healthcare practitioner. There is also a space for notes at the end of each chapter, so you can arm yourself with the book and use it if necessary when you have to make choices related to living well with menopause. If you make notes as you go along they will help you to remember all the questions you need to ask your doctor during your appointments, when you may feel rushed and anxious.

I

What is Menopause?

Prue is tall and slim. She is an ardent sportswoman in her early forties, matter of fact and organised in her daily life, self-contained and extremely down to earth. So it was out of character for her to be laughing hysterically and describing her anxiety and distress during the past few weeks. 'I am so relieved this morning,' she said, 'I've just got my period. I'd missed two months, had unbelievably sore boobs and felt emotional, even slightly sick. I was absolutely sure that I was pregnant – it felt just like it. But it's back again and really heavy.

'The reason I was so freaked out,' she explained, 'apart from my age (she has two children in high school), is that my husband's had a vasectomy and there's no possible way I could be pregnant!'

We all laughed, but what Prue had just experienced could happen to any woman of her age. She is perimenopausal. The symptoms of perimenopause vary widely and can come out of the blue. For some women there are clear, unambiguous signs, for others, the transition from being a fertile woman in the menstrual cycle to being menopausal is so gradual that they hardly even notice.

Because there is so much research into the subject of menopause at this time and because the published findings of the Women's Health Initiative (WHI) at the beginning of 2004

1

turned the accepted ideas about menopause on their heads, it is vital that women understand what is happening to their bodies in the years before the actual moment of menopause so that they are better able to micromanage this often tumultuous time and will be able to look back on those years as fulfilled, healthy and productive.

What does perimenopause mean?

The term menopause actually means the last day of your last period ever. From that point, in medical terms, you are considered menopausal. Until then, your body, as it moves from being fertile, able to produce eggs and bear children, to the moment of menopause when you no longer ovulate, is in a transition period known as the *climacteric*, a word meaning a critical stage in human life; a period which is especially likely to be connected with a change in health. During this time of the climacteric when you are moving towards the menopause, the changes taking place in your body cause certain symptoms, physiological (physical) and psychological changes that are happening to you as the levels of estrogen in your body fluctuate and the levels of progesterone start to decline. We use the word 'peri', which comes from the Greek word meaning 'around, round about and about', in conjunction with the word menopause, because it is a useful way to describe all the things that are going on in your body before, during and after the actual moment of menopause.

Before I describe what happens in perimenopause there is a very important point that you need to understand. Each woman is an individual so her menopause is unique and specific to her and her own body or biochemistry. It is pointless to compare yourself, your perimenopausal symptoms and the way you choose to manage your menopause with anyone else. As a friend of mine who is a preschool teacher points out, 'You always have to remind parents that each child develops differently. I tell parents that just because Jenny is catching a ball at four years old doesn't mean that Susie's ready to do so; she will in time, but she is developing at her own pace.' Don't forget this when you're sitting around discussing your perimenopause with your friends.

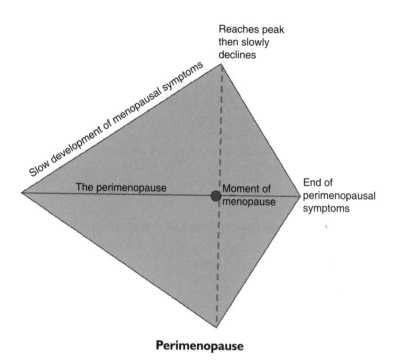

Slow development of menopausal symptoms

Reaches peak then slowly declines

The perimenopause

Moment of menopause

End of perimenopausal symptoms

Perimenopause

Much of the confusion arising from menopause is caused by the fact that for decades women were lumped together as a species and treated as if they were all the same, with no understanding that what was great for one woman might be disastrous for another. The old adage (slightly altered from a feminist perspective) holds good here: 'One woman's meat is another woman's poison'. It is vital to remember that the time leading up to menopause is different for every woman, just as the symptoms listed below are different for every woman.

The changes of perimenopause usually begin in the most subtle way, two to fourteen years before the actual onset of menopause, depending on your own body chemistry, unless you have undergone a surgical or chemical menopause. The diagram of the perimenopause shows how these symptoms build up over a period of time and then slowly decline after the actual moment of menopause. For some women the good news is that they will hardly experience any symptoms or only some of them for a very short time, while other unfortunate women will experience the full range of symptoms and these symptoms may continue for several years after the moment of menopause. So, as you read through the list and recognise some or all of these symptoms, remember that there are millions and millions of women out there going through a similar experience; you are not alone and what is happening to you is part of your life process as a woman. This stage will resolve itself, as did all the other stages in your life.

Some of the main symptoms of perimenopause:

- Hot flushes (You may see books written in America describing them as hot flashes)
- Night sweats
- Forgetfulness
- Undefined anxiety
- Inability to concentrate
- Mood swings
- Weight gain
- Sleep pattern changes
- Loss of libido (sexual desire)
- Change in the type of PMS
- Headaches or migraines
- Irregular periods – either too often or with months in between
- Changes in the type of menstrual periods
- Symptoms that mimic pregnancy; sore breasts, ravenous hunger, tearfulness, fatigue.

Symptoms that may persist after the other symptoms have abated:

- Vaginal dryness
- Persistent loss of libido
- Urinary problems.

The list of perimenopausal symptoms is long, varied and often idiosyncratic (specific to you alone), so although I have only listed the most common symptoms in this chapter, in Appendix 1 on page 265 you will find a list of almost every possible symptom that women complain about during perimenopause, which may reassure you that you are not going mad or suffering from some obscure and life-threatening disease.

The symptoms of perimenopause can mostly be blamed on your changing hormone levels. Your levels of estrogen are fluctuating and you don't have adequate progesterone to balance the estrogen. In fact, when the levels of estrogen stop fluctuating, many of the symptoms that have plagued you throughout the perimenopause will stop. Estrogen is an extremely potent hormone and in Chapter 2 I will explain the physiology of estrogen and why it has such a powerful effect on you.

What happens before menopause: Your menstrual cycle

Once you understand the process of your menstrual cycle and the roles that estrogen and progesterone play in it, it is much easier to understand what is happening to your body during perimenopause. Look at the diagram of your body on page 7 so that you have a picture of what your reproductive system looks like.

You are born with two *ovaries* containing eggs. Each egg is surrounded by a sac-like structure called a *primordial follicle* (this means that the follicle is in a primitive state). The egg and follicle are often called the egg unit and are in a resting state. When you start puberty your ovaries contain about 500 000 eggs but by the time you reach menopause only about 3 000 eggs remain. The chart on page 6 will help you understand how the ideal 28-day menstrual cycle works. This is also a good place to remind you that only about 12 per cent of women have a 28-day cycle, so your cycle may normally be between 24 days and 35 days, or you may be one of those women who has always had irregular periods.

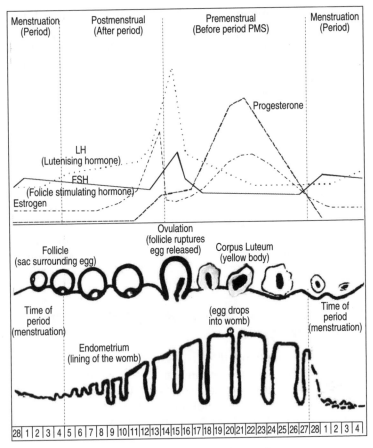

Diagram of reproductive cycle

The build-up to ovulation

Your menstrual cycle begins on the first day of your period. The *pituitary gland* in your brain produces a hormone called *follicle stimulating hormone* (FSH). This is one of the important hormones to note when understanding what is happening to your body, because when women become perimenopausal or go to their doctors complaining about some of the symptoms I have listed above, they often have blood tests which show that their FSH levels are raised.

The FSH causes the egg units to produce estrogen and this increased production level of estrogen causes the lining of the womb (*endometrium*) to thicken. During this time up to 1 000 egg units begin to mature. By day nine, one of these egg units starts to grow much more quickly than the others and becomes the dominant (leader of the pack) follicle. The other egg units, having done their work in supporting the *dominant follicle*, start to degenerate.

As this follicle matures its estrogen production increases and on about day 13 it reaches a level which tells the *hypothalamus*, the part of the brain involved with your endocrine system and thus your menstrual cycle, to send a message to the pituitary gland to reduce the FSH production and to secrete *luteinising hormone* (LH).

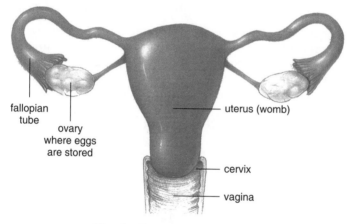

fallopian tube

ovary where eggs are stored

uterus (womb)

cervix

vagina

Simple diagram of the womb

Ovulation

On day 14, which is called mid-cycle in our ideal 28-day cycle, the ripening follicle develops a weak spot caused by a surge of LH and the contents of the follicle are slowly pushed out through this weakened area. This process creates a chemical change around the ovary, which attracts the finger-like extensions at the end of the fallopian tube. These behave very much like the waving fronds of a sea anemone and create a current that draws the egg and the fluid that was in the follicle into the fallopian tube, which leads into your womb. This process is known as ovulation. It can pass unnoticed or it can be painful and many women say they know when they have ovulated because of the physical sensation or pain on one side, which may come from the rupturing follicle.

Sometimes the small amount of fluid or blood spilled when the follicle releases its contents can irritate the pelvic lining, which can cause tenderness. Often women say they know when they have ovulated because they experience some of the symptoms that are caused by rising progesterone which is released during this time. These may be a sudden very bad headache or migraine, a craving for chocolate, tender or very sensitive breasts, or an outbreak of acne or one huge pimple which always seems to appear in the same place.

The ruptured follicle is now known as the *corpus luteum* (Latin for yellow body) and begins to produce small amounts of estrogen and increasing amounts of progesterone, which stabilises the thickened lining of your womb or uterus, so that if the egg is fertilised the lining will be lush and ready to receive the fertilised egg. If you do not become pregnant the corpus luteum begins to degenerate and the levels of progesterone and estrogen it produces begin to drop. Since the lining of the womb needs progesterone to sustain it, when the levels of progesterone and estrogen have dropped far enough the lining begins to crumble and within a couple of days it separates from the wall of your womb and you start to menstruate approximately 14 days after ovulation. This menstrual cycle generally continues in more or less the same way during your fertile years unless you are pregnant, or until you begin to get older, which is when things start to change.

What happens to your menstrual cycle as you become perimenopausal?

As I have discussed above, the ovary is a hormone-producing organ that becomes less effective as you age, but it doesn't just shut down and stop producing hormones. This is where so many doctors were so mistaken in their determination to explain to women how they had 'run out' of estrogen and why they needed hormone replacement therapy (HRT). During your fertile years, the main hormones produced by your ovaries were two types of estrogen (estradiol (E2), which is very potent, and estrone), progesterone and small amounts of androgen (see Chapter 2). As you approach menopause your changing ovaries produce estrogen in lower amounts and increased amounts of androgen. (Testosterone, the main male hormone, is an androgen.) At the same time the balance of the types of estrogen being produced changes and you begin to produce larger amounts of estrone and smaller amounts of estradiol. Your ovaries are still functioning, but less efficiently.

From your late thirties onwards an ageing process takes place. This varies widely among women. Each of us has a biological clock and the rate at which it ticks depends on the different biochemistry of each woman. This means that it can tick faster for some women, so their egg units become less efficient earlier, or more slowly for others, in whom the symptoms and signs of perimenopause appear later. The process can happen in your mid-thirties or in your late forties and can take from two to fourteen years.

As you age your remaining egg units become progressively less efficient, regardless of the rate of your biological clock. Because the egg unit is becoming inefficient, which means that it is less responsive and less functional, the hypothalamus and pituitary gland respond accordingly. The pituitary has been doing its job month in and month out for many years, producing FSH, which means that there is a consistent level of hormones rising and falling during your most fertile years. When the pituitary 'recognises' that the remaining follicles are not responding to FSH as they used to, it increases the FSH production to try to force the follicles to respond, a process that can be slow and subtle in some women, precipitous in others. This is the reason why so many doctors tell women they believe to be perimenopausal to have a blood test to see if their levels of FSH are rising.

Why do hormones fluctuate during perimenopause?

So, why do levels of estrogen rise and fall so erratically during the perimenopausal years? It's quite simple really. The follicles in your ovaries are starting to show their age and are less effective, so their response at the beginning of your 28-day cycle is poorer. The pituitary, responding to the fact that the follicles aren't doing their job, pumps out higher levels of FSH in a desperate effort to stimulate them and some follicles respond by pushing out large amounts of estrogen, sometimes much higher than average. If this happens you may ovulate and experience exaggerated symptoms of ovulation like sore breasts, heightened emotional responses and sugar cravings. If you have ovulated, your levels of pro-gesterone rise and fall and you get a period, which because the high amounts of estrogen have made your womb lining thicker than usual, is very heavy and may be accompanied by large clots.

On the other hand, your follicles may respond to the raised amounts of FSH by producing unusually large amounts of estrogen but you don't ovulate because the maturing egg cannot complete the process. This means that the lining of your womb gets thicker and thicker but you don't have a period because there is no ovulation so the follicle hasn't become the corpus luteum and doesn't produce the proges-terone which helps to control menstruation. This is why you don't have your period at the usual time.

But now, just to add to your confusion, your estrogen level may drop suddenly and this thickened lining may become unstable and shed, causing a heavy bleed, which is not a period, at a time that is entirely unrelated to your 'normal' cycle, perhaps out of the blue after several months of having no period. Or, the lining of your womb may thicken just a bit and then become unstable because of the fluctuating levels of estrogen and you have a funny, light bleed when you least expect it. Or, you may have continued estrogen production without ovulation, which means that the endo-metrium becomes so thick that it cannot be maintained and partially breaks down, causing bleeds that are heavier and last longer than usual.

Another point to remember is that even if you have irregular periods, if your ovaries are still ovulating, even only occasionally, you can still get pregnant, so until you have been confirmed as fully menopausal and haven't had a period for at least 12 months you should still use contraception (unless your husband or partner has had a *vasectomy*).

These irregular bleeds or 'periods' are signs of perimenopause and are caused by fluctuating levels of high and low estrogen which are no longer balanced by progesterone. In a normal menstrual cycle these two hormones balance each other out but now they are out of sync because the levels of progesterone are steadily declining while estrogen production may remain normal or become higher.

Remember, it is these changing levels of estrogen and not simply low levels that cause many of the symptoms of perimenopause: hot flushes, memory lapses, exhaustion one day because the estrogen level has dropped, or wild irritability and tearfulness, bloating and sore breasts on another, because it has risen or because of ovulation. So blood tests showing high FSH and low estrogen may not be useful at the start of perimenopause.

Let's assume that you are showing signs of perimenopause so you go to your doctor, who recommends that you have a blood test. The test results show that you have raised levels of FSH and lowered levels of E2. The doctor then recommends additional estrogen in the form of estrogen replacement therapy (ERT) but despite this, the next week, because your raised levels of FSH affect your remaining egg units and your estrogen levels rise suddenly, you may ovulate and because of the ERT you are taking, your body will have too much estrogen and you will suffer the associated symptoms of excess estrogen.

The problem with relying on blood tests at the start of perimenopause is that a woman can continue to menstruate for a long time in spite of raised levels of FSH. Some doctors may recommend a low-dose contraceptive pill, which inhibits ovulation and controls your fluctuating estrogen. But as with all hormone replacement therapy it is important to find out whether this treatment suits your individual body chemistry and whether it is absolutely necessary.

The prospect of these rising and falling levels of hormones and their consequences may be very depressing, but there is some good news. As you approach menopause the drastic changes in hormones level out and you will probably have the same high levels of FSH and LH and the same levels of estrogen for the rest of your life, if you lead a balanced life. However, estrogen levels can be affected by an increase in or loss of weight, by chemicals or stress, and they can fluctuate. If they are stable though, most of the symptoms of perimenopause will eventually stop and the only symptoms that may remain are those of postmenopause: vaginal dryness, low libido and, sometimes, urinary problems.

How can you test for menopause?

By now you must be thinking, 'how on earth can I confirm that I am actually menopausal?' You can see that a single blood test which looks at your levels of FSH, LH and estradiol, especially in the first few years of perimenopause while you are still menstruating, may not be useful due to the fluctuating levels of these hormones. In perimenopause, your FSH levels can reflect the fluctuations of your estrogen levels. So when your estrogen levels drop, your FSH may be high, but a few days later the FSH may be lower again as your estrogen levels rise. If you have a blood test only to determine your levels of estradiol (E2) and they are less than 50 pmol/L, (pmol/L are the units used to measure the amount of estrogen in your blood), there may still be some doubt as to whether or not you are menopausal.

There are two reasons for this. The first, as we know, is because estrogen levels can fluctuate madly during the early years of perimenopause. The second is that estrogen, progesterone and testosterone are bound to something called *sex hormone-binding globulin* (SHBG), a protein produced by the liver which binds the main hormones and decreases their biological effectiveness. The only hormones that are really relevant are those that are not bound to the SHBGs because these are the hormones that can easily enter the body tissues. They are called bio-available.

Some manufacturers of 'natural' or *bioidentical* hormones, and healthcare practitioners who recommend these products, will tell you that a salivary assay is the only accurate way to test the baseline of hormones, including estradiol, progesterone and testosterone. They may tell you that they can determine what the 'normal' levels of your hormones should be for your age. There is no scientific evidence that this type of testing is accurate or reliable and so far 'normal' levels of hormones in menopausal women have not been established. Another problem with this kind of testing is that in order to establish serum hormone levels from your saliva you need *at least* five daily saliva samples because hormone levels vary greatly in each individual woman throughout the day and from one day to the next. Your doctor will tell you that even the hormone levels in your blood as opposed to those in saliva vary from day to day.

If you are in your late thirties or your early forties, have irregular periods and are experiencing some of the symptoms discussed above, your best bet is to have a blood test which shows your FSH and your E2 levels. There is some discussion about when this test should be done and whether it is an accurate predictor of menopause because FSH levels may remain high despite the fact that estradiol levels appear adequate in blood tests. Two other hormones, *Inhibin B* and *Anti-Mullerian Hormone* (AMH), are involved in FSH levels. Inhibin B is produced by the ovaries to help with the recruitment of eggs (see page 7). As women age, their ovaries produce lower levels of Inhibin B, causing the pituitary to produce higher levels of FSH.

AMH is also produced by the developing follicles in the ovaries and new research suggests that this may also be useful in determining whether a woman still has an adequate number of functioning eggs in her ovaries. So, if you combine levels of Inhibin B, AMH and FSH you will probably have a fairly accurate idea of whether or not you are menopausal. However, currently these tests for levels of Inhibin B and AMH are not usually done on peri- and postmenopausal women. So your doctor should test your FSH levels. Ideally you should have the test between day two and day five of your menstrual cycle while you are menstruating regularly so that you have a baseline level with which to compare any future results.

If you are already perimenopausal and your periods are irregular, it will be more difficult and you should have the FSH levels tested in conjunction with your E2 levels. If the test shows that your FSH is high and your E2 is low, it probably means that you are perimenopausal. However, although there are norms for the hormones levels, results may vary greatly depending on the individual. Also remember that that the actual hormone measurements may vary slightly depending on the methodologies used by different labs.

As a rule of thumb if you haven't had a period for 12 months and you have FSH levels that are greater than 20 U/L and E2 levels lower than 50 pmol/L, you can be pretty confident that you are now menopausal. These results should be interpreted by a healthcare practitioner who understands the subtle changes that are taking place in your body during the time of perimenopause.

Before you are told that you are menopausal, you should have had a thorough physical examination. Also remember that a transvaginal ultrasound, which allows your doctor better access to assess your womb and your ovaries, is now considered an integral part of your gynaecological physical. Using this technique your doctor can rule out any major abnormalities in your womb and ovaries. Depending on the results of that examination your doctor will probably recommend tests to establish your levels of FSH, E2, prolactin and your thyroid function.

The reason I suggest that you have a physical examination and check prolactin levels and your thyroid function is that there may be factors other than the decline of normal ovarian functioning which are influencing your menstrual cycle. So if you don't think that you are perimenopausal, ask your doctor to check your thyroid function, note whether you are on any new medication for other conditions and exclude the possibility of illnesses that may affect menstruation. Excessive weight loss and lifestyle habits like too much alcohol and heavy cigarette smoking may cause menstrual changes, as will chronic or acute stress and sometimes, just travelling through different time zones.

By now you should have a better understanding of how your body works and how you've reached this perimenopausal stage. You also know why you start getting strange symptoms and what the changes signal. Unlike Prue, you won't be freaked out when your periods suddenly stop and think that you are pregnant!

Empowerment points

- It is entirely reasonable and sensible for you to ask your doctor to explain your symptoms and the results of your tests in a way that is clear and easy for you to understand. You should never feel rushed or stupid, or that you are wasting his/her time. You have paid for the consultation and this is your time. If she or he does not do so in a manner that is acceptable to you, then you must seriously question whether she or he is the correct practitioner for you.

- Don't accept it when your doctor tells you that she or he thinks you are too young to be perimenopausal or that you will get your menopause when you're 40. Doctors aren't psychic. Insist that you have your hormone levels tested if you think you may be perimenopausal. There is no harm in being sure. Even if you aren't experiencing the symptoms of menopause you may want to have a record of your levels as a baseline comparison for the future.

- Never feel awkward about asking questions or asking for information to be clarified.

- If you have had tests, the practice should phone you with the results as soon as possible and you should be able to discuss these results in detail with your doctor at a follow-up appointment.

2

All About Hormones

I had just started writing this chapter when my phone rang and a woman asked to speak to me. She told me she was in her sixties. She was obviously well educated, articulate and informed, and had made it her mission to research osteoporosis, with which she had been diagnosed.

She refused to take osteoporosis medicine (bisphosphonates) because she is a firm believer in alternative and complementary medicines. She told me that she had consulted experts in America and the UK, where she had spent time with one of the so-called gurus of natural progesterone, a disciple of Dr John Lee, who practises in London. This doctor had recommended natural progesterone, which she was to apply to her skin in a small 'dollop ... about the amount you would put on a toothbrush'.

She asked me what I thought of natural progesterone. I took a deep breath. It is very confusing when women talk about natural progesterone. What does the word 'natural' mean? Natural progesterone is a product that has been formulated to be biologically identical to the progesterone that is found in your body. Like all the other hormone replacement products, it has been synthesised in a laboratory. Yet this woman, who is very opposed to conventional HRT, was quite happy to put an arbitrary amount of progesterone on her body, without any real understanding of the strength and potential side effects of this hormone, which is, in its own way, as powerful and potentially harmful as too much estrogen.

In Chapter 1 I discussed several hormones that play a large part in a woman's peri- and postmenopausal life. But when you do not understand how these hormones work, it is hard to appreciate just how much they can affect you during the transition to menopause. If you grasp how they function, you can, together with your doctor, make an educated decision about whether or not you want to use hormone therapy.

Hormones are chemical substances that act like messengers. They travel through your body in your bloodstream to different tissues, where they send out signals for organs to react in a certain way. The hormones come from a series of glands which form something called the endocrine system. There are many different kinds of hormones and they behave in a most complex and subtle way to affect our bodily functions. However, I will only write about a few of the main hormones which will affect you most during your menopausal process and the last few decades of your life.

Estrogens, progesterone and testosterone, which I mentioned in Chapter 1, are called sex steroid hormones. All the sex steroid hormones originate from cholesterol and are controlled by the functions of the hypothalamus and the pituitary. In females, many of the sex steroid hormones are produced in the ovaries in a very specific order but some are produced in the adrenal glands, which are the small structures situated on top of your kidneys, and in the fatty tissues of your body. Doctors may refer to these fatty tissues as *adipose tissue*. Most of the hormones that are important to women are produced via a series of steps or pathways known as the adrenal cascade. Hormones and their actions are intricately woven into the functioning of your body. They are like the players in an orchestra. The hypothalamus is the musical director, the pituitary is the conductor and the various hormones are the members of the orchestra. As in an orchestra, if one player is out of tune, the whole piece of music is out of tune, so, if a hormone is not functioning at its appropriate level, the body is out of tune.

A hormone called *pregnenolone*, made from cholesterol, is the basic building block of the sex steroid hormones. The pregnenolone hormone produces *progesterone*, which as you will remember, is secreted by the corpus luteum after ovulation. Other hormones that are derived from pregnenolone and progesterone are the *androgens* and the *estrogens*. Only two androgens, testosterone and *DHEA* (*dehydroepiandrosterone*) are relevant to women in perimenopause.

One of the above-mentioned estrogens, estradiol, is produced mainly in your ovaries and, to a lesser extent, in your fatty tissues. This estradiol is called *17ß-estradiol* and is the most potent estrogen circulating throughout your body during your fertile years. *Estrone*, which is the principal circulating estrogen in your menopausal years, is produced chiefly in your fatty tissues and is stored there and converted back into estradiol or estrone.

But both estrone and estriol can also be formed from estradiol in the liver. So, even if you have become menopausal, you can still be producing greater amounts of estrone than usual. Raised levels of estrone are associated with stroke, breast cancer and cancer of the lining of the womb. Because this hormone is produced from your fatty tissues, the fatter you are the more estrone you will produce. It is therefore very important that you do not gain too much weight during this time. A third estrogen called *estriol* is produced by the placenta in pregnant women because of the interaction of estradiol and estrone, and is the major estrogen in pregnancy. It is also produced from estrone in normally menstruating women but it is not particularly important in menopause. Some research suggests that estriol, which is known as free because it is not bound to a storage or carrier hormone and because it does not convert back into estradiol and estriol, may be a good hormone therapy (HT) option (see Chapter 4).

In discussing estrogens I should mention an enzyme called *aromatase*, which is probably one of the most important enzymes responsible for the formation of estrogen in our tissues. You will read more about this hormone in Chapter 8 when I discuss breast cancer. The aromatase enzyme is found in our fatty (*adipose*) tissues, adrenal glands, muscles and skin. After menopause, when the ovaries become quiet, the activity of this enzyme usually increases and becomes one of the main ways that we continue to produce estrogen when we are postmenopausal. Aromatase can cause our estrogen levels to increase to a degree where our bodies show all the effects of excess estrogen, such as thickening of the lining of the womb, bleeding and even estrogen-positive cancers. Aromatase is also present in our brains and bones, which may be the reason why our cognitive function and bone mass can be maintained after menopause even without HT.

Another group of hormones called *glucocorticoids* is produced in our adrenal glands. These also have pregnenolone and progesterone as their building blocks, but *cortisol* is the only one that is really relevant to menopausal women.

The levels of hormone production are controlled by a feedback loop which resembles a thermostat: when the temperature drops, the thermostat will stimulate the heating so that temperature rises. This is very similar to what happens with your hormone levels. In Chapter 1 I discussed how the hypothalamus sends a message to the pituitary, which initiates the secretion of two hormones, follicle stimulating hormone (FSH) and luteinising hormone (LH). The action of these two hormones leads ultimately to the production of estrogen and progesterone.

Because these major hormones are produced in the ovaries, many women believe that when they reach menopause they no longer produce them, but as I explained in Chapter 1, the ovaries don't stop functioning at perimenopause and menopause, they just operate differently. There are other areas in your body besides the ovaries that can produce the same hormones, albeit in smaller amounts.

There is a very good reason why this happens. The hormones in your body give messages to different organs and tissues to behave in a certain way. They are able to do this because all these areas have special groups of cells which are called *receptors*. Receptors are all different, so the estrogen receptors will respond only to estrogen, while the progesterone receptors respond only to progesterone. A similar process takes place with all the hormones; there are specific receptors for specific hormones, much like locks and keys. The wrong key cannot open the lock.

Each hormone that I have mentioned has carefully defined functions and this is why when the levels of these hormones drop or rise and the receptors are deprived of their specific hormone or inundated with it, there will often be a profound effect on your body.

But here is the good news – because the precursors of the sex steroid hormones are also made in the adrenal glands, and because there are specific hormone receptor sites throughout your body, these hormones continue to be produced, just in smaller amounts. For example, as I mentioned, you can partially compensate for the fluctuating levels of estradiol produced by your ovaries by producing more estrone. So although there are often very noticeable changes in your body during perimenopause and menopause, the small amounts of sex steroid hormones that are still being produced allow your body to adjust to the different hormonal levels and this is when the most aggressive symptoms of the perimenopause tail off.

Each hormone has its own unique function and once you see how it works you will begin to understand that if the amount of a particular hormone drops below or rises above its normal levels, certain symptoms will occur.

Estradiol is the most potent of all the estrogens and is a vital hormone in maintaining a healthy fertile cycle. There are estrogen receptors throughout your body – your brain, skin and hair follicles, your breasts, your skeleton, the fatty tissues of your thighs and buttocks, and other body areas. Thus estradiol adds fatty tissue to your breasts, thighs and hips, mainly during puberty, but this can continue throughout the rest of your life. There are also estrogen receptors in your vagina and your uterus, so estradiol is involved in the growth of your uterus and thickens the lining of your womb in preparation for pregnancy. It also keeps your vagina moist and plump. One of the reasons for this is that the walls of the vagina and the outer areas of the urethra are very rich in estrogen receptors. It makes sense, therefore, that during perimenopause, when the levels of estrogen are fluctuating, or when they stabilise and become lower than the levels experienced during your reproductive years, the lining of the walls may change; become thinner and less elastic. There will also probably be less lubrication, because estrogen stimulates the secretion of vaginal and cervical mucus. Several changes to your vagina during perimenopause can affect your sexuality, but not all of these are the result of reduced levels of estrogen, as I will explain when I discuss sexuality and perimenopause.

Since there are estrogen receptors in the skin, which help to make it look smooth and glowing, you can see how lowered levels of estradiol may impact on your skin's youthful appearance. There are also estrogen receptors in the smooth-muscle cells of your arteries and it is believed that estrogen might play a protective role in preventing heart disease. The issue of estradiol and heart health will be discussed in Chapter 7. There are estradiol receptors in your brain, which appear to interact with different brain chemicals (*neurotransmitters*), so the fluctuating levels of estradiol in perimenopause may cause some of the mood swings and erratic emotions that I discussed in Chapter 1. These interactions are very complicated and further research needs to be done to improve our understanding of estrogen's role in both your brain and your heart.

Estrogen is also very helpful in reducing the risk of fracture in peri- and postmenopausal women because it stimulates the activity of the osteoblasts or bone builders in the bones.

Like the other hormones, estrogen can have some adverse effects on your body. Breast cancer and cancer of the lining of the womb can be caused by excess estrogen, which over-stimulates the estrogen receptor cells in theses areas, but I will discuss these in detail in Chapter 8.

Progesterone is the sex steroid hormone responsible for sustaining a pregnancy by maintaining the thickened lining of the womb. Progesterone comes from the ovaries but is also produced in small amounts in the fatty tissue of the brain and nervous system. One of the main roles of progesterone is to balance the effects of estrogen on the female body. Progesterone helps to limit your blood loss during menstruation. This is one of the reasons why during perimenopause bleeding may be heavy and you may have longer periods than usual.

Progesterone can also cause fluid retention during the second half of your menstrual cycle and often causes weight gain and adult acne. Raised progesterone levels also stimulate the breasts so that they feel heavy and sensitive. The progesterone receptors in the brain and nervous system may react to falling levels of this hormone by causing heightened levels of anxiety and depression. It is also interesting to note that excess amounts of progesterone can unmask and enhance depression. Too little progesterone may affect your body's production of cortisol because, as I mentioned above, progesterone is a building block for cortisol.

Progesterone has sedative properties, which may help to calm you and to promote deeper sleep. So when levels of progesterone drop during perimenopause your sleep patterns may change and you may experience 'panic attacks' or palpitations. Progesterone helps to build and maintain bone, and it can affect your thyroid function. A lack of progesterone may cause endometrial cancer because there is uncontrolled stimulation of the lining of the womb by estrogen.

Testosterone is an important male hormone which is also produced in small amounts in women. Like the other sex steroid hormones, it is derived from cholesterol and is produced in the ovaries and the adrenal glands. It can also be produced from estradiol in the liver and fatty tissues. It is one of the male androgenic hormones. In puberty, testosterone has a similar effect on girls to the effect it has on boys, though to a lesser extent, causing increased body odour, pubic hair, an oilier skin (which can lead to acne), and bone growth. Testosterone may be intricately intertwined with a woman's libido (sexual desire), but as I will discuss further on, there are many other issues that affect your sex drive in perimenopause. And since there are testosterone receptors in areas other than your ovaries, even if you have had a hysterectomy you will still produce small amounts of this hormone.

Testosterone also affects the quality of your muscle tone and energy levels. If your estrogen levels drop below your levels of testosterone, this imbalance can affect your hair growth, and the hair on your head may become thinner, sometimes mimicking the way men go bald on the top and front of their heads. You may also develop facial hair and an oilier skin, which can lead to adult acne.

Cortisol comes from the adrenal cortex in the adrenal glands and is one of the hormones most important to maintaining a healthy body. A hormone called *adrenocorticotropin* (*ACTH*) is secreted by the pituitary gland and stimulates the adrenal glands to produce cortisol. If you are stressed, either physically or emotionally, the pituitary gland increases its production of ACTH, resulting in raised levels of cortisol, which cause all sorts of problems. This is why, later in the book, I will discuss the importance of dealing sensibly with your stress levels.

Cortisol is a very powerful hormone; it is the watchdog of your immune system because it helps it to respond to stress, extreme temperature changes and allergic reactions, and has a strongly protective effect in slowing down the inflammatory reactions of your body. It plays a vital role in helping to maintain blood pressure and cardiovascular activity. Because it is instrumental in balancing the action of insulin in breaking down sugar, it helps raise your energy levels and ensures the appropriate metabolism of protein, fats and carbohydrates, which is why raised or lowered levels of cortisol can alter this delicate balance. Higher than normal levels of cortisol slow down your metabolism, which means that you gain weight. Too little causes you to lose appetite and weight and feel sluggish, exhausted and weak.

Normal levels of cortisol help to stabilise your emotions because certain sections of your brain that are involved in your emotional functioning are rich in cortisol receptors. However, extreme emotional stress appears to raise levels of cortisol and the effect of these higher levels is often to cause emotional upheaval and impaired memory function.

Cortisol can fluctuate because of raised levels of stress, illness and fever, and although it plays such an important role in maintaining the intricate hormonal working of your body, cortisol levels that are raised over a length of time because of factors such as long-term stress can have some very undesirable effects. These include the weight gain that I mentioned earlier, extreme fatigue, very low levels of energy, and a lowered immune system. Raised levels of cortisol can also lead to the suppression of the hormone known as *DHEA*.

DHEA is a milder form of cortisol and derives from cholesterol in the adrenal glands, where it, and a similar hormone called *DHEA-S* can be building blocks for both testosterone and estrogen. It is thought that DHEA has many of the beneficial effects of cortisol without being as potent. Research into this hormone is still in its infancy, but it is thought that DHEA helps to strengthen the immune system and maintain bone density, assist normal sleep patterns and is involved in protecting heart health by controlling the levels of LDL cholesterol (the more dangerous or 'bad' cholesterol). Research suggests that DHEA improves levels of vitality and energy, the ability to cope with stress, and the general sense of well-being and of being on the ball.

Thyroid hormone is one of the most significant hormones in the menopausal process because so many middle-aged women suffer from some kind of thyroid dysfunction, which can cause symptoms that may mimic those that you may experience during your perimenopause.

There are two main thyroid hormones, *thyroxine* (T4) and *triiodothyronine* (T3) which are produced in the thyroid gland when the pituitary secretes a hormone called *thyroid stimulating hormone* (TSH). The best way to describe the action of thyroid hormones is to compare the functioning of your body to the idling of a car engine. If the engine idles too quickly (an overactive thyroid – hyperthyroidism) or too slowly (an underactive thyroid – hypothyroidism) we can expect engine problems. Thyroid hormones are essential to the promotion of healthy cell functioning in the human body; they help your body to function well and healthily.

The reason thyroid dysfunction is an important factor to be aware of in perimenopausal women is that many of the symptoms of too much or too little thyroid hormone may mimic the symptoms of perimenopause. If you have too little thyroid hormone circulating through your body you may experience, among others, the following symptoms, which are very similar to those experienced in perimenopause: fatigue, sensitivity to cold, memory problems, depression, menstrual disturbances (irregular or erratic periods) and weight gain. These menstrual problems may be caused by raised levels of *prolactin*, which can result from an underactive thyroid. If you are producing too much thyroid hormone you may find that you are very hyped-up, anxious, have palpitations, lose weight and experience irregular periods. This is why, in Chapter 1, I wrote that if you are having symptoms of perimenopause you should ensure that they are not, in fact, signs of thyroid problems.

Prolactin is secreted in the pituitary gland in response to high levels of estradiol and nipple stimulation during breastfeeding. It is responsible during pregnancy for helping to prepare your breasts to produce milk. Another of its functions is to repress ovulation after your baby is born. However, some women find that if they are not pregnant or breastfeeding and their prolactin levels are higher than normal, they may not menstruate. High levels of prolactin are called *hyperprolactinemia*. There are several reasons why prolactin levels may be inappropriately high, including a small tumour on your pituitary gland (*microadenoma*), medications like certain tranquillisers, antidepressants and blood pressure medication, greater amounts of estradiol, extreme stress and an underactive thyroid.

Insulin is a hormone secreted by the area of the pancreas known as the islets of Langerhans. By maintaining steady levels of glucose in your body, insulin ensures that primarily the sugars and, to a lesser degree, the fats and proteins you eat, are properly broken down (metabolised) and used to make new tissue. Insulin ensures that these foods are used efficiently and that food energy that is not needed is properly stored and then released when it is needed. It also controls the way that fat is stored in your body. However, if your insulin levels are raised, all sorts of problems can be expected and, as many women gain weight in midlife, they may start to experience them.

When you are overweight, eat the wrong foods and/or don't exercise, your insulin doesn't work as well as it should. Your doctor may call this insulin resistance. There is a lot of talk among menopausal women about insulin resistance and type 2 diabetes. Many healthcare practitioners suggest that insulin resistance causes obesity, but it's actually the other way around. So take care! It has become fashionable, when a woman has insulin resistance, to diagnose her as having something called the 'metabolic syndrome'. Many midlife women think that taking a medicine called glucophage will keep their weight down, but as with all magic bullets, there are problems related to this. The best way to prevent insulin resistance is not to gain weight, or if you are already overweight, to lose weight. This is a very complicated and important subject, and I will discuss it at length in Chapter 10.

The way in which hormones send instructions to the various tissues and organs and keep our bodies working at optimum levels of health is miraculous. It is important to remember that this process is incredibly intricate and complicated. You can see from the extremely simplified description that I have given of the major hormones involved in perimenopause that an imbalance in these hormones can cause all sorts of physical and psychological changes, illnesses and problems. This is why you need to be both educated and exceptionally careful before you make decisions about hormone therapy, so that you don't upset this delicate balance.

Empowerment points

- Because so many women in their fifth decade suffer from some kind of thyroid dysfunction, it is vital to eliminate this possibility when you experience what you and your doctor may assume are the symptoms of perimenopause. If your doctor does not recommend that your thyroid function be tested, ask for a test.

- In midlife many women find that their lives have become exponentially more stressful for a wide variety of reasons: the 'empty nest' syndrome, changing relationship patterns, bereavement, self-doubt and angst over lifestyle choices, and a partner who may also be suffering from a midlife crisis. As a result of these stressors, you may be suffering from raised levels of cortisol. If you know that you are unduly stressed and have been for any length of time, ask your doctor to prescribe a test to check your cortisol levels. Raised levels of cortisol can cause huge physiological and emotional problems. If you think that you have these symptoms you are probably not imagining them.

Notes

3

A Brief History of Hormone ~~Replacement~~ Therapy

'I need to see you!' Jenny sounded furious. I asked her what was wrong and she replied: 'I'm so angry I can hardly talk'. She explained that she had gone for her annual gynaecological check-up and had been informed by her doctor that she was now menopausal and that he would like to have a consultation with her and her husband.

Slightly mystified and more than a little anxious at this turn of events, Jenny and her husband came to the appointment. The doctor proceeded to list the woes of menopause, ending with these dire words: 'I'm not prepared to sleep with a dried-out old woman and that is why my wife is on HRT and you should be too!'

Jenny was appalled at this thunderbolt. Apart from the fact that she had no menopausal symptoms, she was not particularly keen to go on HRT and she and her husband enjoyed a happy and fulfilled sex life. She felt that this little interview had thrown a spanner into the works of their relationship and made her feel anxious and guilty. Was she in some sense shirking her wifely duty by not agreeing to take HRT?

She was also furious that the doctor had felt it necessary to tell her husband what she should be doing, as though she was an errant, rather ignorant child who could not make up her mind about her own treatment. She felt that if she had needed her menopause explained to her husband she would have been quite able to either explain the options to him herself or to make an appointment for him to meet her doctor on her own initiative.

In the past 40 years, many women have been 'bullied' by their doctors in similar ways. This particular doctor probably thought it was his duty to help this poor estrogen-deprived woman; to prevent her from becoming a miserable dried-out old crone who would cease to be attractive to her husband. For the doctor, the benefits of estrogen replacement therapy were so apparent that he literally couldn't understand why a woman wouldn't feel the need to be on it.

HRT or HT?

I think it is very important to be careful about the terminology we use when discussing this subject. Recent publications have taken to calling this therapy *hormone therapy* (HT). The phrase *hormone replacement therapy* (HRT) is a misnomer. As we saw in Chapter 1, you don't actually need to replace your estrogen, although you might need to balance it. Therefore the phrase HRT emphasises the commonly held misconception that women in peri- and postmenopause are estrogen deficient and need to have their estrogen replaced. So when you see a doctor who uses the phrase HRT ask yourself why she or he is doing this and be careful that she or he is not expressing outdated views. In this chapter I use the term HRT when I am discussing the historical perspective but once I move to the present I use HT.

This is probably the most complicated chapter in the book. But if you want to understand why this subject is so bewildering and why it seems so difficult to get simple answers to your questions, it is necessary to plough through some of the history and see why we have reached the confusing point we are at today. Understanding the dynamics surrounding the controversy about HT is really empowering, so persevere. In writing this chapter I have chosen the bits that seem most significant to me and have focused on the main issues.

Of all the topics surrounding the perimenopause, hormone therapy is the most controversial and difficult for laywomen to grasp. There are so many factors that need to be taken into consideration, so much conflicting research and, it must be said, huge commercial interests at stake. So in the interests of understanding this subject better here is a brief history of hormone replacement therapy; how we got to this place and why the whole topic has been turned on its head in the past few years.

Feminine Forever

In 1966, a book called *Feminine Forever* by Dr Robert Wilson radically changed the medical profession's perspective of menopause. The book, which was a paean of praise to the virtues of estrogen, became the gospel for those who touted the theory that menopause was a disease; that menopausal women were hapless victims, deprived of miraculous youth-providing estrogen, doomed to live as miserable, embittered, old women. The book was written in a powerfully smug, didactic and hectoring style. Women were described as 'de-sexed, unstable, frigid, cow-like, castrates'. Dr Wilson saw the state of menopause as a kind of purgatory: 'no woman can be sure of escaping the horror of this living decay'. And secure in his belief in his role as saviour of these desperate middle-aged women, he set out to save them from their fate. So deep was his conviction that estrogen would be the salvation of women that he managed to convince not only the average woman of the validity of his theory – over 100 000 copies of his book were sold in the first year of publication – but many of the most respected members of the medical fraternity agreed with him, particularly after he had published several articles on the subject in medical journals.

Dr Wilson's sexist and paternalistic views might have died a natural death if the doctors of the time had not agreed with them so wholeheartedly. His opinions gathered such momentum that the unappealing image he drew of menopausal women was perpetuated and the ensuing 35 years spawned a plethora of research, all showing the extraordinary benefits of estrogen replacement.

Even today pharmaceutical advertising perpetuates the myth of estrogen deficiency and its effects on 'desperate' middle-aged women. It is not uncommon to page through medical journals and see pictures of a well-preserved woman smiling beatifically at the camera. An advertisement from the June 2004 edition of *Update: The Journal of Continuing Education for General Practitioners* shows an attractive middle-aged woman coyly clutching a large wooden giraffe. The caption reads: 'She's entering menopause and she still loves the wild life.' The text continues: 'Growing older makes living in Africa no less exciting. The symptoms of menopause can make daily activities difficult and uncomfortable. Replacing oestrogen with low dose 17β estradiol, identical to woman's natural oestrogen, is the most effective way to treat and eliminate these symptoms. So that her life doesn't need to change.'

Premarin

The most popular of these magical antidotes to the 'disease' of menopause was a hormone treatment called Premarin. This wonder drug had been synthesised from the urine of pregnant mares, hence the name *pre*gnant *ma*res' u*r*ine, and consisted of an equine (horse) estrogen called equinol. The main ingredient of Premarin is *conjugated equine estrogens* (CEE). It was the gold standard of HRT.

A gynaecologist friend of mine, recalling lecturing medical students in the 1970s, says ruefully: 'We thought that nothing was as good as Premarin.' Because Premarin appeared to solve all the problems of menopause, it was accepted throughout much of the Western world. However, in December 1975 a dark cloud appeared on this rosy horizon. The prestigious *New England Journal of Medicine* published an article stating that there was a greatly increased risk of cancer of the lining of the womb in women who were taking Premarin.

In Chapters 1 and 2 I explained how estrogen was responsible for the build-up of the lining of your womb (your doctor will probably talk about *endometrial hyperplasia*). I also said that if there was no progesterone present to control menstruation, the presence of unopposed estrogen (estrogen used by itself without other agents to balance it) causes the womb lining (*endometrium*) to become thicker and thicker, increasing the presence of abnormal cells, which means that cancer may develop. So it is logical that peri- and postmenopausal women who were taking high levels of unopposed estrogen without shedding that thickened lining were going to be prone to endometrial cancer.

As you can imagine, there was a tremendous outcry about the article and, in spite of the fact that the main pharmaceutical companies tried to show that the statistics were overstated, the research that followed thick and fast on the heels of the original results not only confirmed the findings, but showed that the risks of endometrial cancer if you were taking a hormone like Premarin were even greater than had originally been suggested. So, it was decided to add synthetic progesterone to the treatment and Provera, which is Medroxyprogesteroneacetate (MPA), saved the day. Doctors felt that if they prevented the build-up of the uterine lining they could continue to give women all the miraculous benefits of estrogen.

Over the past 40 years there have been literally thousands of publications devoted to explaining why HT is so beneficial to women – it protects our bones, our hearts, our brains and our colons; it keeps our skins young and glowing; and gives us plump, moist vaginas and superb memories. In short, it seems that there is no reason, apart from some concern about the risks of breast and endometrial cancer, why women should not be taking HT. The statistics showed that of the hundreds of thousands who took HT, only very few were at greater risk for breast cancer than their counterparts who were not on HT, and appropriate doses of *progestogen* (synthetic progesterone, see page 60) for women with wombs solved the problem of endometrial cancer.

In 1999 I asked representatives of a giant pharmaceutical company, a leader in the field of HT, if they had any medical information for me on the risks and benefits of HT. They were delighted to help and I was stunned to receive an enormously thick volume citing more than 334 abstracts of research articles which had been published in a wide range of prestigious medical journals, all of which, to a large extent reinforced the perception that HT was beneficial to women's health. This is not surprising since the company had funded the bulk of the research – there were almost no examples of independent research in that volume. It is important to remember that good medical research is very expensive.

Where's the catch?

In spite of all the evidence that HT was so great for women, I felt a bit sceptical. I knew that the information that I was gathering from the women I spoke to was anecdotal, but I couldn't understand why so many battled on HT; felt bloated and overweight, suffered from painful and hypersensitive breasts, had breast tissue that was so dense that it was hard to do effective mammograms, had bad headaches, adult acne and raised cholesterol levels, and struggled with insulin resistance, sugar cravings and depression. I also knew that I wasn't alone in these doubts and that many feminists were complaining about the fact that menopause was seen as a disease and that doctors' attitudes undermined women and manipulated them to be on HT.

In addition to these critics, there were the natural proges-terone gurus like Dr John Lee, who Leslie Kenton praised in *Passage to Power*, or those, like Dr Jonathan Wright, who extolled the virtues of biologically identical hormones in a combination called Triple Estrogen, which contained estradiol, estrone and estriol, and reinforced the theory that estrogen should never be taken unopposed, whether a woman has a uterus or not.

Although some of the findings of these doctors seemed to make sense, there were aspects of their thinking that still concerned me. I didn't understand why they didn't put their theories to the gold standard of medical tests, the double-blind randomised controlled study. Some of them refused to debate with other healthcare professionals in the public, academic arena and once again I was wary of the claim that any hormone, bioidentical or not, was a 'magic bullet'.

So, while it made sense to me to add some progesterone to the mix, I couldn't understand why so many women thought that 'natural' progesterone was the Holy Grail and I felt that claims that 'natural' progesterone could cure everything from depression to porphyria were a little exaggerated.

I also found the boasts of complementary or alternative practitioners worrying; for example, black cohosh or don quai seemed miraculous until, on closer examination, it was found that many women using it were battling with tender, dense breasts; sometimes experiencing some nipple secretion and, in a recent article, concern was expressed that women taking it might have problems with liver function.

Research and HT

This is probably a good place to explain the complications associated with the research findings on HT. I have found that most women, even those who have discovered the joys of surfing the Net, don't have the medical expertise to read and interpret statistics. So they hear reports on the radio or television, read sensationalist articles in magazines, or listen to a number of statistics during the 15 minutes allotted to them by their doctor, which make sense to them at the time, but which are incomprehensible later. I am not suggesting that you now take a course in statistics or read complicated medical articles, but when you see an article you should have some tools to help you evaluate whether it makes medical sense and whether you can use the information in it to make an informed decision.

How to recognise good research

What makes a good study, one that doctors are prepared to accept when deciding whether or not to recommend a treatment? Many doctors believe that long years of medical experience, during which they have had many opportunities to observe the effects of HT, qualify them to recommend a treatment, but as medicine has become more and more scientific and it has become possible to test different medicines and understand the risks and benefits better, we can make decisions which are more informed. Medicine that is based on good research is forcing doctors to look differently at the treatments they prescribe. They are now beginning to see that many of the trials on which they had based their opinions were not properly controlled and so the results, which they were using as gospel truth, were incorrect.

As a rule of thumb, a good study should be carefully controlled, using a large sample group, which is divided into two groups. One of the groups, the control group, is on a placebo treatment (an inactive treatment that the people taking it believe is a specific drug), so it can act as a basis of comparison with the group actually taking the treatment. The words 'double-blind' mean that neither the people conducting the experiment nor the subjects taking part in it knows who is receiving the actual treatment until the research has been completed, so that their information is unbiased. The next time you read some information on HT or look at a pamphlet telling you how good the results of a study were, see if it has the following criteria:

- A large sample number
- A control group
- Is it a double-blind study?
- Has it been carried out over a reasonable period of time to show some significant results?
- Have the researchers declared their interests? The manufacturer of the drug under review may be funding them. Dr Robert Wilson's research was heavily funded by several pharmaceutical companies, including Ayerst, which we know today as Wyeth Ayerst, and which was the sole manufacturer of Premarin.
- Read the research with a healthy dose of scepticism: just because something is in print doesn't mean that it's correct. Remember that no study can cover all the different types,

age groups, different hormone treatments and regimens. So what might suit you may not suit another woman. Don't take the printed word as an absolute truth.

- You can also appear to be very knowledgeable by asking your healthcare practitioner whether the research is rated. Studies are usually rated Level I, Level I-1, Level II-2, Level II-3, Level III. If it is Level I it is a properly randomised controlled trial; as the levels drop the study becomes less and less good until it is rated Level III, which means it is based on anecdotal opinions, descriptive reports and experiences of respected clinicians; in other words it is not evidence-based medicine

So, what was one of the main things that went wrong with the early research on HT? In many of the earlier studies, the researchers didn't take into account the kind of woman who wanted the 'benefits' of HT. She wasn't just any menopausal woman. She was probably someone who worried about her figure, so she would eat properly and exercise, which would be good for her cholesterol and for her general health.

She would also be the sort of person who would visit her doctor regularly, so her practitioner could pick up any pending problems or medical conditions before they became too severe. She was the kind of patient that doctors call compliant; she takes her medicine and she listens to instructions. So when researchers showed how healthy women taking HT were, they were ignoring a very important factor in the research; that the kind of woman taking HT would probably be healthy anyway.

Another problem was that while doctors were saying that HT was good for women's hearts, they were basing their research on studies that had used only men! Or they were basing it on observational data which seemed to suggest that women got coronary heart disease much later than men – only when they become menopausal. So it seemed logical to their doctors that estrogen was protecting them.

As with other aspects of HT and its presumed benefits for women, there had been a plethora of research data showing the benefits of HT in the cardiovascular system of women, but I wondered why, if HT was so good for their heart health, so many women who were on HT were also taking choles-terol-lowering drugs (*statins*). And inevitably, in the late 1990s, a conflict between these shiningly hopeful results and other newer results surfaced. By 2000 there was clear evi-dence that there was an increased risk of blood clots (*venous thromboembolic disease*), as well as stroke. The Heart and Estrogen-Progestin Replacement Study (HERS) found the opposite of what doctors had expected; instead of improving heart health, estrogen and progestin did not appear to pre-vent heart disease. In fact there seemed to be an increase of coronary incidents in the first year of taking HT. So, where women had been told for many years that it was practically their duty to take HT to prevent heart disease, more recent results seemed to disprove these claims.

The Women's Health Initiative

These rumblings came to a head in May 2002 when all the previously accepted wisdom about HT was shattered by the results of a very large, well-constructed study, the Women's Health Initiative (WHI). The WHI was a 15-year multimillion-dollar research programme, established in 1991 by the National Institute of Health, to address the most common causes of death, disability and poor quality of life in postmenopausal women – cardiovascular disease, cancer and osteoporosis.

It was not primarily a study of menopause, the intention was to investigate the risks and benefits of HT to postmeno-pausal women of 50 and over who were not experiencing perimenopausal symptoms and who were taking either a combination of estrogen and progestin, or estrogen alone. So the results of the WHI would not necessarily be relevant to younger women who had premature menopause and took HT at an early age. The WHI wanted to see the differences between those taking the treatment and those who were on the placebo. The medical profession awaited the results with interest, although generally, they believed that their faith in the benefits of HT would be justified.

They were destined for a shock. The results were so alarming that the accepted attitudes of the medical fraternity towards HT were forced to change. The first disturbing fact was that although the study was scheduled to last until 2005, the Data Safety Monitoring Board (DSMB) involved, which had set down certain guidelines relating to the safety of the study, recommended that it be stopped in July 2002 because it appeared that in relation to stroke, the risks of HT outweighed the benefits. A DSMB is an independent committee composed of community representatives and clinical research experts who review data while a clinical trial is in progress to ensure that participants are not exposed to undue risk. It may recommend that a trial be stopped if there are safety concerns or if the trial objectives have been achieved.

The trial of estrogen alone continued, since many doctors felt that it was the progestin that had caused the problem and that the continuing trial would confirm their belief. This was not to be. In February 2004 this trial was also terminated early because of the increased risk of stroke and the fact that there appeared to be no benefit in relation to heart disease. In this case it was the National Institute of Health in America that decided it would be unethical to continue the study.

The outrage provoked by this termination was fascinating to behold. I was at the gala reception of the South African Menopause Conference on Friday 27 February when Dr Wolf Utian of the North American Menopause Society (NAMS) announced that he had been informed that the second arm of the trial had been terminated. It was as though the ideals dearest and closest to the hearts of the assembled doctors and gynaecologists had been assaulted. And indeed they had. These doctors had spent most of their professional lives recommending HT and swearing by its benefits; to have their beliefs challenged by a very large and well-designed study was humiliating. The fallout from the termination of both arms of the study was enormous. When the first arm was terminated terrible rows broke out between the different menopause societies in different countries. Dr Jacques Rousseau, who headed the research at the National Institute of Health (NIH), became a pariah in the eyes of many gynaecologists and the publications that came out of the WHI data were attacked from all sides.

What did the WHI say?

The study shocked doctors because the initial results of the estrogen/progestin part of it showed that for every 10 000 women taking HT there would be eight more cases of breast cancer than among those on the placebo treatment, seven more cases of cardiac events, 23 more cases of dementia, 18 more cases of blood clots (*venous thromboembolism*) and eight more strokes. On the upside there would be six fewer cases of colon cancer and five fewer hip fractures.

The estrogen-only part, which was halted in February 2004, showed an increased risk of stroke; eight more women out of 10 000 would be at risk for stroke and it seemed that there was no effect, either good or bad, on heart disease. The NIH decided that the risks outweighed the benefits, in spite of the fact that after an average of seven years into the study the women involved appeared to be at no increased risk for breast cancer.

Looking at these numbers you might say to yourself: 'Well, eight more cases of women per 10 000 women a year doesn't sound so bad.' The factor that halted the trials was not the absolute but the relative risk. On the downside, this relative risk showed that there was a 29 per cent increased risk of heart attack (a significant figure), a 26 per cent increased risk of invasive breast cancer and a 41 per cent greater risk for stroke. But on the upside, the risk of hip fracture decreased by 39 per cent.

The next paragraph may seem complicated but it's vital that you understand this complex concept because, in medicine, information about absolute and relative risk is essential to any decision you might make about whether or not to take hormones. It is also a very complex concept, which took me a long time to grasp and I will try to explain it as clearly as possible.

Absolute and relative risk

You may go to your doctor and say: 'I read in the WHI study that there was an increased risk of my getting breast cancer or having a stroke.' Your doctor might reply that the absolute risk is still small, about eight more cases of stroke per year per 10 000 women taking HT. This doesn't sound too bad, except of course, if you happen to be one of those eight, but still, in the greater scheme of things, why should those figures have caused such concern? The answer is relative risk. In the WHI study, the NIH decided that the continuing relative risk for stroke was not acceptable in a prevention trial for healthy women, given that HT appeared to offer no benefit to offset the risks – it did not protect women against heart disease.

So what exactly is relative risk? If we do a study of middle-aged women at risk for heart disease and we find that it occurs frequently, for example, 20 middle-aged women in every 100 have a heart attack, but when we give them certain medication, like a cholesterol-lowering drug, which reduces the number of those women who have heart attacks to 10 out of 100, the absolute number reduction would be 10 women per 100 (a relative risk decrease of 50 per cent, which is meaningful). However, if the event happens only rarely, for example, 20 middle-aged women in every 100 000 have heart attacks, and giving them the medication reduces the number to 10 in 100 000, the absolute risk reduction is only 10 per 100 000, but the relative risk reduction is still 50 per cent.

This is why relative risk is the big problem for many doctors, who feel that it is a tool for people who 'play' with statistics. They feel that sometimes the relative risk is widely overstated, causing a panicky reaction from the media and, subsequently, from their patients. In other words, what opponents of the WHI are saying is that although the statistics in the WHI show a significant relative risk, the absolute risk is small. However, despite this small absolute risk, because so many women worldwide were, until recently, on HT, the number of women who were at increased risk for a stroke or breast cancer was large. If the events occurring are rare, relative risk makes these rare events look much more dramatic, so it would be more sensible to look carefully at the absolute risk revealed by the study.

Why all the fuss?

Given these facts, why was there such a panicked reaction? Well, firstly the media picked up on the increased relative risk as a result of HT, didn't understand it properly and had a field day. Then, many women felt that if they were one of the eight women in 10 000 who might be at increased risk for stroke and became one of those statistics, when it might have been prevented by not taking HT, that would be one woman too many. Although the absolute results from the WHI looked reassuring, with only eight more cases of breast cancer per 10 000 women, if we do some simple maths and take these figures to their quite startling conclusion, the scenario would be very worrying. For every one million women on HT there would be 800 more incidences of breast cancer, so that in countries like America for example, where millions of women are on HT, it could mean that if 25 million women were taking HT there would be 25 000 more cases of breast cancer. So, if you play with these numbers they look quite meaningful. If there are 100 million women on HT worldwide, we are looking at 80 000 more women with breast cancer because they took HT, and this number in any terms is huge!

Finally, with myriad treatments and interventions on the market today, the WHI showed that old-fashioned, observational medicine was no longer good enough. Evidence-based medicine has now become the order of the day. Evidence-based medicine means that in evaluating a clinical decision, doctors should make use of the best available evidence from the most current, academically sound research. Many women today are more aware of their rights and are better educated, and the Internet has given them new, though often suspect, sources of information. These liberated women demand to know and feel more comfortable about asking their doctors questions, and these questions need answers. Drugs and interventions must be tested and doctors and patients must have access to the results of the tests in order to decide whether the risks outweigh the benefits. Good research will have factored in all sorts of issues: family history, weight, nutrition, alcohol intake, smoking, amount of exercise and general health. Conscientious doctors will use the research to help women decide whether it will be good or bad for their specific health profile in the long run to take the hormones.

Where is the WHI in 2007?

Research about how gynaecologists felt about the WHI in 2007 showed that older male gynaecologists were more sceptical than younger practitioners, both male and particularly female, about the results of the WHI. The younger group were probably better trained to understand and respect evidence-based medicine and so may have had less of a problem changing their preconceptions.

It is comforting to note that the research shows that in spite of this scepticism on the part of the older men overall, the way they prescribe HT has definitely changed and only a few recommend HT to lower the risk of heart disease or for disease prevention in general. Interestingly, research showed that in France, where the most common kind of HT used is transdermal estradiol and micronised progesterone, the manner of prescribing HT did not change after the WHI. (I will discuss this type of HT in Chapter 4.)

Some important and conclusive answers were produced about the risks and benefits of HT in relation to women who generally were at least 10 years past their menopause. However, some believe that the WHI did not provide definitive answers about the use of HT among younger menopausal women (between the ages of 50 and 59), because of data emerging from subgroup studies. (A subgroup study is one where a smaller group of subjects from the main study are chosen by different characteristics such as age or sex to see whether these characteristics would change the overall results shown in the main group.)

This data from the WHI subgroup study was called the 'timing hypothesis', which suggested that younger menopausal women would benefit from ET. It showed that potential benefits of ET, especially in relation to heart disease, may be related to the time that estrogen is given to postmenopausal women – that is, whether it is given at the onset of menopause or later.

One of these studies, the WHI-Coronary Artery Calcium Study (WHI-CACS), came out strongly saying the earlier younger women are given ET, the greater the long-term benefits (see Chapter 7). This is still being hotly debated, although some studies show there appears to be no risk for heart disease when HT is given to young, healthy, menopausal women and it may even protect against it in the long run. However, there is still not enough research to show if the risk of heart disease is increased or decreased in younger women who are taking ET or HT (estrogen and progestogen together). There needs to be urgent ongoing research to try to provide more satisfactory answers.

Caveat emptor! Buyer beware!

The WHI gave doctors throughout the Western world a wake-up call. It showed that HT appeared to have no effect on reducing heart disease in menopausal and postmenopausal women. It showed that in some cases, whether or not there was consensus about the way the statistics had been interpreted, the risks of HT might outweigh the benefits. It showed that much of the previously accepted research and conventional wisdom about menopause and HT was incorrect. It showed doctors that HT should be prescribed with care and caution, and that it was not a universal panacea for all menopausal ills. It showed that HT did not necessarily represent the fountain of youth for middle-aged women and that all the alleged benefits may not have been founded on solid research. It showed that much of the previous data might have been skewed or based on incorrect, observational evidence. It showed that we didn't know as much about HT as we thought we did and that there were other treatments and interventions that needed to be properly tested. It showed that equine estrogen in combination with synthetic progestin may cause problems.

So, even though there are problems with the way some of the data from the WHI research was interpreted, the study was large enough, long enough and well designed enough to sound a warning both to women and to their healthcare practitioners.

Empowerment points

- When your doctor quotes a bunch of statistics to show you the benefits of a hormone treatment, don't be overwhelmed. Ask him or her to explain the statistics to you. Ask whether the risk is relative or absolute. Ask about the research, check out the sample numbers and find out whether the research is recent and whether it has been published in a prestigious journal such as the *New England Journal of Medicine*, *The Lancet* or the *Journal of the American Medical Association*.

- Don't get carried away when searching the Internet. Recent research has shown that much of the information on the Internet may be incorrect and also dangerous because the sites may belong to those whose commercial interests are paramount or who may have developed crackpot theories which look sensible but have absolutely no substantial medical basis. Remember, just because it's on the Net doesn't mean that it's correct. So follow the same rules that you would when evaluating printed information. Are the authors identified and have they declared their commercial interests? Ask your doctor to recommend some good sites. He or she should be delighted to help you get the most useful information.

Notes

_____

_____

_____

_____

4

What Now? Hormone Therapy Explained

A tale of three treatments

Tale 1

Louisa is an attractive, intelligent woman of 54. She explained that she felt fine on the hormones she was taking – a combined oral contraceptive and an estrogen supplement every day – but wanted to know more about them.

I asked her why she was taking both the contraceptive and the hormone therapy (HT).

'Because of my age, my doctor tested me while I was on the contraceptive; he wanted to know if I was perimenopausal,' she said. 'He found that my hormones were a bit low, so he told me to add some hormone therapy to the oral contraceptive. Six months later I went back for my check-up and he told me that at my age I must be menopausal and tested my E2 (estradiol), which was a bit low, so he said it was time to go on to proper HT and gave me combined HT. I felt terrible on it and got night sweats for the first time ever. So I asked him if I could

go back onto the previous combination for another six months.'

I was a little perplexed by this story. Her gynaecologist had tested her hormone levels while she was still on the oral contraceptive, which meant that the results would be inaccurate. As a woman of 54, it was almost impossible that she would still be fertile, so why was she still on birth control tablets?

Furthermore, her levels were a bit low because she was either peri- or postmenopausal. It was not clear why her doctor supplemented her hormone levels. He should have taken her off the contraceptive, waited for it to clear from her system and done a proper hormone level test before he prescribed HT, which may or may not have been necessary.

Tale 2

Colleen had had a total hysterectomy when she was 33 and had been put on to conjugated equine estrogens (CEE) (unopposed estrogen; no progestogen, because she no longer had a womb). Today, some 24 years later, she is still taking it. On Mondays, Wednesdays and Fridays she takes 1.250 mg; on Tuesdays and Thursdays she halves the dose and takes 0.625 mg.

She is very unhappy about her weight but is terrified to come off the estrogen because she is worried that she will instantly shrivel up, look old and feel miserable. A few years ago, when she had been on CEE for nearly 20 years, she stopped it cold turkey and felt so dreadful that she immediately went back on it.

Again, I was perplexed. Why should she be taking the stronger dose at all? Since the WHI most doctors and indeed the manufacturers, were recommending a much lower dose of estrogen for a shorter amount of time and in the form of a gel or a patch, not a pill.

Even more worrying was that Colleen had not been monitored and had not had her levels tested for more than three years. Whenever she mentioned her concerns to her healthcare practitioner, he was very non-committal; his attitude was: 'If you're okay don't worry', and because she'd had a total hysterectomy he didn't feel there was any problem with her continuing this dose. He did not bother to explain to her any of the risks associated with taking high doses of estrogen, which include increased risk for breast cancer, heart disease and strokes.

The reason she felt so awful when she stopped the estrogen cold turkey was that no one had explained to her that her body would've become used to the hormone and it might have been better for her to taper off the estrogen gradually, allowing her body to adapt to the new situation. She had asked her pharmacist and he knew so little that she started scouring the magazines and newspapers for answers but came away feeling more confused than ever.

Tale 3

Rosie hated the idea of HT but had, for a while, used a transdermal estradiol patch and bio-available progesterone to maintain her womb's healthy lining. 'I felt good on it,' she said. 'I didn't have any hot flushes, I had more energy and I didn't feel so down, but because of all the media hullabaloo about the dangers, I got anxious and came off all the hormones.

'After a while I started having hot flushes again and I didn't feel great, so I thought I would try the natural route and went to see one of the local alternative medicine gurus. Everyone was singing his praises. He was

very eager for me to try all sorts of exotic treatments but I wasn't too keen, so I said no.

'This doctor then referred me to a homeopath, who told me that my estrogen levels were low but my progesterone levels were fine, so I was given an estrogen cream.'

The cream was in a squat white plastic jar. It had a label with very little information on it. Melilotus – homaccord. Ignatia Homacord apply ¼ tsp to skin daily for three weeks estradiol 0.5 mg, estriol 2 mg.

What is interesting about this story is that while Rosie's estradiol level was low, it was less than 37 pmol/mL, her progesterone level was very high – 12 pmol/mL, which is the same level as in an ovulating woman.

I didn't understand how a fully menopausal woman could have a progesterone level that high if she wasn't taking additional progesterone. In fact, on further questioning, it transpired that Rosie was using a body cream which contained progesterone, although it wasn't on the list of ingredients.

The homeopath, however, hadn't bothered to find this out, even though it was hormonally impossible that Rosie would have such high levels of progesterone naturally when her estrogen levels were so low. Although the homeopath recommended the estrogen cream, which contained a high amount (2 mg) of estriol, which is meant to be a less powerful estrogen, the cream also included 0.5 mg of estradiol, which is a powerful and active estrogen, and in fact many manufacturers are suggesting that women use even lower levels of estradiol since they are able to find symptom relief with this dosage.

When you read the above stories are you surprised that women are so confused? For each of those tales there are a hundred others. Each story shows how women were subjected to different hormone regimens and in each one the women were not given the requisite information by their doctors to allow them to make sensible choices. They were not properly tested, family histories and health histories were not carefully taken and the doctors ignored the most recent medical research, doing what they thought was best, without much regard for the consequences of their actions and often paying no attention to the wishes of their patients.

As we saw in Chapter 3, the problem is that we know a bit about HT but not enough. Research is costly and lengthy, and it is difficult to set up credible studies. What research there is may be flawed because there is often bias, conflicting financial interests and skewed data. There is also a flood of data being released which is full of contradictory information. Because the situation is so confusing, it is very hard for women, even those who are well informed, to know what to do.

Doctors are also confused and sometimes anxious about prescribing something that may be harmful to their patients; a product that might look okay today but will prove to be a health risk tomorrow. Of course, there are also doctors who prefer to rely on their own clinical experience, don't believe in evidence-based medical research and continue to give their patients large doses of estrogen. This chapter should help you clarify your options and make some sensible choices that are appropriate for you and your individual menopause.

Position statements

When the estrogen/progestin arm of the WHI trial, followed by the estrogen-only arm, was terminated, menopause societies throughout the world convened boards of experts to help their confused members and to give them some guidelines about prescribing HT.

These guidelines are reviewed on an ongoing basis. The experts are some of the best and most experienced in the field of menopausal medicine and they reviewed a wide body of literature on the subject. They debate among themselves, consider the options carefully and, where the research data seems clear, use their clinical opinions and expert knowledge to write up comprehensive position statements on HT that they hope will clarify the confusing research and make sense of the hype in the media.

Because these statements are often lengthy and written in medical language I have summarised and drastically simplified the positions of five of the most powerful and influential menopause societies in the Western world. Many doctors may not agree with these statements but you can read them and draw your own conclusions.

The North American Menopause Society (NAMS) has brought out four position statements, the last one published in March 2007. NAMS is much more conservative than the European Menopause and Andropause Society (EMAS), the International Menopause Society (IMS) and the British Menopause Society (BMS), in the sense that their position statement regarding the use of HT in the treatment of hot flushes associated with menopause is more cautious and comprehensive than those of the latter three.

In their most recent position statement, NAMS suggests that all women should have a thorough medical history and examination before deciding to use HT, which they term ET (estrogen-only therapy) or EPT (combined estrogen and progestogen therapy). ET/EPT should be given to women to treat moderate to severe hot flushes and not for the prevention of heart disease in younger or older women.

Women older than 65 should not take EPT to prevent dementia or declining mental function since there is not enough evidence to suggest that ET/EPT benefits or harms women who take it during menopause or at the onset of early menopause. If vaginal atrophy (dryness) and the related symptoms are the main indicators of menopause, NAMS recommends the prescription of a local vaginal estrogen preparation.

In the event that a woman decides to take ET, NAMS suggests the lowest effective dose of estrogen should be taken for the shortest possible time in conjunction with progestogen if the woman has a uterus. They say that transdermal ET/EPT may offer some benefits over oral prescriptions such as a lower risk of blood clots if a woman uses transdermal 17β-estradiol.

There are certain indications for extended use of ET/EPT, if women are aware of the risks and are carefully monitored. This recommendation would apply to women with severe ongoing symptoms who feel that the symptom relief outweighs the risks, especially where they have tried to stop taking HT and failed, women who have moderate to severe symptoms and are at risk for fractures, and to women who cannot take first line treatments for prevention of bone loss.

NAMS believes that practitioners should work with their patients to determine the best treatment for each woman's particular lifestyle, and suggests that women be carefully monitored if they are on ET/EPT, and that ET/EPT use is reviewed regularly. NAMS also identifies the need for further research in all areas of HT.

In July 2007 the South African Menopause Society (SAMS) bought out a revised position statement which incorporated new evidence and re-evaluated evidence they had used in their 2004 position statement. It gave its members very practical advice and agreed with NAMS that it was essential for HT to be specific to each individual.

Before starting a regimen of HT all patients should be given a thorough physical examination and a mammogram; in fact, all menopausal women, whether taking HT or not, should have regular mammograms. Systemic HT should only be given to treat specific conditions such as hot flushes and associated sleep disorders and/or dry vaginas and in early menopause to prevent bone loss. Women should use progestogen if they have a womb to protect the lining and it should not be used in women who have had a hysterectomy.

Once a woman has decided to be on HT, she should take the smallest possible effective dose for relief of her symptoms and this decision should be reviewed on an annual basis. All types of hormone therapies should be considered to have the same risks and benefits. It is suggested that a women who has been on HT for a period of more than four years should stop the treatment to see how she feels without it.

SAMS gives a very clear directive to doctors treating menopause to be well-informed about the latest research and developments regarding the status of HT so they can help their patients make informed decisions about its risks and benefits.

In the 2006/07 updates on clinical recommendations on postmenopausal hormone therapy, the EMAS says that its previous point of view and recommendations have not altered. It agrees that some women may be at risk for blood clots but believes that HT is the best option for women with climacteric (perimenopausal) symptoms, and that since it improves their quality of life, the benefits of HT far outweigh the risks.

EMAS feels that the type of treatment prescribed should be individualised and that the lowest dose should be prescribed for a maximum of two to three years. HT should not be prescribed to prevent heart disease or to improve mental (cognitive) function, and that a healthy lifestyle is important to improve quality of life and to prevent heart disease, osteoporosis and breast cancer.

In 2007 the IMS updated recommendations on postmenopausal therapy that suggested that HT is still the most effective therapy for hot flushes, dry vaginas and other menopause-related complaints. It argues that HT, when prescribed to suit each particular individual, improves both quality of life and sexuality in menopausal women.

Like other European societies, it feels that HT is effective in preventing bone loss in menopause and decreases fracture risk, and unlike NAMS, it suggests that HT is a first-line treatment for postmenopausal women, especially those under 60 and those who have become surgically menopausal.

IMS argues that HT, when started in recently menopausal women who are younger than 60, does not cause early heart disease and in fact reduces the risk of heart disease and death. In addition, it states that HT given at the onset of menopause or to younger menopausal women may reduce the risk of Alzheimer's disease. In its statement, the risks for HT focus mainly on breast cancer, blood clots, stroke and coronary disease.

However, IMS argues that the degree of association of HT and the risk of breast cancer remains debatable. In addition, that risk is very small and may depend on different types, administration and kinds of HT. Women with a womb should take a progestogen with ET. IMS suggests that women taking continuous EPT have a lower rate of thickening of the lining of the womb than those who do not. Low and ultra-low doses of estrogen and progesterone may stimulate the lining of the womb less, and cause less bleeding.

Transdermal estrogen may prevent the risk of heart disease and blood clots, which may occur with oral HT. Further study is required to determine whether complementary and alternative therapies are safe and effective. Research has shown that non-hormonal therapies like antidepressants and anti-epileptic medication (gabapentin) are effective in alleviating hot flushes in the short term, but further study is needed to determine long-term safety.

The quality and purity of bioidentical hormones have not been tested, nor have they been scientifically proven safe or effective. Salivary assays are not useful. Ultimately the safety of HT depends on age, and generally, the benefits of HT when it is started within a few years of menopause are greater than the risks for most women.

The BMS also produced a consensus report and, like the European society, it is more sceptical than the American and South African societies about whether the risks of HT out-weigh the benefits. It agrees with the other societies about the risk of blood clots. Since, in the opinion of the BMS, HT is the best treatment for relieving hot flushes and other related menopausal symptoms, it feels that estrogen should still be used as the treatment of choice. The merits of long-term use should be assessed annually for each individual.

The BMS also believes that estrogen may be to be the best treatment option for osteoporosis. Like all the other societies, the BMS says that unopposed estrogen should not be given to women who still have their wombs and that treatment should be individualised. Ultimately, the BMS believes that the benefits of HT may outweigh the risks if the therapy is appropriate.

As you can see from the plethora of data and the different opinions, the debate rages on and is not likely to abate. Read carefully, make use of the information that is available to you, and keep an open mind about the risks and benefits of HT.

My position

I am not a medical doctor, but I have been consulting with menopausal women for many years and during this time I have followed the extensive research on menopause. I have read as widely as I could on this subject and listened to the opinions of many different experts in the field. I have sat in conferences and talks and tried to weigh up and think carefully and logically about what I have heard. I have looked at the financial interests of those who were passing out the information and I have spoken to different experts in the field. What I write may well be proved wrong by future research, but here is my personal position.

Before you even consider taking HT...

Before you decide to start taking HT I think that you should take a careful look at your lifestyle. As I explained in Chapter 1, not everything can be blamed on menopause. You need to re-evaluate how well you are caring for yourself. Are you eating healthily? Do you smoke or drink in excess? Are you exercising regularly? How is your mental health? Are you dealing well with the stresses of middle age? Once you can honestly say that you have considered these issues and believe that you are doing your best to live a healthy, balanced life, you should spend some time with your healthcare practitioner discussing the risks and benefits of HT and whether it is suitable for you.

You already know that before you decide to take HT you should have a thorough medical examination. This can be time-consuming and expensive, but it is worth it. Commit to caring for yourself; don't go blindly into it.

Your doctor should ask you about your family history, paying special attention to whether you had a mother, or maternal or paternal grandmother, who had breast or any other cancer and whether other close family members died of cancer, heart disease or a stroke. Specific tests should be performed to see if you are at risk for blood clots. Your doctor should make a record of the medication you are taking and whether you had a thrombosis or risk of one when you were pregnant. If this is so then you might need specialised testing, called a thrombotic screen, which involves a number of tests and includes a clotting profile. This should be done if your doctor feels that you are at risk for blood clots.

Your doctor should also be aware of whether you smoke, whether you drink and how much you drink daily. In my opinion, if you are a very heavy drinker or you smoke, it is too risky to be on estrogen. Your weight must be checked. Overweight women are at greater risk for heart disease, and this is increased when they take estrogen. A body mass index of 25 to 30 or greater than 30 should be a warning flag.

Any medical problems should be noted and you should tell your doctor if you suffer from migraines. If he or she doesn't ask you any of these things, bring them up yourself. Levels of cholesterol, fasting glucose and your thyroid should be checked.

Before you decide to start taking HT you should have a mammogram, an endometrial scan and a bone density scan. Most importantly, you should have your hormone levels tested, but be sure the measurements that are being taken are accurate. One of the most glaring errors that occurs in the care of menopausal women is the confusion that arises when doctors measure hormone levels. It is accepted that you can't measure the estrogen of women on oral contraceptives or non bio-available hormones. The serum estradiol levels you measure can *only* be from bio-available hormones. So what often happens is that a doctor tests the hormone levels of a woman who is on conjugated equine estrogens (CEE) but because he or she is only measuring one type of estrogen, and the CEE has not been converted into that estrogen, it looks as though the woman's estradiol levels are low and so the dose of her hormone therapy is increased. This is why women on HT often have the symptoms of excess estrogen.

When should you have HT?

I think it is important to stress here that women who, because of surgery or cancer treatment (see Chapter 6) are plunged into premature menopause before their chronological menopause is due should, subject to their doctor's consent and if HT is not contraindicated, have hormone therapy. There can be some debate but only about the length of time for which they should take the hormones and about the type of hormones that will be most effective and offer the highest benefits and lowest risks.

Once you have had all the appropriate tests, it is my opinion that you should take HT if hot flushes are affecting your quality of life. If you get a hot flush once in a while or only a couple of hot flushes or temperature changes during a day and are coping well with these, there is no need to take HT. You may want to try alternative remedies or just live with this small, transient change in your life.

But ... it is time to take HT if you wake up during the night drenched in sweat; if night sweats are disturbing your sleep patterns with the result that you feel ratty, weepy and depressed the next day. It is sensible to take HT if, during the day, you are immobilised by hot flushes and if you find that summer has become unbearable. If the accompanying symptoms of the hot flushes are nausea, giddiness, a ringing in your ears, a pounding heart, intense heat, and/or a very red face, and if all or any of these symptoms are affecting the way you live your life and the way you feel emotionally, it would be a good idea to take some form of HT.

Another reason to take HT would be if your vagina is so dry that sex is miserable, or that your dry vagina is causing all sorts of urinary infections and problems. But if you are experiencing these symptoms and are not plagued with hot flushes, I would suggest that you take HT in the form of a local vaginal estrogen product.

Some doctors feel that women who are at risk for osteoporosis in the first years of menopause should take HT to prevent fractures, but if these women don't have severe menopausal symptoms, there are other products on the market which may be a better option, and I will discuss these options in Chapter 9.

When not to take HT

You are not a candidate for HT if you are very overweight, have high blood pressure, and are at risk for stroke, heart disease or blood clots. Smokers or heavy drinkers should not take HT. Neither should women who may be at risk for breast cancer or have had or currently have breast cancer. If you have liver disease or have any known or suspected estrogen-positive malignant tumours, HT is not a wise idea.

Be careful if you have any genital bleeding. The cause should be diagnosed before you begin any HT regimen. If you suffer from severe migraines, unless it has been clearly indicated that they are not due to fluctuations in your hormone levels, you should be careful when you take HT. If you have a skin disease known as *porphyria cutanea tarda* you should also not take HT.

What kind of hormones should you take?

There is no need to suffer from hot flushes and a dry vagina when we know that estrogen helps these symptoms. Choose the type of estrogen carefully. You have probably heard a lot about 'natural' progesterone and estrogen. There's nothing really natural about them. The word natural used in this sense means that they are exactly the same (*bioidentical*) as the hormones in your body. But whether they are bioidentical or not, they have been manufactured (*synthesised*) in a laboratory.

There are many different hormones available containing estrogen. They have names such as estradiol hemihydrate, estradiol valerate, ethinyl estradiol, estropipate, sodium estrone sulphate, conjugated equine estrogens, estriol, estradiol and 17β-estradiol. The last three are *exactly* the same as the estrogen found in your body. The others may be very similar but they are not identical.

You know that the active estrogen in CEE is equinol. Although it has a similar effect to human estrogen, this equine estrogen is stronger than your main circulating estrogen, which is called estradiol and is bio-available, and it doesn't have the same molecular structure as estradiol. So, when your body breaks CEE down (*metabolises* it), it doesn't do it as effectively as it would a bioidentical estrogen and the estrogen stays in your system for longer.

So logically, wouldn't you rather use a product that your body has been processing for years? There are thousands of women using bioidentical hormones in different forms – creams and gels – but as yet there are no large compelling studies, like the WHI, on the risks and benefits of these hormones, so much of the information about them is anecdotal. However, until we have better research, logic seems to say that this is the way to go.

At this time there is a lot of discussion about bioidentical products (see page 63) called Tri-est and Bi-est, which are meant to have the same composition as the estrogen in your body (*endogenous estrogen*). In other words, they are made up of estriol, estradiol and estrone, and/or estriol and estradiol, respectively. Now, in Chapter 2, we discussed these three main estrogens and the theory is that if you are going to balance your hormones, why not use a mix identical to the one that is in your own body? It certainly sounds very persuasive and researchers are beginning to look more closely at the benefits of estriol, which as you will remember, is a free hormone and won't convert back into estradiol or estrone. But there are a few issues here that concern me.

By the time we reach menopause the estrogen composition in our bodies has changed. The main estrogen is no longer estradiol but estrone. Research into breast cancer indicates that concentrations of estrone, estradiol, and estrone sulfate are high in women with breast cancer, despite low levels of circulating estrogens. So I am concerned about adding more estrone in a cream like Tri-est, when estradiol and progesterone in peri- and postmenopausal women are more likely to convert into more estrone anyway. However, like everything else in the field of HT, there needs to be a lot more research to find out the precise role that estrone and estrone sulfate play in the role of breast cancer in peri- and postmenopausal women who are taking HT. Also, although the advocates of Tri-est and Bi-est would have you believe that estriol has the same effects as the stronger estrogens without the risks, one would wonder why estradiol and estrone need to be added, given the risks we know they involve.

The claims for estriol are that it is much less potent than estradiol and it may have fewer of the risks commonly associated with estrogens. Although it can never be given in the same doses as estradiol, estriol still carries certain risks – it can cause the lining of the womb to thicken and it can stimulate certain breast cancer cells. On the upside, when taken vaginally, it can help alleviate dryness in the vagina and is often prescribed for women who have breast cancer and suffer from vaginal dryness. We need longer and better research to show that estriol, when used over a long time in the higher doses that seem to be necessary for it to work, will not produce the same risks as estradiol. Take the emotion out of the equation and examine the facts.

Progesterone

Here is the big question: what about progesterone – to add or not to add? The terminology relating to this hormone is often very confusing for women. So for the sake of clarity, the word 'progesterone' is usually used to describe bioidentical progesterone, which is the same as your own endogenous progesterone (the progesterone that your body produces). When you read about progestins or progestogens they are usually synthetic products, but all three – progesterone, progestins and progestogens – have the same effect on the lining of your womb, causing it to be shed when it is ready. And just to add to your confusion, the term progestin can also refer to progesterone. In this book when I write about progesterone, I mean the hormone that is identical to your own progesterone, and when I refer to progestins I am referring to all the others.

The WHI and other recent research seem to suggest that the addition of MPA and other more androgenic progestogens to hormone therapy may increase the risk for cancer, stroke and heart disease. There may also be other effects, like bloating and water retention, although some new-type progestogens like *drospirenone*, *dydrogesterone* and micronised progesterone can dampen the effect of *aldosterone*, a hormone that controls the levels of fluid in your body and which, when combined with estrogen, may prevent water retention and may be a better choice.

There is also research showing that synthetic progestogens can contribute to depression in women, while micronised progesterone is often helpful in combating depression and maintaining sleep patterns. Some research suggests that bio-identical progesterone does not appear to have the damaging effect of synthetic progestogens on the thin, flat cells called the endothelium that line the inside of the blood vessels of the entire circulatory system. When the endothelium is damaged it can lead to heart disease and stroke. More research is required in this area.

A lot has been written about 'natural' progesterone, which I want to emphasise once again, is not natural, but is synthesised in a laboratory like all the other progestins. The big difference is that it is identical to your own body's progesterone. I also don't believe that slathering on progesterone is a good idea. 'Natural' or not, it is still a powerful hormone and overdosing with it can cause a lot of bad side effects.

If you are keen to use a 'natural' progesterone make sure that it is one that has been passed by a medicines regulatory body. There are good micronised progesterones available, although to control bleeding you may need higher doses, which may then cause other side effects. Many of the brands of so-called 'natural' progesterone have not been tested and the doses they contain are not standardised, so even progesterone packaged with the same brand name may differ in quality and in the amount of bio-available progesterone it contains. It may also not control bleeding or the thickness of the lining of the womb. So be careful if you are using this cream in conjunction with estrogen therapy.

Some healthcare practitioners recommend 'natural progesterone to alleviate menopausal symptoms. Their rationale is that there are progesterone receptors throughout your body and progesterone is a precursor or building block hormone for estrogen and testosterone, as I discussed in Chapter 2. They suggest that if you take progesterone, it may give you high enough levels of those hormones to maintain a healthy hormonal balance, but there is just not enough hard research on this method of HT to be sure it does not carry too many risks and undesirable side effects. In addition, some of these creams contain wild yam, which is useless, because human beings do not have the necessary cofactors to convert this into anything useful. It is also not disclosed that these creams sometimes contain progesterone, which be a safety issue, especially if a woman is at risk for or has had breast cancer.

> *Remember Rosie from the cautionary tale at the start of this chapter? She complained that she was sleepy all the time and felt listless and depressed. When I questioned her closely I found she was happily applying a body lotion that contained large amounts of progesterone. She had absolutely no idea how much she was taking; she bought the cream from a health food store as a good product for the symptoms of menopause. When she had a blood test, she found that her progesterone levels were constantly as high as the levels in an ovulating woman, and remember that level only peaks in a normally menstruating woman, it doesn't remain as high on an ongoing basis.*

At this time some studies suggest that certain progestogens may cause problems in the long run. But once again, more research is needed to give definitive answers. So at present if you haven't got a womb, you should probably not take progestogen. If you have a womb, you will definitely need to take a progestogen because if you do not, you could be at risk for cancer of the lining of your womb.

Some small studies suggest it may be safe not to take a progestogen, or to only take it intermittently if you are taking low-dose or ultra-low-dose estrogen, but the problem is that although this very low dose of estrogen appears to help prevent osteoporosis, it may not alleviate menopausal symptoms. More research is needed to establish whether taking progesterone intermittently is safe in the long term and whether it is preferable to taking a continuous combined dose. If you and your doctor decide to go this route, you must understand the risks and be closely monitored by a transvaginal ultrasound scanner.

The big discussion is when you should have your progesterone – only in what would have been the second part of your cycle when you were a menstruating woman (the luteal phase) or a small dose daily? Some people believe that if you still have your womb you should give your body a break at the time your period would have happened in your cycle when you were still menstruating normally. Others believe that women should take progesterone continuously.

An alternative to an oral progestogen or cream is a loop (intrauterine device) containing a progestogen (Mirena). This type of loop, containing 20 mcg of a progestogen called *Levenogesterol*, appears to control bleeding and prevent the lining of the womb from thickening. It may also not have the suggested adverse effects of an oral progestogen because it is local, so the amount of progestogen that enters your system is lower, though a fair amount of this progestogen is still absorbed. More research is needed to establish whether its effects on the breast or heart differ from those of other available progestogens. There have been cases of postmenopausal women who use this device experiencing spotting or breakthrough bleeding.

There is also the option of taking a progestin after few months of estrogen-only treatment to ensure a bleed. You have to see which regimen suits you best. Discuss your options with your doctor and make sure that you have the lining of your womb monitored regularly to see that it isn't getting too thick. Don't forget too, that if you have had an endometrial ablation (see Chapter 6) you will still need a progestogen if you are taking estrogen because small pockets of the endo-metrium (lining of the womb) may remain.

Bioidentical hormones and compounded bioidentical hormones

Both compounded bioidentical hormones and manufactured bioidentical hormones are available on the market, although most of them have not been approved by medicine control boards. However, some doctors do prescribe them, and the best way to find where they are available, is to hit the Net. When you find them, this chapter should have given you enough information to present to your doctor and to help you decide whether she or he will monitor you.

In the aftermath of the WHI, with heightened awareness and fears about the risks of HT, women began to investigate alternatives to commercially produced hormone products. Searching for relief from menopausal symptoms, they became aware of bioidentical hormones, which are marketed as safer and more effective. However, although there is an increasing tendency to use compounded, bioidentical hor-mones for individual hormone therapy, the term bioidentical therapy, which was coined by marketers, has no scientific meaning and is neither defined nor standardised. However, the term bioidentical means that these hormones are struc-turally identical to the hormones produced by a woman's ovaries. Bioidentical hormones can be both manufactured and compounded. Women are told that these products are 'natural', which, as I indicated above, is simply not true.

If you are told that the bioidentical hormones you are using are compounded, this means that a doctor has asked a pharmacist to combine, mix or alter certain ingredients to create a medication that has been customised for you. These hormones are made from plant derivatives and are then pre-pared, mixed, assembled, packaged, or labelled as drugs.

The whole point of compounded, bioidentical hormones is that they should be specific to the person for whom they were prescribed. Unlike commercially manufactured hormone therapy, bioidentical hormones claim to replace hormones rather than treat specific menopausal symptoms. There is a great deal of hype about returning hormone levels to 'normal', so proponents of bioidentical hormones say that they are actually 'replacing' hormones, while traditional HT is used to treat transitional menopausal symptoms.

In fact, it has not been established what the 'best' or most 'normal' hormone levels in postmenopausal women are and a woman's physical comfort may not even be related to her hormone levels – you often simply need a small amount of HT to help your symptoms rather than a whole regimen to replace your hormones. So, with the aim of 'replacing' your hormones, these products usually include estradiol, estriol, estrone, progesterone and testosterone. Many bioidentical hormone products have not undergone rigorous clinical testing for safety or efficacy, and issues regarding purity, potency and quality are a concern.

In addition some bioidentical hormone products on the market are not compounded but still believed by many women to be safer than so-called artificial hormones. But don't be fooled. Patients often receive incomplete or incorrect information about these products. Bioidentical hormones are not necessarily safer than the so-called artificial or synthetic hormones. A hormone IS a hormone, though different types have different levels of potency, so there are the same safety issues with compounded bioidentical hormone products as there are with hormone therapy medications that have been approved for use by various regulatory bodies. There is no scientific evidence to support claims of increased efficacy or safety for individualised estrogen or progesterone regimens. It is clear that all hormone regimens, whether bioidentical or commercially manufactured, should be subject to the same stringent controls.

Unlike manufactured hormone products, bioidentical hormones generally have no package insert describing their risks and benefits, and have not been approved through rigorous testing or Level I research. The people who sell these products quote all sorts of research and also do what I discuss in Chapter 5, which is to pick sentences out of research, edit them and use them out of context. So an article criticising bioidentical hormone use may actually be quoted as supporting it, using the edited quote next to the source. Many of the studies of bioidentical hormones are short term, carried out on animals, are not placebo-controlled or use very small sample numbers. Most do not meet the criteria set out on page 36 for Level I evidence, which is the crème de la crème of research. As one doctor said to me: 'If a menopausal rat walked into my consulting room, I'd know exactly what to treat it with!' The trouble is we're not rats, we are menopausal women, and should demand that anyone recommending bioidentical hormones should produce adequate evidence.

Studies done on bioidentical hormones have revealed that fewer than half the samples contained the ingredients claimed or the amount of active hormone they promised. Because the amount of estrogen or progesterone in many of the products is not clearly indicated, it is easy to take more estrogen than is necessary. Just because the estrogen in a product is bioidentical doesn't mean it is safer.

Suzanne Somers of the television sitcom *Three's Company* recently wrote a book about bioidentical hormones called *The Sexy Years*, which has taken America by storm. While what she says makes some sense, the fact that she is taking 1 mg and sometimes more of estradiol a day means that she is putting herself at unnecessary risk. As you read at the beginning of this chapter, recent research has shown that that this dose is simply too high.

Remember that hormones that have been passed by a regulatory body must be consistent in their quality, purity, potency, efficacy and safety. The products from compounding pharmacies are not regulated in the same way and their quality can vary. As I said earlier, a hormone is a hormone, and in my opinion, it is criminal for health food shops and people who are not experienced in reproductive endocrinology or in the field of menopause, to sell creams or gels containing these very potent hormones to unsuspecting women. They are *not* harmless because they are bioidentical!

If you are keen to take bioidentical HT do it sensibly; enlist the help of your general practitioner, gynaecologist or physician. Find out exactly how much of the particular hormone you are taking in each dose and be sure that it is the correct amount. If you have a womb, make sure you have annual endometrial scans to see that the lining is not becoming dangerously thick. Have annual mammograms and have your hormone levels monitored. I must stress the point though, that if you decide to use these hormones, it is a case of 'buyer beware'. Don't forget that compounding pharmacies also promote their products and are well aware of their market.

Hormone therapy is not anti-ageing medicine

There is also a tendency among some of the proponents of HT and those who advocate bioidentical hormone therapy to tell women that they must take hormone therapy because it will keep them young. This is, in my opinion, an extremely dangerous stance. Beware of the healthcare practitioner who is in love with this idea and overenthusiastic about the perceived benefits of HT! Estrogen is not the elixir of life; there are many other medications for disease prevention, which may not carry as many risks. There is NO robust evidence at this time to show that HT should be used for anything other than the alleviation of menopausal symptoms, and the data indicates that it should be taken in the lowest possible dose for the shortest possible time.

The jury is still out as to whether ET protects against heart disease and two long-term studies, KEEPS and ELITE, will address this. I discuss this issue in Chapter 7. There is no evidence that ET improves your mental ability or protects against dementia. In fact, a recent study showed that once the effect of general ageing is taken into account, there is no association between blood serum estrogen levels and mental function. There is an urgent need for more research in this area but ageing is genetically programmed into our bodies. You will get older but the way in which you age is *your* responsibility. There is no magic bullet to keep you young and long-term or high-dose HT or bioidentical therapies may carry all sorts of risks that will outweigh the benefits. HT has not yet not been proven to prevent disease or retard ageing. It is vital to eat sensibly, exercise religiously, deal with your stress and watch your weight. These are the things that will keep you looking younger and feeling better. At this time research suggests that HT should not be used for disease prevention or as anti-ageing medicine.

Testosterone

Currently a lot is being written about women in menopause and their decreased desire for sex. I have my own ideas on this subject, which I will deal with in the section on sex and menopause, but since some doctors recommend testosterone when prescribing HT to perimenopausal women, I will try to give you the low-down on it. Some doctors have been using testosterone implants for years but this testosterone is not bioidentical, it is usually *methyltestosterone* – a synthetic type – and is often given in quite a high dose that may well upset your delicate hormonal balance and create unpleasant side effects like aggressiveness, greasy skin, unwanted facial hair, adult acne and weight gain. It may also impact badly on your cholesterol levels because it is an androgen and can drive up your LDL (bad cholesterol).

Some women really battle with low sexual desire and have had blood tests showing that their levels of testosterone are very low indeed. But this in itself is a problem because serum testosterone levels reflect only a tiny amount of the total testosterone available in your body, so measuring total and free testosterone may only give a limited picture of a woman's testosterone levels. Interestingly, new research has shown that testosterone continues to be produced by the cells in the ovaries (*stroma*) for some time after the onset of natural menopause, so low levels of testosterone in menopause may not be a cause of low libido.

On the other hand, women who have had surgical menopause often find that the dramatic removal of their ovaries causes a sharp drop in sexual desire even if they are taking estrogen. Newer research has shown that these women had improved sex lives when using a testosterone patch, which gave them a daily dose of 300 mcg of testosterone in conjunction with transdermal ET.

Other research into a low-dose patch with bio-available testosterone showed that after four weeks of use there was a marked rise in sexual desire and after six months all the women using the patch were very satisfied with their sexual encounters. The good thing about this patch was that there were very few of the usual side effects – a slight increase in facial hair and some very minor cases of acne, and all agreed that the sexual satisfaction far outweighed these disadvantages. If you are very keen to use some testosterone, I would suggest you stick to the rule of using one that is bioidentical.

DHEA

Because DHEA is the main building block hormone for so many of the steroid hormones, including estrogen, progesterone and testosterone, certain healthcare practitioners like to prescribe a bio-available DHEA. It was banned by America's Food and Drug Administration (FDA) in 1985 as a medical treatment but is now available in the USA and many other countries as a dietary supplement.

There are many products which are called DHEA, one of which is a pharmaceutical product that has exactly the same molecular structure as your own DHEA. However, take care, as there are many other preparations, found mainly in health shops, which are labelled DHEA and may contain some of this bioidentical DHEA but may also include many different kinds of additives and hormones which could be harmful. If you are determined to take DHEA, you should never take more than 5 mg daily and never for longer than three months at a time.

DHEA is touted as a miracle hormone with myriad helpful effects, including burning fat, building muscle, strengthening your immune system, boosting your libido, energising you, preventing memory loss and helping to diminish stress. Studies have shown that DHEA can improve testosterone levels in women but it doesn't usually relieve symptoms or improve cognitive functioning. Research into DHEA is ongoing but has not yet verified these claims.

Make no mistake, like all other hormones DHEA is very potent and if you decide to take it you should be aware of the problems that can be caused by overdosing. These include sleep pattern interference; increased masculine characteristics like lots of hair growth on your body and face, while your hairline recedes; a greasy, porous skin and an increased risk of heart disease because DHEA lowers the level of good cholesterol (HDL) and raises that of bad cholesterol (LDL); and weight gain, because it increases insulin resistance. (The two types of cholesterol are described fully in Chapter 7.) Just because it is one of the main building block hormones doesn't mean that adding DHEA to your system, where you hope it will metabolise in such a way that your hormone levels will be the same as when you were in your twenties, will solve your perimenopausal woes. I would suggest that you only add DHEA to your HT regimen if you are under the care of a very experienced endocrinologist who has the expertise to monitor you and to understand the correct dosage.

How should you take your hormones?

I think that the best way to take HT is through your skin (*transdermally*). The reason is that when you take HT in the form of a pill it must first pass through your liver (*hepatic first pass*) in order to be absorbed by your body. This is believed to interfere with a very important hormone called *insulin-like growth factor 1* (IGF1), which has a good effect on your bones and helps to maintain bone density. IGF1 also has an insulin-like effect.

When you take oral estrogen it interferes with the delicate production process of IGF1, resulting in raised levels of insulin, which means that your metabolism slows down, your blood sugar drops and you crave sweet things and carbohydrates. On the other hand, when you apply estrogen to your skin it is absorbed and, like the estrogen that is manufactured in your own body (*endogenous estrogen*), it is carried to your heart and from there, as I explained in Chapter 2, it is distributed to the estrogen receptor sites before it gets to the liver.

Research has shown that when you are menstruating normally you produce between 100 and 200 mg of estradiol over a period of 24 hours, but when you take estrogen orally a larger amount is often delivered to your body in one go and reaches the liver within a few hours, which means that your body has to deal with metabolising this rapidly instead of in its normal steady way.

In Chapter 2 I likened the complex and subtle way the hormones in our body are programmed to the instruments playing in harmony in an orchestra. If one member is out of tune the whole melody is discordant. Logically, it seems to me, this is what happens when you take estrogen orally.

When you take the estrogen through your skin, especially through a slow-release patch, or by applying measured doses of the cream or gel, your body is getting its estrogen in a way that is almost identical to the way it is received it when your own body was producing enough estrogen. Allowing for very stable continuous hormone levels. It seems that this is generally a safer way for your body to receive HT.

Recent research has also shown that unlike oral estrogen, transdermal estrogen had no effect on IGF1 levels or those of *C-reactive protein* (CRP), a protein that is produced by the liver only when your body is experiencing severe inflammation. This is important because once again it shows that transdermal HT does not interfere with the way the liver works. Research has shown that although CRP levels may be raised when you have a heart attack, it is not clear what role it plays in heart disease; whether it is just a marker of this disease or whether raised levels may be a risk factor in heart disease.

Women taking transdermal estrogen had lower levels of estrone sulfate than those taking their HT orally, and the estrone sulfate levels in those using the patch were similar to the levels found in menstruating women. This is important because it is thought that increased levels may be implicated in breast cancers. Researchers also found that women prone to migraines suffered far more when taking oral HT while there was no increase in the frequency and severity of migraines in women using the patch. Data from the ESTHER (Estrogen and Thromboembolism Risk) study showed that there may also be a lower risk of blood clotting with transdermal estrogen, micronised progesterone and less androgenic progestogens.

There are also more and more products containing 17β-estradiol that you can take through your skin. Some women who don't have wombs are very happy with a 20 mg estradiol implant, which is bio-available estrogen, appears not to affect cholesterol levels or to add to the risk of stroke, and is available throughout the day without causing the problems that occur when you take one dose at a time. Once again though, you need to discuss all the pros and cons of this implant with your doctor. I personally prefer being able to change the dose at a moment's notice if I have to.

What is the safest and best dose of hormones?

In their position statements NAMS and SAMS suggest that women take the smallest amount of estrogen possible to alleviate the symptoms of hot flushes and dry vaginas. So I would suggest that you begin with the lowest dose available and increase it if you find it isn't making a difference.

It is interesting to note that as soon as the results of the WHI were published and the media were having a fine time panicking the public, hundreds of thousands of women stopped taking their HT 'cold turkey' and profits of companies like Wyeth, who manufacture Premarin, plummeted by 30 per cent in one year. Suddenly all the big companies started advertising hormones with very low doses of estrogen and progestins.

Look at this comparison, I selected the most relevant points and I have highlighted important words and numbers in italics.

In *Menopause* in 1997, Prempro advertised like this:
- Simplicity of a single tablet
- One prescription for you, one tablet for your patients

- The most prescribed HRT regimen in America
- Proven endometrial protection with a *low* dose of only *70 mg* of progestin over four weeks of therapy. One PREMPRO tablet contains *0.625 mg* of the conjugated estrogens found in Premarin® tablets and *2.5 mg* of medroxyprogesterone acetate.

In *Menopause* in 2004 things had changed somewhat:

- Today, menopausal symptom relief starts here *0.3/1.5*. The *lowest effective* dose. Proven efficacy with the *lowest* starting dose
- 52 per cent less estrogen, 40 per cent less progestin
- Manage patients at the lowest effective dose. Women should be started at *0.3 mg/1.5 mg* daily
- Wyeth – our commitment to women's health continues
- 'Go *low* with Prempro'

Suddenly there is a plethora of low-dose estrogen products on the market, all of them paying attention to guidelines which suggest that much lower doses of estrogen and progestin are as effective and much safer. In your doctor's waiting room you will notice a series of pamphlets advertising these new 'low-dose' products. So you can be sure that no matter how much the manufacturers of hormones argued against the results of the WHI, they took notice of the FDA recommendations and the fact that women had woken up to the risks of large doses of HT, and reacted by lowering the amount of estrogen in their products.

Many very low-dose estrogen patches and creams are already available and more will be coming on to the market, so keep your eyes open for them and ask your pharmacist to let you know as soon as they become available. Start with the lowest dose you can – you can always increase it if it isn't effective. Research has shown that women using products with doses as low as 0.025 mg no longer battle with hot flushes. But for a rule of thumb, 0.3 mg of the CEE tablet, a dose of oral 17β-estradiol ranging from 0.25 mg to 0.50 mg and 0.025 to 0.050 mg for transdermal estrogen (the patch, creams or gels) are all acceptable doses.

I am a great believer in the mantra 'less is more', as you will realise when you read the chapter on vitamins and supplements. Be moderate with your hormone therapy. Another important point is how you take your HT. Because bioidentical hormones metabolise quickly, it would probably be sensible to take your daily portion in divided doses even if the manufacturer suggests only one application daily. Rub the cream or gel on in the morning and the evening for the best results. Try to mimic your body's rhythm. If you are using the patch you need to split up your week exactly. So apply it on Tuesday morning and then replace it with a new patch on Friday evening.

For how long should you take HT?

Most doctors believe that women can safely stay on HT for up to five years. If you are taking HT for that length of time, the rule about having regular check-ups and being carefully monitored by your doctor applies even more strictly. Today the consensus is that if you still have bad menopausal symptoms after five years, have tried to stop HT but can't because these symptoms are making you miserable and you are not at risk, you can continue HT as long as you are very carefully monitored and understand all the risks and benefits.

I would suggest that you re-evaluate how you feel after a year. If you don't have hot flushes and the other symptoms have disappeared, you could slowly taper off the HT. What often happens though, is that the flushes have stopped but your vagina still doesn't feel great. This is when I would suggest you try vaginal estrogen. Some healthcare practitioners prefer vaginal estrogen creams, tablets or *pessaries* (small oval shaped pills that you can put into your vagina). An estriol cream can be very helpful and doesn't have any side effects. It can be applied three times a week and really seems to work, though some women don't like the mushy feeling of the cream.

The method I think is most convenient and least invasive is an estradiol-releasing vaginal ring. This is a thin rubber ring impregnated with estradiol which is tucked securely behind your cervix where you don't feel it and stays there for three months, alleviating the problems of a dry vagina by giving out small amounts of estradiol.

Eleanor's sex life had been put on hold because, as she told her GP, sex had become so painful that she found it almost unbearable to make love to her husband and they were both, understandably, feeling very frustrated. Her doctor recommended the estradiol-releasing ring and Eleanor started using it. Within two weeks she found that her vagina had stopped feeling dry and painful and that sex was fine again. But when she went to her gynaecologist for her annual check-up he told her to stop using it. When she asked him why, he replied that he didn't like it, but gave her no further explanation.

Many doctors only prescribe the estradiol-releasing ring for much older women who are suffering from some of the urinary tract problems, like urinary incontinence and urinary tract infections, which often accompany a dry vagina, rather than to alleviate the problem of a dry vagina that comes with menopause, but it seems to me to be a safe and uncomplicated way to beat this problem too. As Eleanor's story illustrates, some doctors do not like it, but many women have found that their vaginal problem improves markedly with the use of the vaginal ring. The ring can remain in place for three months and should be changed after that, which means that four rings should be used each year.

It is thought that the ring can be used indefinitely, even if a woman has a uterus, and up to now it has been believed that the effects are almost entirely local, which means that the estrogen that is released is confined to the vaginal area and doesn't circulate throughout the body. However, some of the latest research has shown that the vaginal ring not only relieves vaginal dryness but may alleviate hot flushes. This means that some of the estrogen released from the ring circulates throughout your body, which is known as a systemic effect, rather than just a local effect. So although much less estrogen is absorbed systemically with both the ring (and the tablet), some research has shown that there are changes in the cholesterol levels of some women who are using these, which means that specialists have still not decided whether the amount of estrogen absorbed systemically is safe for cancer survivors.

More research is needed to find the lowest most effective dose of vaginal estrogen that would only work locally. So, if you are at risk for breast cancer or any other estrogen-positive cancer and decide to use the ring, you must discuss all the risks and benefits with your healthcare practitioner and continue to be carefully monitored. Other local vaginal estrogen preparations such as an estriol cream, which have been found to be effective, might be safer in this case (see above page 73). This debate aside, research on the ring shows that it generally has no adverse side effects and women find it comfortable and easy to use.

Designer hormones

Some hormones used in HT have been specifically manu-factured to try to overcome some of the problems found in regular estrogen and progestogen products. There has been a lot of research into these products but more is needed, especially using larger sample groups to try to understand their risks and benefits more fully.

SERMs

Selective Estrogen Receptor Modulators (SERMs) are hor-mones with an estrogen effect on certain areas of your body that will benefit you and block unwanted estrogen effects on other parts of your body so that the amount of active estrogen in your body is not increased.

The best-known SERMs are *Tamoxifen* and the second gener-ation SERM *Raloxifene*. Although Tamoxifen has been used for nearly 30 years to treat women with estrogen-positive breast cancer, and millions of women have done well on it, it does have some unpleasant side effects. One of the most serious of these is that it doesn't relieve hot flushes, it sometimes aggravates them. It is thought that this happens because Tamoxifen blocks the effects of certain estrogen receptors in the body, including in the brain. Research has shown that after more than five years on Tamoxifen there is increased risk of endometrial cancer and strokes.

Raloxifene was developed to help prevent osteoporosis in women and has been very effective in this area. Like its predecessor, it has an anti-estrogenic effect on breast tissue and it doesn't stimulate the lining of the womb. It appears to lower the bad cholesterol and triglycerides, although it doesn't raise the levels of good cholesterol. Like Tamoxifen, it doesn't alleviate hot flushes and may make them worse. The risk of blood clots is the same for women on this hormone as for those on regular estrogen preparations. Because it is a relatively new designer hormone, much more research needs to be done before doctors can say with certainty that the long-term benefits of Raloxifene will outweigh the risks.

In my opinion you should not take a SERM as a substitute for HT. SERMs should only be taken for a specific medical condition such as the control of breast cancer and severe osteoporosis. There are now some third generation SERMs on the market which are showing some very promising results.

Tibolone, a designer preparation, has a combination of weak estrogenic, androgenic and progestogenic effects on your body. It reduces hot flushes and is recommended for women with osteoporosis because it increases bone mineral density. It also has several additional positive effects, including the fact that it does not appear to lead to thickening of the lining of the womb and the estrogen in it is tissue-selective, which means that it has a beneficial estrogenic effect on certain tissues, including those in the vagina and bone, but not on breast tissue or the lining of the womb. It does, however, have some unpleasant side effects which include breakthrough bleeding if you still have a womb, weight gain, bloating, and water retention, and more worrying, it seems to cause an increase in LDL, the bad cholesterol, and a reduction in the level of good cholesterol.

In 2006 a trial to determine the effect of tibolone on new vertebral fractures in elderly women – Long-term Intervention with Fractures (LIFT) was stopped prematurely as the

Data Safety Monitoring Board (DSMB) found that there was an increased risk of stroke in the group taking tibolone as opposed to the control group. In May 2007 another randomised placebo-controlled clinical trial designed to assess the safety and efficacy of tibolone, when used for the relief of menopausal symptoms in patients with a history of breast cancer, was discontinued ahead of schedule because the DSMB found that there were more breast cancer recurrences in the group of women who were randomised to receive tibolone.

The results of these long-term studies are still awaited, so tibolone should be regarded as having the same risk profile as regular ET/EPT. Once again, my personal preference is for bio-available hormones, which metabolise as nature intended them to, though many doctors are happy to prescribe tibolone and their patients feel good on it.

Different kinds of HT regimens

As discussed above, there are different ways to take HT and it's important for you to decide which regimen is best suited to your lifestyle and body chemistry. Some women loathe the patch; they may be allergic to the adhesives on it or find that it peels off when they are exercising and, of course, it's useless for those women who do daily water aerobics. Others like it and feel really good on it. They may find that they get an ideal dose if they cut the patch in half and they don't like the problem of remembering to add hormones daily. Other women are more comfortable with a gel or cream.

If you have a womb you need to decide, with your doctor, whether you want to take progesterone daily in conjunction with your estrogen or only sequentially, and there are also different options here. You can take it every two weeks. If you are taking a very low-dose estrogen you may find that the lining of your womb doesn't thicken and you may only need progestogen intermittently, but in this case you must understand the risks and be closely monitored by a doctor who is skilled in the use of transvaginal ultrasound.

How to find out what's best for you

Sometimes it's hard to know which HT regimen is best for you. But it's here that you have to take responsibility for yourself. You will know if you feel good on something. You will know when your hot flushes have stopped, you are sleeping better and sex is no longer uncomfortable. You are allowed to start an HT regimen and then stop it if you start experiencing uncomfortable symptoms.

Whatever you choose, it may not work immediately. In fact, with most products it is at least two weeks before you feel a difference, but if after you have started a new hormone you feel bloated or nauseous, your breasts are tender, you feel symptoms of PMS or become very moody or irritable, the product you are trying is not for you or you may need to try an even lower dose or a different combination. Work with your healthcare practitioner; ask your doctor for all the options and work out carefully what is best for you. It's your right to feel as good as possible and you may need several attempts before you find the hormone therapy and hormone regimen that really suits you.

The terminology of HT regimens

HT	Hormone therapy (either ET or EPT)
ET	Estrogen therapy
EPT	Estrogen progestogen therapy
CC-EPT	Continuous combined estrogen progestogen therapy (you get progestogen and estrogen daily)
CS-EPT	Continuous sequential estrogen progestogen therapy (estrogen daily with progesterone added in a set sequence, for example, every two weeks)
Systemic ET/EPT	Preparations that work throughout your system, not just on your vagina

Local ET   Preparations that work mainly in your
                  vaginal area

As I write this there are several very low, transdermal estrogen products in the pipeline, so keep your eyes open and ask your doctor or pharmacist to let you know when they arrive on the shelves. When you are deciding on a hormone treatment read the product insert carefully. There are many viable products, but in my opinion, those that are closest to the bio-available hormone, those that are low-dose and are taken transdermally, are preferable.

Empowerment points

• When you are having a check-up before you go on HT or when you return to your gynaecologist for your annual check-up, make a point of telling him or her if you are on any new medication or if you have had any illnesses or medical incidents during the year. For example, you can't expect your doctor to be psychic and intuit that a cardiologist has put you on a blood thinner or that since your last appointment you have been diagnosed with high blood pressure. It's not up to you to decide what is and is not relevant about your medical history. Let the expert decide. If you don't impart the information you can't blame your doctor for making a bad decision. Everything that relates to your medical history during the intervening months is important if you are to have a successful partnership and not put yourself at unnecessary risk if you are on HT.

• Think for yourself and use your own judgement. The fact that your doctor's wife is on 0.625 mg of CEE doesn't mean that it's okay for you.

• When you decide to stop your HT, you should probably wean yourself off it slowly. The way in which you do it depends on the type of HT you are taking. Discuss this with your doctor. I believe that it is better for your body to become accustomed to having low levels of estrogen. If you stop it abruptly you may experience the same sort of symptoms that come from fluctuating levels of estrogen in perimenopause.

- HT Pointers:
  - Sensible lifestyle
  - A full check-up
  - HT should only be taken to alleviate hot flushes, night sweats and a dry vagina
  - Hormones should be bioidentical
  - HT should be applied transdermally
  - The dose should be as low as possible
  - HT should be taken for the shortest possible length of time
  - Taper off the HT after one year and check whether your perimenopausal symptoms have abated
  - If your only remaining symptom is a dry vagina, try a local vaginal estrogen product
  - If you are on HT you should have regular check-ups, including an annual transvaginal examination and a mammogram.

Notes

_____

_____

_____

_____

_____

_____

_____

_____

_____

_____

5

If I Shake You, Will You Rattle?
Vitamins and Minerals in Menopause

Laurie is an attractive 58-year-old brunette who came to see me because she felt terrible: 'I'm nauseous and my head aches. I feel very tired and I can't remember things. It's strange, because, although I feel exhausted, at the same time I feel nuts, like I'm wired. And if that's not bad enough, I recently lost a lot of weight and now I've put it on again. I can't seem to keep it off no matter what I do.'

Laurie's symptoms fitted right in with those of perimenopause, but they seemed to be unusually bad. She explained that she was very aware of her health and was taking several vitamins and supplements daily. She was also drinking three to four litres of water a day because she had been told it was healthy. She could not understand why, when she took such care of herself, she should feel so awful. She told me that she was nervous about taking HT and was a great believer in alternative medicine, which she thought would help her through menopause.

I asked Laurie to show me all the supplements she was taking and was horrified to discover that she was swallowing a daily dose of 16 different vitamins, supplements and homeopathic tinctures. In addition, she was taking at least six painkillers daily because she had such bad headaches. From a purely logical point of view, given the number of supplements Laurie was taking, it seemed to me that her liver was working overtime.

She was obviously having rebound headaches from the painkillers and drinking far too much water, so she was flushing large amounts of the supplements down the drain and putting a lot of stress on her kidneys. In addition, it didn't seem that the products she was taking were alleviating her perimenopausal symptoms; they were making them worse!

Many peri- and postmenopausal women are firm believers that vast quantities of vitamin and mineral supplements will not only get them through menopause but will also keep them healthy and eternally young. This is a very thorny topic. In fact, as I read the extraordinarily wide selection of literature and media advice on the subject, I felt more confused than ever about HT. For all the passionate outpourings from the conventional medicine industry denouncing supplements, there were equally passionate refutations, claims and denials from the producers and proponents of supplements in the complementary and alternative medicine industry.

Once again, we women are caught in the crossfire. We buy into the idea that by not taking specific vitamins and minerals we are abdicating responsibility for our own health and well-being and compromising our chances of a healthy life and old age, yet we are worried by reports that not only may we be wasting our money on these supplements but they may actually be harmful.

A friend who arrived from America carrying plastic bags brimming with different vitamins, knowing that I was sceptical about their efficacy, brought me eight different newsletters and glossy magazines on the subject. While I was reading them I suddenly realised why women are conned into believing that supplements are vital to their future health. The articles in these publications are written by medical doctors; they use medical terminology and speak with consummate authority on the subject. They recommend various supplements in self-assured, breezy, consumer-friendly language.

They offer hope and certainty that we can prevent ageing and ill health; once again, they offer a quick fix. Just as the pharmaceutical companies played on women's fears about ageing when they sold us that magic bullet HT, the producers of supplements are hooking into the same anxieties and we are buying into the hype.

The problem is that many of these so-called medical practitioners, although they are often pictured in white lab coats with stethoscopes draped casually round their necks, may not be licensed and may have degrees that are not recognised by conventional medical authorities. Many of them are sponsored by the producers of vitamins and mineral supplements and, just as I warned you to be wary of research articles on HT which did not declare their interests, I am warning you to pay attention to the hidden interests behind the information you read about supplements. Most of the 'practitioners' are selling the supplements about which they write so glowingly, so their advice is not impartial!

I know that medical science is not perfect and I know that 'there are more things in heaven and earth than are dreamed of ', and that there is still enormous research to be done into this subject, but in order to remain true to my belief that knowledge is power and that women's fears should not make them vulnerable to voracious commercial interests, I am going to hang my colours to the mast and tell you how you might be able to negotiate the supplement dilemma.

A giant industry

Let's begin with some facts. The alternative medicine and vitamin and mineral supplement industry is a giant one. In America alone last year there were more than 29 000 different supplements available. Women, in a desperate quest for health and youth, spend billions annually on products that have usually not been subjected to the rigorous research and development that conventional medicines must undergo.

Most conventional medicines take at least 12 years to develop before the controlling bodies of their respective countries allow them to be manufactured. Their efficacy has to be proved and their side effects stated before they appear on the market. Supplements can be sold as soon as the manufacturer has produced them. There is no onus on manufacturers to give any information on the label other than the ingredients, no need for them to clarify the efficacy and safety of the products or make any reference to the side effects that these products may cause.

Supplement manufacturers are also allowed to make structure-function claims. In other words, they can't say that calcium cures osteoporosis but they can say: 'Calcium makes bones strong'. Because these products are not carefully controlled they may be contaminated with toxic heavy metals like lead, mercury and arsenic, and the amount of the ingredients stated on the label may be misrepresented, so that you may be taking more or less of a supplement than you believe, or even taking something that has not been listed. The doses suggested on the label may not be correct and may have bad effects; for example, many supplements are said to slow down the rate at which something in your body decays or breaks down because of its interaction with oxygen (*antioxidant*) but certain vitamins in the wrong amounts may actually speed up the decay (an *oxidant* effect).

Some of these products may very well be effective. It is just that as yet there is not enough rigorous scientific data available that shows clearly that they really do what they claim. In the past, government bodies like the Food and Drug Administration (FDA) in the USA, the Medicine and Healthcare Products Regulatory Agency (MHRA) in the UK and the Medicines Control Council (MCC) in South Africa classified supplements as foods, so anyone could put a supplement onto the market.

The producers of these unregulated supplements could then make extravagant, perhaps unjustified, claims about the efficacy of the product, not bother to supply data about its safety and label it in such a way that you could not rely on the ingredient information but would get hooked by phrases like 'younger skin at your finger tips', or statements using complicated medical language which give an impression of superior knowledge. For example: 'The cell protective effects of Indole-3-Carbinol help to maintain proper function of estrogen receptor sites on cell membranes, help maintain p21 suppressor gene function, help detoxify pesticides and other environmental pollutants including dioxin, aid in the conversion of 16-α-hydroxyestrone to 2-hydroxyesterone, promote the health of prostate and breast tissue.'

When these statements appear on labels or in advertisements for American products they must also carry a box (which is often in minuscule print) saying 'These statements have not been evaluated by the Food and Drug Administration. This product is not intended to diagnose, treat, cure or prevent any disease.' This is all well and good but very few of us read the tiny print, and the claims made, when taken at face value, sound very impressive. Furthermore, the onus is on the FDA to prove them wrong. In the circumstances, there is absolutely no need for the manufacturers to subject their products to rigorous, well-designed, scientific studies.

Another problem with the information we receive on supplements is that the claims are not substantiated. The trials that are cited have small sample numbers, are not properly controlled, and are often of short-term duration; usually not more than six months. They may often be based on anecdotal information or testimonials (letters that say: 'Since taking x supplement I have lost 15 kg and feel younger and healthier than ever').

Many of the people who sell supplements have not been properly trained in the field and aren't able to understand the complicated biochemical processes whereby food is digested and our bodies obtain the vitamins and minerals essential for our health and well-being. They also don't understand the complicated interactions that can occur between so-called natural substances and conventional medication.

When someone in a health food store or pharmacy offers me ginkgo biloba, telling me authoritatively that by taking it I will improve my memory, I feel like shouting: 'Who says?' I would be delighted if careful scientific research proved this to be true. Which of us menopausal women have not sat with a blank look on our face, trying to retrieve some information or bemoaning to our friends the loss of our memories? It would be great to get some help in this area, but a recent rigorous study of more than 200 healthy adults taking recommended doses of ginkgo showed there was absolutely no difference between the memories of those who took the ginkgo and the control group who didn't.

So why do we, when we are peri- and postmenopausal, think that we need to take vitamin and mineral supplements and *nutraceuticals* (products taken from foods and said to have proven medical benefits, especially in the prevention of heart disease)? I think it is because we want to be responsible for ourselves and our health, and that in some sense we have bought into a concept that has become the rallying cry of complementary and alternative medicine in the 21st century – anti-ageing and preventative medicine.

While I believe that it is very important that women take responsibility for their own wellness and live the kind of lifestyle that helps to prevent illness and disease, I think that we get too hooked into a mindset that promises eternal youth and immortality. Ultimately, most of the anti-ageing claims that the complementary and alternative medicine industry make have not been proved in well-designed, scientifically proven clinical trials. What we do know is this: we will age and we will die.

The best we can hope for and take responsibility for is that to the best of our ability, we will try to live a balanced, sensible life that will ensure a happy and healthy old age. However, we are bombarded with advertisements, information and hype from the media, entreating and beseeching us to take more of this or that supplement.

It is true that we live in a world where our crops are fertilised with all kinds of chemicals and pesticides, that we eat eggs and chickens that are produced in inhumane batteries and that our meat may be pumped full of hormones and antibiotics. Much of the food we eat has food colourants and preservatives and some of us are hooked on fast foods that are high in sodium and saturated fats.

But here's the good news: most of us generally eat enough good, quality foods to ensure that we get most of the supplements we need. In fact, the vitamins that you get from foods probably act more efficiently than a single dose of a particular supplement. Our bodies have been synthesising foods for thousands of years and are very efficient. If our diet is well balanced there is no reason to believe that we won't be getting enough of the right vitamins and minerals. In the chapter on weight, you will see some recommendations for a really healthy and nutritional food plan.

In spite of this knowledge, many healthcare practitioners are eager to prescribe large doses of supplements. I have read of menopause experts who unashamedly suggest that women can easily take 10 or more capsules and tablets daily. I personally think that's an awful lot of supplements to remember to take daily, especially since stress is one of the conditions that adds to our vitamin depletion. In my book, once we feel we should be taking those supplements, it is just another thing to remember and to feel bad about if we don't.

However, I must make a confession. For several years before I really woke up and started looking at the available research, I was a great advocate of supplements. I bought into all the propaganda and, looking back to my client files of six years ago, I see that I generally suggested at least seven or more supplements daily. Today I am convinced that less is more and nothing is better for middle-aged women than taking responsibility for a healthy lifestyle.

Another problem with taking a wide variety of supplements is that many of them contain small amounts of other supplements in addition to the main ingredient. So you may think you're only supplementing with glucosamine because that is the main product listed on the front label but what you are taking may also contain vitamins C, E, B1, B2, B6, B12, nicotinic acid, pantothenic acid, zinc, selenium, boron, silicon and manganese. So you have the additional responsibility (and stress) of being aware of the amounts of the different vitamins in each of the supplements you are taking, in order to keep your dosage within the safe upper limits suggested.

Definition of vitamin and mineral supplements

Vitamins are organic substances that the human body needs, in varying but usually small quantities, in order to grow. They help to break down and use (*metabolise*) the food we eat in the most efficient way, ensuring that our bodies grow and develop, and that we have healthy, functioning cells. Because the body cannot produce all its own vitamins, these organic substances work together with other substances called enzymes, which are special proteins that help the chemical processes in the body, so that the vitamins are used in the most appropriate way. Each vitamin has a number of specific functions in the human body and a deficiency of one or more can result in illness. For example, in the old days, sailors on long sea voyages who didn't have access to fresh vegetables developed scurvy from a lack of vitamin C.

There are two groups of vitamins: those that are water-soluble (vitamin C and the B-complex vitamins) and those that are fat soluble (vitamins A, D, E and K). The former are found throughout the body's tissues, where they interact with enzymes to ensure that your body functions in a healthy and life-enhancing way.

Excess amounts of water-soluble vitamins are eliminated from your body in your urine, but make no mistake, too much vitamin C or too many B vitamins can be toxic, so pay careful attention to the amounts you are taking. Remember, if you are taking several supplements daily you may be getting extra amounts of any one vitamin. Two of the fat-soluble vitamins, A and D, can be very toxic but even too much of vitamins E and K is not wise. Your body, as we discussed in previous chapters, is a finely tuned machine, and moderation is everything. Just as too much of a particular hormone can upset the body's delicate balance, too much of any one vitamin can cause problems. In the case of supplements more may *not* be better.

Like vitamins, supplements can contain amino acids, which are the building blocks of proteins; herbs; and/or botanicals, which are any of the parts of a plant that can be synthesised and used in the product in a variety of ways; and enzymes.

I keep talking about the importance of a healthy diet but many women are not sure what this means, so I have included a list on the next page describing the function of each vitamin, where it is found in the foods you eat, and most importantly, what amounts of it are safe. Most of the antioxidants the supplement manufacturers are promoting are found naturally in these foods. If we can obtain our vitamins and minerals from foods they are cheaper, truly natural and are better absorbed, since the body, developed over thousands of years of evolution, will know how to synthesise them.

The vitamins that come from foods come combined with other vitamins and minerals, and interact in the body in an intricate way, providing the healthiest, most effective results. If you do decide to take mega doses of supplements, you should be aware that many of the trials done on these substances have not been long-term and the long-term poisonous effect (*toxicity*) of the products may not be properly known or understood. Many of these products may also interact powerfully with any conventional medicines that you may be taking. Remember, just because a supplement is said to be natural doesn't mean that it's harmless.

The lists below are intended as a guideline to show you that many of the supplements we are told to take are present in a sensible and varied diet. You should only need to supplement your diet if you don't get enough of a particular vitamin or mineral; have been ill or chronically stressed; have an eating disorder; or eat fast food morning, noon and night. There are healthcare practitioners, like registered dieticians, who have been properly trained and can assess your diet to see whether you might be deficient in one or more of the supplements listed below.

Approach supplementation with caution and never go above the safe upper limit – the highest dose of a particular supplement you can take before it becomes poisonous and you suffer from one or more of the many side effects associated with too high levels of any particular vitamin or mineral.

If you eat a really varied diet containing lots of fruit, vegetables, wholegrains, the right kinds of protein, nuts and dairy products, you should get more than adequate amounts of vitamins and minerals for healthy living. The suggested amount of fruit and vegetables is at least five to nine servings daily.

Vitamins

Guidelines for the daily dose are for women 31-70 years old. The suggested daily dose is called the average intake (AI) and the safe upper limit (SUL) is the highest amount you can take safely.

Also note that mg means milligrams, and mcg means micrograms. 1 mcg equals 40 IU so, by way of example, the label may read either 400 IU or 10 mcg.

Vitamin A (also known as retinol)

Function: Is vital for healthy skin, teeth, bones, tissues and vision.

Food source: Liver, egg yolk, butter, cream, fish-liver oils.

Guidelines for daily dose: AI = 700 mcg; SUL = 3000 mcg.

Beta-carotene

Beta-carotene is a precursor of vitamin A (the body can make vitamin A from this vitamin)

Function: Powerful antioxidant which may lower CRP levels and control or help lower the level of homocysteines in your blood (homocysteine is an amino acid which can be toxic in high amounts and may be a risk factor in heart disease. An amino acid is a chemical messenger in your body).

Food source: Dark leafy greens, yellow and orange vegetables and fruits.

Guidelines for daily dose: 5-6 mg. This dose has not really been established but the above amount is estimated to be safe.

Carotenoids

(including lycopene, zeaxanthin lutein, alpha-carotene, cryptoxanthin)

Function: Powerful antioxidants; also help with healthy vision, skin and lining of blood vessels and help to protect the skin from sun damage and cancer.

Food source: Yellow and orange vegetables, dark leafy vegetables, avocado and red and pink fruits like tomatoes, watermelon and pink grapefruit.

Thiamine (B1)

Function: Vital for the maintenance of healthy nerve cells and the central nervous system; important for growth and digestive functioning; helps in the body's conversion of carbohydrates to energy.

Food source: Wholegrain products, seeds, wheatgerm, meat products, dairy products, legumes, eggs and some fruits.

Guidelines for daily dose: AI = 1.1 mcg; no SUL established.

Riboflavine (B2)

Function: Maintains the growth of cells and is involved in red blood cell production; important for the metabolism of carbohydrates, proteins and fats; maintains the mucous membranes of the skin, eyes and nervous system; involved in the production of adrenaline by the adrenal glands.

Food source: Milk, eggs, enriched cereals, grain, ice cream (the real kind), liver, some lean meats and vegetables.

Guidelines for daily dose: AI = 1.1 mcg; no SUL established.

Folic acid

Function: Plays a vital role in the production of DNA; can prevent birth defects like spina bifida; involved in the formation of white and red blood cells, and may reduce homo-cysteine levels.

Food source: Green leafy vegetables, beans, orange juice, liver, yeast extract, some fruits.

Guidelines for daily dose: AI = 400 mcg; SUL =1000 mcg.

Niacin (B3)

(nicotinic acid and nicotinamide are the active forms)

Function: Maintains healthy skin and nerves; maintains lowered cholesterol levels; converts food to energy; oxidises fats and proteins.

Food source: Beef, pork, eggs and cow's milk, peanuts, chicken, fish and yeast.

Guidelines for daily dose: AI = 14 mg; SUL = 35 mg.

Pyridoxine (B6)

Function: Helps with the synthesis of protein in the body; formation of red blood cells and normal brain functioning, and aids the digestive system; involved in the formation of antibodies and boosts the immune system; involved in regulating moods and relieving depression.

Food source: Fish, pork, eggs, milk, wheatgerm, brewer's yeast, brown rice, soybeans, oats, wholewheat grains, peanuts and walnuts.

Guidelines for daily dose: AI = 1.5 mg; SUL = 100 mg.

Vitamin B12

Function: Vital for the red blood cells and central nervous system; important for the normal metabolism of all cells, especially in the gastrointestinal tract, bone marrow and nervous tissue.

Food source: Eggs, dairy products, animal proteins, liver and kidneys.

Guidelines for daily dose: AI = 2.4 mcg; no SUL established.

Pantothenic acid

Function: Food metabolism, involved in the manufacture of hormones and cholesterol.

Food source: Chicken, beef, cereals, liver, egg yolk, kidney, yeast, broccoli, wholegrains, mushrooms, avocado, milk, sweet potato, salmon.

Guidelines for daily dose: AI = 5 mg; no SUL established.

Biotin

Function: Metabolises protein, fat and carbohydrates; regulates insulin hormones and cholesterol (cholesterol is the building block for most hormones and functioning of cell membranes, especially in the brain).

Food source: Liver, egg yolk, kidney, muscle and organ meats, most leafy vegetables, some fruit, milk and the bacteria in your gut.

Guidelines for daily dose: AI = 30 mcg; no SUL established.

Vitamin C

Function: Healthy teeth and gums; promotes healing; involved in the body's absorption of iron; is a powerful anti-oxidant.

Food source: Ripe fruit, especially citrus fruit; vegetables, especially red peppers.

Guidelines for daily dose: AI = 75 mg; SUL = 2000 mg.

Vitamin D

Function: Body manufactures this after exposure to sunlight. Promotes absorption of calcium, so is vital to the development and maintenance of healthy bones and teeth; regulates the body's levels of calcium and phosphorus.

Food source: Exposure to sun; also found in fatty fish, fish-liver oils, liver, eggs, butter, cream.

Guidelines for daily dose: AI =10 mcg/800 IU; SUL = 12.5 mcg /1 000 IU

Vitamin E

Tocopherol (d-alpha-, beta-, gamma-, and delta-tocopherol are excellent, but beware of synthetic vitamin E).

Function: Powerful antioxidant; protects red blood cells from being destroyed in too large numbers and keeps membranes healthy.

Food source: Nuts and seeds, wheatgerm, leafy vegetables, legumes, egg yolk.

Guidelines for daily dose: AI = 15 mg; SUL = 1000mg.

Vitamin K

Function: Vital to blood clotting; also involved in brain functioning and may help to maintain strong bones in the elderly.

Food source: Broccoli and leafy green vegetables, vegetable oils, small amounts found in eggs, dairy products, meat.

Guidelines for daily dose: AI = 90 mcg; no SUL established.

Minerals

A mineral is a natural inorganic substance with a specific chemical make-up that is vital for healthy body functioning. The minerals I have listed below are those that are most important for a healthy diet. You may know of others. If your eating plan is sensible, you will be getting traces of all of them, which should be enough to maintain general good health.

Guidelines for the daily dose are for women 31-70 years old. Sources are given at the end of the chapter.

Calcium

Function: Essential for bone formation and for cardiovascular, nerve and muscle functioning; maintains cell structures.

Food source: Milk and milk products, especially cheese; sardines with bones; dark leafy greens like kale and broccoli; sesame seeds and oranges; soybean products. Low-fat milk and plain low- or non-fat yoghurt.

Guidelines for daily dose: AI = 1200-1500 mg; SUL = 2500 mg.

Iron

Function: Iron in red blood cells carries oxygen, which is necessary for the production of energy, the functioning of the immune system, and cognitive performance. Iron is an important component of some enzymes.

Food source: Red meats, liver, fish, and poultry. Dark leafy vegetables, cocoa, molasses, wholegrains, oysters, lentils and dried beans, prunes, raisins and some fruit.

Guidelines for daily dose: AI = 18 mg; SUL = 45 mg.

Magnesium

Function: Magnesium is essential to maintain both the acid-alkaline balance in the body and healthy functioning of nerves and muscles (including the heart), as well as to activate enzymes to metabolise blood sugars, proteins and carbohydrates. It is essential for metabolising vitamin D.

Food source: Seeds, unrefined grains, beans and leafy vegetables.

Guidelines for daily dose: AI = 320 mg; SUL = 350 mg.

Potassium

Function: Together with sodium it maintains normal cell functioning, water balance, acid-base balance, muscular and neural functioning, and is important for cellular growth.

Muscle mass and glycogen storage is related to potassium content of the muscles and it works with various enzymes in helping the pancreas to secrete insulin.

Food source: Most fruits, root vegetables like potatoes, milk, beef, liver, chicken, soy, turkey, shellfish and dark leafy greens.

Guidelines for daily dose: 2000 mg = EMR (estimated metabolic requirement); no SUL established.

Selenium

Function: Works in conjunction with vitamin E to provide a powerful antioxidant.

Food source: Seafood, eggs, liver, kidneys, red meat and chicken. Depending on oil content, wholegrains, brazil nuts.

Guidelines for daily dose: AI = 55 mg; SUL = 400 mcg.

Zinc

Function: Supports the health of the immune system; helps to synthesise protein, lipids and carbohydrates, and maintains the health of reproductive organs and cell division. Zinc is a component of insulin.

Food source: Meats, fish, beans, wholegrains, pumpkin seeds, mushrooms and brewer's yeast, oysters, shellfish and herring.

Guidelines for daily dose: AI = 8 mg; SUL = 40 mg.

Trace Minerals

Chromium

Function: Involved in metabolism of carbohydrates; fat and protein metabolism; involved with insulin action; may benefit triglyceride levels.

Food source: Brewer's yeast, oysters, liver, seafood, wholegrains, meat, broccoli.

Guidelines for daily dose: AI = 20 mcg; no SUL established.

Copper

Function: Involved in maintaining the immune system, healthy red and white blood cells, brain development, cholesterol and glucose metabolism.

Food source: Wholegrains, nuts, shellfish, liver and dark green leafy vegetables.

Guidelines for daily dose: AI = 900 mcg; no SUL established.

Manganese

Function: Important in activating different enzymes to help healthy body functioning; crucial in healthy thyroid functioning, digestion and central nervous system functioning, as well as for the formation of connective and skeletal tissue, growth and development, reproduction, and carbohydrate and fat metabolism.

Food source: Grains and cereal products, nuts, green vegetables, tea, legumes, blueberries.

Guidelines for daily dose: AI = 1.8 mg; no SUL established.

Molybdenum

Function: Helps to regulate iron stores in the body and interacts with different enzymes to metabolise carbohydrates, oxidise fats; helps keep teeth healthy.

Food source: Meats, fish, legumes, wholegrains, pumpkin seeds, leafy vegetables, cauliflower, mushrooms and brewer's yeast.

Guidelines for daily dose: AI = 43-45 mcg; no SUL established.

Vanadium

Function: Ultra trace element on which much more research needs to be done. It may be helpful in lowering cholesterol levels.

Food source: Wholegrains, meats and dairy products, seafood, spinach, parsley, mushrooms, oysters.

Guidelines for daily dose: 1.8 mg estimated requirement since the daily requirement is undefined.

In addition to these, peri- and postmenopausal women are offered other supplements, mainly by complementary and alternative healthcare practitioners. Unfortunately, there have not been enough rigorous, scientific trials on these supplements for me to say with absolute certainty that they will be beneficial to you or will help to improve your symptoms.

But women continue to be hugely interested in complementary and alternative medicine, possibly because we have been 'burnt' by conventional medicine and often find that conventional healthcare practitioners are dismissive, stingy with their time and frequently patriarchal. The WHI report and the subsequent scare about HT further encouraged us to look to complementary and alternative medicines as a solution to our problems. Even before the WHI scare, we were uneasy with the side effects that many of us experienced with conventional hormone therapy.

Women are particularly susceptible to the lure of complementary and alternative medicines because we tend to look at things laterally, trust our instincts, be less suspicious of difference and more prepared to accept that life is complex. We think there may be solutions other than conventional ones to problems. We also long for the eternal youth that complementary and alternative medicines promise us. What we don't realise is that we may also be 'burnt' by these products and, because we are susceptible to the lure of promises that we can prevent ourselves from ageing, we need to have a very clear idea of the risks and benefits of the different supplements that are available to us.

The Web is very useful for accessing information, there are literally thousands of sites devoted to this subject, but remember to apply the same critical approach to these sites that I suggested when you are accessing information about hormones:

- Check who runs the site. Is it a reputable government, medical or academic institution? And are the writers qualified – a string of letters or some technical sounding name doesn't mean that they are bona fide; the degrees may come from bogus institutions.
- Is the purpose of the site to sell you something? Does it have advertisements and sponsors, and are there all sorts of links that lead you to products that are for sale?
- Check that there are sound references. Much of the information on dietary supplements uses the trick of selecting a line of information from a study and repeating it out of context, or using a phrase from a study without citing the study or its reference anywhere in the publication.
- Watch out for overly scientific language categorically stating the effects of a product without citing the study or the reference from which it comes
- Check the date of the information on the site. Improved research may mean that something that was a breakthrough in the 1990s has changed radically in the intervening decade.

You should apply the same stringent criteria to articles on the subject. I have just been shown a newsletter written by one of the so-called gurus of complementary medicine, which says the following (*the italics are my comments*):

> Vitamin A deficiency reduces immune function by diminishing the function neutrophils, macrophages and natural killer cells (*says who?*). Normally I suggest 10 000 to 25 000 IU. But if you're working on an infection, such as influenza, I recommend a loading dose (*What does this mean? How will your liver cope with it?*) for three days at 300 000 units daily. Then drop to 25 000 units daily thereafter (*look at my table for the daily safe upper limits of vitamin A – 1 500 IU*). If you're worried about toxicity – don't be (unless you're pregnant). The Merck manual says that you must take 100 000 units for several weeks to months before you reach toxicity with vitamin A.

Whitaker, J. 'Other Supplements to Boost Resistance'. *Health and Healing* December 2004, Vol 14, No 12, p3

All the reading and research I had done had led me to believe that a supplemental daily dose of no more than 1 500 IU would be safe. So practising what I preach, I looked up the Merck manual, which says: '*Chronic toxicity* in older children and adults usually develops after doses of >33 000 mg (10 000 IU)/day have been taken for months' (my emphasis), but on the same page concludes with the following: 'Prolonged daily administration of large doses *must be avoided* because toxicity may result' (my emphasis).

So I went to the Natural Medicines Comprehensive Database http://www.naturaldatabase.com/ which is updated regularly and is the closest I have found to a physicians' reference book (which lists all the information, side effects, benefits and so on of the conventional medicine you take). It says that vitamin A is safe in adults when used in doses of less than 10 000 units per day and gives the following reference: Food and Nutrition Board, Institute of Medicine. *Dietary Reference Intakes for Vitamin A, Vitamin K, Arsenic, Boron, Chromium, Copper, Iodine, Iron, Manganese, Molybdenum, Nickel, Silicon, Vanadium, and Zinc*. Washington, DC: National Academy Press, 2002. Available at:www.nap.edu/books/0309072794/html/.

The above serves to illustrate my point. Be very careful what you read and who you believe; eat and live as healthily as possible and don't go wild with huge doses of any one supplement. There is, as yet, no clear scientific evidence that more is better.

Supplements frequently prescribed for peri- and postmenopausal women

There are hundreds of different supplements in the market-place but those I list below are the ones most commonly prescribed for peri- and postmenopausal women. I have tried to give you an overview of each of them: their risks, efficacy and benefits. In some cases I have given the scientific name with the herbal supplements, so that if a homeopath prescribes a tincture for you, you will know what you are taking.

The first four supplements are thought to act like the hormone estrogen. Much research has been done into these but there are still not enough long-term, well-controlled, double-blind, randomised studies. However, because of the interest in these supplements, good trials are under way and it may not be too long before we can say with much more certainty that they do what they claim to do and are safe as well as beneficial.

Because of the huge interest in complementary and alternative medicine, your healthcare practitioner should be aware of the growing number of products that have been tested which may be safe and effective in relieving symptoms. Your doctor is well trained and qualified enough to understand the research documents so don't be afraid to show him/her information or ask his/her opinion, so that you can have an informed discussion. Your doctor should always ask you if you are taking any complementary or alternative medicines and this should be included in your medical history.

Many women swear that a particular supplement has helped reduce hot flushes, but this is often the result of what is called the 'placebo effect', the situation in which those in the control group believe so strongly that the substance they are taking is going be good for them that they actually exhibit the same physical changes as the experimental group.

The following point is so important that although I wrote about it in Chapter 4 I'm going to repeat it. In a good double-blind, randomised trial there are two groups: an experimental group, which is taking the product being tested, and a control group, which is taking a harmless but ineffective substance called a placebo. The people in the control group believe that what they are taking is the substance that is being tested. Neither of the groups knows whether it is the control group or the experimental group. Much of the research that has been done into plant estrogens up to now has not been of long enough duration to eliminate this reaction, but it does show how powerful the mind can be in controlling symptoms like hot flushes.

Plant estrogens

A word of warning here: because so little is known about the way these plant estrogens interact, be careful of taking two or more in combination. One of them may be fine for you but many of the supplements that health food shops recommend to peri- and postmenopausal women contain all or some of these. Remember, just because they're herbal doesn't mean they're harmless. If you are taking these, you should be monitored as closely as you would be on HT.

Soy isoflavones

Soy protein, which comes from soybeans, is a very important dietary supplement because soybeans are rich in calcium, iron, potassium, amino acids, vitamins, and fibre, and soy also contains all the essential amino acids necessary in a healthy human being. This last point makes it an excellent source of replacement protein for vegetarians.

Most peri- and postmenopausal women know about soy because it contains plant estrogens, which are called phytoestrogens, and in soy are known as soy isoflavones. The best known of these are genistein and daidzein. It is thought that soy has a hormonal action in women because daidzein is metabolised to an estrogenic compound known as equol. The flora in your gut help this process and this is why some women convert daidzein better than others, because we all have different levels of flora. Some women are not able to metabolise daidzein to equol at all, which is why there are women who complain that the soy isoflavones supplements don't help their menopausal symptoms.

Another problem is that the amount of soy isoflavones may differ from soy supplement to soy supplement. The type of soy isoflavone may be significant; recent research has shown that a daily dose of 15 mg of genistein significantly reduced hot flushes in some postmenopausal women.

There has been an enormous amount of research into and discussion of the role that soy plays in helping to alleviate menopausal symptoms, as well as about the many benefits claimed by healthcare practitioners. Different practitioners recommend different doses, but it appears that a daily dose of between 35 mg and 110 mg of soy isoflavones is safe for up to six months. Long-term trials are under way to provide better information about the safety and efficacy of soy isoflavone supplements.

One of the worries about soy is that because it appears to act like estrogen in helping to reduce hot flushes, some researchers think that in the long term it might act like estrogen on breast tissue and on the lining of the womb, but a recent one-year study of women taking genistein found that it had no apparent effect on the lining of the womb. However, women who are at risk for estrogen-related cancers and are sensitive to estrogen should be very aware of any estrogen-like symptoms when taking this supplement, if they decide to risk taking it at all. Because the research in this area is still fairly new, some information suggests that soy isoflavones may protect breast tissue from estrogens, while other evidence shows that they may stimulate it.

Soy also seems to be helpful in reducing bad cholesterol, but research has shown that it is better to take actual soy protein, like lecithin powder, for this purpose rather than capsules or tablets. Other research shows that soy may have a very strong antioxidant action. There is ongoing research to determine whether soy isoflavones are helpful in maintaining or building bone density; some double-blind, randomised, controlled trials have shown that soy isoflavones are effective in maintaining the bone mineral content in women who are in late menopause, while other double-blind research shows that they do not protect against bone loss in women with early menopause.

Black cohosh (*cimicifuga racemosa*)

Many of my clients have been given this in tincture or tablet form by alternative and complementary healthcare practitioners to alleviate the symptoms of menopause. The best-known brand product is Remifemin, which is manufactured in Germany, where it has been available for more than 50 years and has been carefully regulated. Trials have shown that a daily dose of 40 to 60 mg can be used safely for about six months but longer term studies are still needed.

There has been some non-conclusive evidence that the substance may have some adverse effects on the liver. Of even more concern is the possible long-term effect of black cohosh on breast tissue. Although several trials have already shown that it does not really have significant estrogenic effects, in fact it acts like the selective estrogen receptor modulators (SERMs) I wrote about in Chapter 4, except that black cohosh is a plant (*phyto*) SERM. This is precisely why there is a need for well-designed, long-term, controlled clinical trials of this product, with substantial sample numbers. As I write, there are several good randomised trials under way at prestigious academic institutions which hope to determine whether black cohosh acts in the long term like estrogen on breast tissue and the lining of the womb and whether it has beneficial effects on heart health or bone formation.

Red clover (*trifolium pratense*)

A safe dose of red clover appears to be 40 to 160 mg daily and the best-known brand is Promensil, an Australian product containing isoflavones. Some of these are found in soy: *biochanin A*, and *formononetin*, which then metabolise to form the isoflavones *genistein* and *daidzein*. Promensil's website promises that the product will do the following: relieve the symptoms of menopause, hot flushes and night sweats; help improve general well-being; maintain bone health and cholesterol. However, in randomised, double-blind, placebo-controlled trials of menopausal women, red clover has not been shown to be clinically effective in reducing hot flushes over a period of 12 weeks and much more evidence is needed to support all those claims.

So it is unlikely that red clover will reduce your menopausal symptoms, but as in the case of black cohosh, large, well-controlled clinical trials are currently under way and once they are completed we will be better able to rate the efficacy of red clover and establish whether it has an anti-estrogenic effect on breast tissue and on the lining of the womb, and is beneficial to heart health and bone formation.

Some other research has shown that red clover may have an anti-inflammatory effect on the arteries, so a lot of work needs to be done there as well. I myself have recommended that women try red clover or black cohosh to alleviate their meno-pausal symptoms and if either of these supplements works for you, there is no harm in trying it for a while, but be alert for sensitive, tender breasts, have a scan of the lining of your womb annually and be aware of any changes in your body.

Until more research has been done I would suggest that you avoid taking products that combine these two herbal supplements because we don't know how they react together. Novogen, the manufacturers of Promensil, have a website with a link for professionals, but if you're interested in checking out the clinical trials, forget it. They only want clinical professionals to read about them and I wonder why. Luckily the Natural Medicines Comprehensive Database is available and, although you need to pay a small subscrip-tion, if you are really concerned about what you are taking and if your own healthcare practitioner doesn't have this manual, I would highly recommend that you subscribe to it and take a look for yourself.

Don(g) quai (*angelica sinensis*)

Don quai is also a plant estrogen and is thought to be safe in 400 mg daily doses in powder form. Complementary and alternative healthcare practitioners are enthusiastic about prescribing it to help with menopausal symptoms, but like the other substances in this group, its safety and efficacy has not yet been adequately proven and it appears to have estrogenic effects, which may be why it seems to alleviate hot flushes in some women.

Flaxseed or linseed

A type of plant estrogen, this is covered in detail in the section on omega-3 fatty acids on p 108.

Glucosamine

This supplement is recommended for the aching joints and arthritis that often plague us as we get older. A dose of 1 500 mg daily seems to be safe, with no bad reactions, and long-term research has shown that this daily dose does relieve symptoms of osteoarthritis. You will find that glucosamine is often combined with a supplement called chondroitin. Once again there is no evidence to show that they work better together than alone.

As with many products, glucosamine supplements are not carefully regulated so you should try to buy a reputable brand name to ensure that you are getting glucosamine sulphate and not glucosamine hydrochloride with added sulphate. Because there is so much interest in this product there are some very good double-blind, randomised, controlled trials under way to determine how safe and beneficial it is (see page 200).

Coenzyme Q10

This is similar to a vitamin. It is thought that the amounts of CoQ10 in your body begin to decline as you get older, which is the reason why so many complementary and alternative healthcare practitioners recommend it to middle-aged women. Supplements may be recommended in doses ranging from 30 to 100 mg.

Although small amounts of CoQ10 are obtained from certain foods, particularly seafood and meat, the body produces almost all we need for healthy living. It is fat-soluble and is found throughout the body in almost all the cells, with high levels in the major organs of the heart, pancreas, liver and kidneys, but these amounts are not bio-available to (*metabolised or utilised by*) the body.

Interestingly, the CoQ10 found in soybean oil has been found to be bio-available, which reinforces my belief that soy protein may act as an antioxidant. CoQ10 maintains healthy cell function and plays a vital role in the production of *adenosine triphosphate* (ATP), which is essential to the storage and production of energy in the muscles in a process by which all the energy and nutrients in food are released to ensure that they are assimilated by the body.

Because of the role CoQ10 plays in cell respiration and the release of energy it is thought to be a powerful antioxidant, which may play a protective role in the human body as it begins to age, especially in relation to heart disease. The results of several well-designed research studies over the past few years seem to bear this out. Trials have also shown that CoQ10 may help to lower blood pressure, reduce insulin levels and LDL cholesterol, and increase levels of some important vitamins and HDL cholesterol.

Ginseng

Ginseng is called an adaptogen by complementary or alternative healthcare practitioners. This means it is believed to play a specific, beneficial role in the body where, they say, it helps to regulate certain functions before it is harmlessly absorbed or eliminated.

The problem with ginseng is that there are several different kinds, including Siberian, American and Panax. Ginseng has been used for thousands of years in traditional Chinese medicine but because there are varying kinds and varying doses, and because it is extracted in different ways, the supplements you buy may have varying results.

There are all sorts of claims made about ginseng. It is said to improve flagging energy levels, the immune system and the libido. Some practitioners believe that it reduces stress. Since many peri- and postmenopausal women complain of many of these symptoms, it seems logical that they are offered ginseng supplements, but once again, well-designed clinical trials have offered no evidence to back up these claims or show that ginseng is safe in the long term. In fact, it may have some very harmful effects on women who are suffering from high blood pressure, migraines or heart disease.

Fatty acids

Most of us know by now that the omega-3 and omega-6 fatty acids are absolutely essential to good health. They are vital fats, crucial for the efficient functioning and maintenance of every single cell in our bodies. The main fatty acids that we know about are *linoleic acid*, which is the omega-6 fatty acid, and *alpha-linolenic acid* (ALA), which is the omega-3 fatty acid.

In our 21st-century diet we get more than adequate omega-6 fatty acids from different vegetable oils, nuts and seeds, and from grain-fed meat and poultry, but our diet doesn't usually provide us with enough of the omega-3 fatty acids, so the ratio of the omega-3 to omega-6 fatty acids in our bodies is often unbalanced, leaning heavily on the side of the omega-6 fats. Without going into a confusing description of the body's biochemistry, it is vital for optimum health that the two be balanced. Omega-3 fatty acids appear to be powerful antioxidants, help to prevent inflammation and thrombosis (*antithrombotic*) and they may also help to lower blood pressure. Some research suggests that they may help to lower triglycerides and LDL (bad cholesterol).

In the chapter on weight and diet I will write about 'good' and 'bad' fats, but since we are discussing supplements, I would suggest that most middle-aged women should supplement their diets with omega-3 fatty acids, which come from flax-seed oil, fish oil, flaxseeds, hemp seeds and purslane; oily cold-water fish like herring, mackerel, salmon and sardines; soybeans and walnuts and walnut oils. If you include any of these in your diet in decent quantities you may be getting enough omega-3 fatty acids, but if you are like most of us and can't be bothered to eat enough oily fish each week, you can supplement using fish oil.

If you are taking a fish oil supplement, be careful of the brand you use; some fish oils may be contaminated by toxic chemicals, so you should be comfortable that the manufacturer is reputable and can back up its quality claims. A downside of fish oil supplements is that they tend to 'repeat' and can cause a fishy taste, but today there are many highly refined fish oil supplements and if you take these with food it shouldn't happen and fish oils are an excellent source of omega-3 fatty acids.

In some cases, vegetarians who don't want to take fish oil or women who have a religious objection can use flaxseed oil. However, alpha-linolenic acid (ALA) in flaxseed must be converted in our bodies to the two important fatty acids: EPA and DHA. There is new research suggesting that only a small amount of ALA in flaxseed is converted to EPA and DHA. This is because ALA is often broken down very quickly in our bodies and because of the high content of omega-6 fatty acids in our typical Western diets. So it is probably better to supplement omega-3 fatty acids in the form of fish oil, where the EPA and DHA are already converted from ALA.

You should have a daily minimum of 1 000 mg of omega-3 in your diet. A 1 000 mg capsule of fish oil provides 180 mg EPA and 120 mg DHA (300 mg together). Two to three of these capsules daily should meet your needs. There are lignans in flaxseed, which are a type of plant estrogen, and these may help to improve menopausal symptoms, and the quality of your hair and skin, so that some flaxseed in the form of oil, seeds or one or two capsules may be a good addition to the diets of peri- and postmenopausal women.

Gingko biloba (*adiantifolia*)

This is mainly prescribed for middle-aged women who find that they are battling a failing memory. Poor memory is a frequent symptom in peri- and postmenopausal women and many of us use or try out this supplement. Although ginkgo is prescribed for a wide variety of ailments, the claim that it can help poor memory is of most interest to menopausal women.

Ginkgo biloba is one of the oldest known plants in the world and has been used in traditional Chinese medicine for thousands of years. A daily dose of 240 mg seems to be safe, but once again there is no consensus on how risky or helpful it is. There is currently a five-year study under way, conducted by NCCAM, to establish whether a daily 240 mg dose will prevent Alzheimer's disease or age-related dementia. Gingko is often combined with ginseng in supplements said to improve memory, but once again there is no hard evidence about whether this combination is helpful or safe.

My opinion

Now that you have read the vitamin and mineral tables you are probably thinking that your diet and lifestyle are such that you are not getting some or all of the supplements that you think you need. For example, very few middle-aged women get enough calcium from dietary sources and I would think it unlikely that they would be getting enough omega-3 fatty acid.

While I do not advocate huge amounts of supplements, I am definitely a believer in moderate amounts. I think that women who want to take supplements should speak to an expert, someone who is properly trained and registered, and not an assistant in a health food shop or someone who is selling supplements as part of a pyramid scheme.

I have recommended the following supplements over the years:

If your diet is poor or your lifestyle is unhealthy, I would recommend a good multivitamin supplement. Some practitioners don't like these combination vitamins, others swear by them, but if you decide to take them I would suggest you lean towards those that come in a food state form (a form that is very similar to the natural form the vitamin in food comes in) because your body will metabolise them more quickly and better.

Calcium – Although you get calcium from your diet, your lower levels of estrogen mean that you don't absorb it as well, so I would recommend that all middle-aged women take 1 200 to 1 500 mg of elemental calcium daily. The doses should be divided either three times a day or morning and night. (There will be more about calcium in the chapter on osteoporosis.) It is vital to see that you combine this supplement with correct amount of vitamin D (800 IU) for maximum absorption.

A *vitamin B complex* supplement – Many middle-aged women are very anxious or stressed and battle with low energy and a good vitamin B complex seems to be helpful. On a biased anecdotal note (just what I told you to beware of), a great uncle of mine who was a very famous physician and way ahead of his time in many of his theories, was a great believer in vitamin B. He lived to a ripe old age and his widow, who is in her late eighties, healthy and exceptionally bright, has been taking a large daily dose of these vitamin B supplements for more than 30 years.

If you are taking a multivitamin that has the appropriate amount of *folic acid*, that's fine. If you are not, I would recommend that you take 400 mcg daily as a precaution against heart disease and to protect against breast cancer.

Flaxseed capsules in a dose of between 1 000 and 2 000 mg daily – Flaxseed oil contains plant estrogens and seems to have an antioxidant effect, is good for hair and skin, and may help alleviate menopausal symptoms. A helpful side effect is that it seems to prevent constipation.

Many practitioners and some women swear by an *antioxidant* supplement containing CoQ10 or a supplement containing *selenium* and *vitamin E*. Recent research has shown that some antioxidants like beta-carotene, vitamin A and vitamin E may help with disease prevention, although more research is needed on vitamin C and selenium.

If you are battling with menopausal symptoms and don't want to take conventional HT, you could try one of the plant estrogens I have mentioned, with soy isoflavones and black cohosh probably being the best researched. Remember that there is no definitive long-term research into the risks and benefits of these and they may not be safe if you have had or are at risk for breast cancer. Don't combine these supplements.

Empowerment points

- Always tell your healthcare practitioner what supplements you are taking. Many of these supplements have been shown to cause side effects and others may react with medicines that you may be taking, interfering with them or causing unwanted reactions. A good doctor will have taken the trouble to make him/herself aware of the latest research on supplements and should be able to advise you. If your practitioner can't help you in this regard, find a certified dietician or a specialist physician who has this knowledge and spend some time discussing your lifestyle, especially your daily diet, with him or her. She or he will soon pick up areas where you may be lacking in vital supplements or be able to tell you that you are on the right track.

- Don't be gullible or naïve. Always ask yourself about the self-interest of the person who is trying to sell you the supplements.

- Be sure to buy your supplements from someone who is truly knowledgeable about them. A person who is selling supplements as part of a pyramid group just can't be as knowledgeable as an expert, and once again, his or her advice may be biased by a profit motive.

- Eat a healthy, varied diet. You will see from the information in the lists that you will be able to get most of the vital nutritional supplements you need from a sensible, well-balanced meal plan.

Sources

I referred to many articles and books while I was collating this information and also found the following particularly helpful:

Medline Plus, a service of the US National Library of Medicine and the National Institute of Health.

The Expert Group on Vitamins and Minerals [EVM] report 2003, published by the Food Standards Agency© Crown Publishing.

NICUS (Nutrition Information Centre, University of Stellenbosch).

DRIs (Dietary Reference Intakes). National Academy Press 2003.

Krause's Food, Nutrition & Diet Therapy 11th edition. Mahan, K. Escott-Stump, S. Saunders. Philadelphia: Elsevier 2004.

If you are interested in keeping up with the latest research on complementary and alternative medicine by reading some of the leading medical journals you may have to subscribe to them, but you can always find the abstracts of the articles on a site like the PubMed, which is the National Library of Medicine's database. The interest in this field is now so great that you can look for new research on this subject at CAM at http://www.nlm.nih.gov/nccam/camonpubmed.html. Here the National Council for Complementary and Alternative Medicine (NCCAM) has paired up with PubMed. Abstracts from this site will give you the gist of the study and the conclusions the researchers reached.

Notes

_____

_____

_____

_____

_____

_____

_____

_____

_____

_____

6

Hot Flushes and Hysterectomies

'I'm sitting in the middle of really important presentation,' said Ilana, 'and things are going well. Suddenly
I feel a strange feeling; almost out-of-body. I feel sort
of disassociated and then I know it's going to happen.
I feel this wave of heat travelling up me, growing in a
rush. I know that my face is turning blood red and I
start to pour with sweat. I feel like I'm in a sauna. My
colleagues, mostly men, are looking at me in astonish-
ment and usually I find myself rushing out of the room
to mop up!'

Nicki smiled sympathetically. 'I know just how you feel.
Mine aren't as bad as that, though I feel terribly hot.
They seem to come in waves throughout the day and
they get worse if I drink my soup or coffee hot. Nowadays
everything I drink has to be lukewarm or I find myself
reaching boiling point. I also often feel incredibly anxious, sometimes even panicky, when this happens.'

Chris shook her head. 'That doesn't happen to me at all.
I feel a sort of humming in my ears, a tingling feeling
like pins and needles in my fingertips, then there's this
wave of giddiness. I feel like I'm going to keel over but
I'm not much hotter than usual.'

'Yes,' says Sara. 'It's not that I feel burning hot, it's
just that for the past few months I've felt that my whole

*body temperature is higher. I hardly ever feel chilly now
and it seems to me that summers have become much,
much warmer than they used to be.'*

*'I agree,' nodded Jo. 'But though the days feel warmer,
it's the nights that really bother me. I don't even sleep
with a duvet any more, even on the coldest winter nights.
My husband has had to get his own blanket. Sleep has
become a rare commodity. Even if I fall asleep feeling
reasonably comfortable, I wake several times during the
night drenched in sweat. Sometimes I've had to change
my nightdress and put a bath towel underneath me; the
sheets are so wet and I don't want to wake my husband
up to change the bed.'*

The conversation of this group of middle-aged friends is
typical of that of women who are in the throes of perimenopause. They are all experiencing the result of fluctuating
levels of estrogen on the hypothalamus in their brains. In
other words, they are getting hot flushes. But because they
are all biochemically different individuals, the kind of hot
flushes they are experiencing vary widely.

Because hot flushes are the red flag of menopause, an
enormous amount has been written about them; of all the
symptoms of menopause it is hot flushes that women obsess
about most. As I wrote earlier, many writers in a backlash
against the old anti-feminist mindset that menopause was
a disease, tried to reframe these symptoms by calling them
power surges. Leslie Kenton wrote a bestseller called *Passage
to Power*, which was one of the first works to suggest that
menopausal women were strong and functioning, desirable
and desirous, not dried-out old crones. Other feminists had
ceremonies where they honoured the menopausal woman
as a wise woman or shaman.

I'm not so sure the answer is to rename a hot flush or have
a ceremony. I think this puts additional stress on a middle-
aged woman by making her feel that she should be honouring
her menopause, believing that these flushes are empowering
her, when all she longs for is to feel cool again or have a good
night's sleep and not wake drenched in sweat. But I do think

that the way you handle these flushes has a lot to do with how you perceive them. I believe that knowledge is power. If you know what's happening to you physiologically and you have some handle on how to deal with them, hot flushes will become a tiresome part of the perimenopausal process; often uncomfortable, terribly disruptive, sometimes unbearable, but ultimately transitional. We know that except in incredibly rare cases, hot flushes do eventually stop.

As I discussed in Chapter 1, there may be a variety of reasons for hot flushes including early ovarian failure, various medications, a sensitivity to alcohol, thyroid or endocrine problems, and fevers that may be caused by viral or bacterial illness, so if it's unlikely that you're perimenopausal you should ask your doctor to investigate other reasons. Hot flushes may begin a couple of years before menopause and, it is believed, can last between two and fourteen years. Some fortunate women never have a hot flush, or their hot flushes don't last longer than six months, while some unfortunates, especially those who have had an abrupt transition into menopause following removal of their ovaries, have them well into their eighties.

Hot flushes that follow surgically induced menopause are often very severe and more frequent than the flushes of the natural menopause. Women who become menopausal as a result of chemotherapy or radiation treatment may battle with hot flushes, as do those who are taking SERMs or aromatase inhibitors (see Chapter 8). Hot flushes may start gradually and build in intensity over the months as a woman's levels of estrogen drop. Some women experience a month of hectic hot flushes, then they peter out and recur after a few months. Others have a few unpleasant months and never have another hot flush. Still others suffer only from night sweats or get a hot flush when they are very stressed, while some battle morning, noon and night, and feel that they are constantly on fire. There are also women who find themselves chilled and shivering uncontrollably once the hot flush has passed.

Hot flushes come in many guises and combinations, and it is thought that at least 70 per cent of women who are undergoing natural menopause experience some kind of hot flush. They can last for as little as 30 seconds or build in intensity and then go on for as long as five minutes or more. Women usually experience the hot flush in their upper bodies and it seems to sweep upwards in a wave. Most women have said that they know when they are about to have a flush, either because they experience strange tingling sensations, a growing feeling of warmth, or even a strange disassociated, out-of-body sensation. The permutations seem endless, but I have found that once women have decided how they want to handle their hot flushes and taken control of the process, they cease to be so important.

In spite of all the research, the way in which hot flushes occur is still not properly understood. What we do know is that all human beings have something known as core body temperature. The normal average body temperature of a healthy person is usually 37°C. The body is an amazing machine which maintains this temperature by ensuring that the heat it produces balances the heat it loses or gains in its environment.

The area that maintains this temperature control and helps your body maintain a normal temperature is in the hypothalamus, which is situated in your brain, and which I wrote about in Chapter 2. The hypothalamus sends a message to the pituitary, which initiates the secretion of FSH and LH. In addition, your nervous system keeps your hypothalamus in constant touch with what is happening to your body's temperature. It is then the job of your hypothalamus to ensure that your body has the appropriate physical responses which will keep you cool or warm, depending on your environment. So sometimes your blood flow is increased and sometimes it is decreased. Sometimes the way in which you metabolise food is sped up and sometimes it is slowed down, sometimes you start shivering, which makes your muscles contract so that you become warmer, and sometimes it makes you sweat so your body cools down as the sweat evaporates.

Researchers think that a hot flush may be caused by a sudden rise in your body's core temperature which can take place at any point from two minutes to 17 minutes before the actual hot flush. When the hypothalamus detects this sudden rise in the core temperature, it sets into action those physical changes that have been designed to cool the body down – sweating, a change in heart rate and an increased flow of blood to the skin, which happens because the small blood vessels become wider so that the blood can flow through them more quickly.

It is believed that the temperature control area in your hypothalamus responds to the interactions of several of the special chemical messengers (*neurotransmitters*) in the brain, as well as to *endorphins*, which are substances your body produces when it is stressed, and hormones.

Two of these neurotransmitters are called *serotonin* and *norepinephrine* and are especially important to the way in which hot flushes occur. It seems that both before and after a hot flush the levels of norepinephrine in the blood are higher. We know that norepinephrine is responsible for an increase in our core body temperature and it is also involved in the way our bodies respond to this rise in temperature.

Now it is thought that appropriate amounts of hormones like estrogen, androgen and testosterone keep the levels of norepinephrine under control. In perimenopause when the levels of these hormones fluctuate or drop suddenly, the levels of norepinephrine increase and cause a rise in your core body temperature, so the cooling off reactions start up and you begin to sweat, your heart pounds, and you get all the symptoms of a hot flush. It seems that it is not the low levels of estrogen that cause hot flushes but the sudden drops in estrogen levels that occur in perimenopause. In postmenopause, when your estrogen has stopped fluctuating and levelled out, the hot flushes usually stop.

In another twist to this tale, researchers have worked out that the neurotransmitter serotonin seems to be involved. It is thought that when estrogen levels drop, levels of serotonin in the blood drop too, and the serotonin receptors in the hypothalamus increase. This, as you can imagine, is a very complex interaction and when it happens the body usually cools off. Remember that serotonin is the 'feel good' transmitter and special medicines that are called *selective serotonin re-uptake inhibitors* (SSRIs), like Prozac, are used to combat depression when serotonin levels drop. The reason I point this out is that when we come to the chapter on menopause and depression in middle-aged women it will give you a head start in understanding what happens when levels of estrogen and serotonin fluctuate or drop in peri- and postmenopause.

Another thing to look at is when hot flushes are most prevalent. The fact that they are linked to your core body temperature means that they are also linked to your body's biological clock. This biological clock is regulated by a structure which is also situated in your hypothalamus, so everything is interconnected. In the early evening, a few hours after your core body temperature reaches its highest point, hot flushes seem to increase in intensity. This is why when perimenopausal women who are suffering from hot flushes travel, they experience a variation in their hot flushes – the biological clock may be upset by time zone differences.

The issue for many women is how to handle their hot flushes; whether they can stand them or not. Do they interfere with your quality of life or are they just a minor inconvenience, which you can cope with because you know that this stage in your life is transient? As I wrote in Chapter 4, HT is recommended for women with moderate to severe hot flushes – more than eight hot flushes a day. I have seen some women who laugh off the discomfort and others who feel quite desperate about it. There are those who have had mothers or family members with breast cancers, or have even had their own bout with cancer, who are terrified to take HT and really battle, and those who say they don't care, they will take the risk because they refuse to put up with hot flushes. Each woman handles hot flushes in her own way. Here are my thoughts and recommendations on how to deal with them.

Dealing with hot flushes

Lifestyle

There is not much good clinical research available on how lifestyle changes may help your hot flushes, but I think that common sense is the watchword here. I often wonder how our mothers and grandmothers dealt with the problem;

perhaps they just suffered in silence. Of course, synthetic fabrics were much less common, which may have made a difference, so it may be sensible to wear natural fibres and sleep on cotton sheets and use cotton blankets.

Wear fabrics that breathe! Anything that makes you feel constrained, uncomfortable and hot may precipitate a hot flush. Wear layers during this time and clothes that float rather than those that are tight and clingy, especially tight waistbands or elastic that cuts into your waist. Remember too that most women put on weight during perimenopause so make sure your clothes are loose fitting. Even in winter wear cotton as well as wool and be able to remove layers in a very warm room before your core temperature responds to the heat. At night turn down the heat in your bedroom (but provide your partner with a heating pad or a hot-water bottle and an extra blanket; he or she shouldn't have to freeze because you're hot).

Some women find that as the warning signs preceding a hot flush start they can pre-empt the actual hot flush by dabbing cool water on their pulse points: their wrists, the back of their necks and the backs of their knees. I know that some women carry small spray bottles of water in their bags for this purpose. Do you remember seeing old ladies splashing the back of their necks before entering the sea to lower their body temperature? Strange as it might seem, this can help.

Many women find that if they eat spicy or very hot food they precipitate a hot flush, and the same happens when they drink very hot drinks or soup. It may not help, but it can't hurt during this time to have lukewarm drinks and bland food. Too much alcohol may trigger a hot flush, as may a bout of overeating and too much coffee. But because all women are individuals, hot flushes can be triggered by different factors depending on your biochemical make-up.

Smoking and exercise

Stop smoking. Research shows that women who smoke have worse hot flushes than those who don't because smoking interferes with your estrogen production, so that your levels of estrogen will be much lower and you will have less circulating estrogen available in your body. In any case your health will improve exponentially if you stop smoking and, in my view, any woman who smokes is putting her health at risk – period.

On the same track, it may help reduce your hot flushes if you exercise. Even if it doesn't, the benefits of regular exercise, as I will discuss later, are so great that it's worth it. Research shows that women who exercise probably have fewer, less severe hot flushes. This may have something to do with the endorphin levels. Of course, as with everything in menopause, nothing is straightforward and the rise in your core body temperature when you exercise may precipitate a hot flush, but even then those are usually shorter and less severe.

Weight loss

Staying on the subject of health, one benefit of weight loss may be a reduction in hot flushes. It seems that women who carry more weight suffer more. Although women who have higher body mass probably have higher estrogen levels than very thin women, we know that fatter people often battle with temperature, so losing some weight may be helpful; you know it will be healthier in any event.

Stress

There is no research that suggests that stress precipitates hot flushes or makes them worse, so I will just have to rely on anecdotal evidence here. I think that many middle-aged women often get hot and bothered, and when they do they have a hot flush. Whether the 'hot' in the above phrase refers to a rise in your core body temperature, I don't know, but I do know that many women have told me that when they are stressed they have more hot flushes. So on the off-chance that stress is one of the triggers for hot flushes, try to de-stress.

Exercise is a good option and other ways to reduce stress are discussed further on in this chapter. If you do experience a hot flush, don't panic, especially if your heart is pounding and there is a ringing in your ears. Breathe in slowly through your nose for a count of seven, hold your breath for four counts and breathe out very slowly through your mouth for eight. Repeat this routine a couple of times. Research has shown that controlled breathing either at specific intervals during the day or when a hot flush begins may be very helpful and I can say without reservation that this treatment has NO adverse side effects.

Hormone therapy

The most effective help for hot flushes, especially if your symptoms are produced by surgical menopause, is HT, unless otherwise indicated. This subject has been thoroughly discussed in Chapter 4. Remember the guidelines: if possible, bioidentical estrogen, in the lowest, most effective dose, should be taken through the skin (*transdermally*) for the shortest possible time. You need a progesterone if you still have a womb and, in any event, may want to add a little even if you don't have a womb, but whatever you decide to do, do it with your own individual profile in mind.

Non hormonal treatment of hot flushes

In certain women, especially those with breast cancer, hormone therapy may not be suitable to help ease severe hot flushes, so other remedies may be suggested. Some of these remedies were not specifically designed to counteract hot flushes, but women using them found coincidentally that they seemed to help.

Unfortunately studies conducted on these products to see if they alleviate hot flushes are not large enough to establish whether these treatments are safe and effective in the long term. They may be helpful in treating menopausal women who cannot take estrogen therapy but the absence of sufficient information means they are not the treatment of choice for women where HT is the first option. Among these products are the following:

Clonidine was originally used for women with high blood pressure (hypertension). Although research has shown that clonidine in high doses can be effective in reducing the frequency, length and severity of hot flushes, these doses can cause side effects such as insomnia, a dry mouth, constipation, drowsiness, rash, nausea and gastrointestinal disturbances (stomach upsets). So without further and more robust research at this time, it is hard to establish the most effective dosage or for how long this medicine should be given to women battling with hot flushes. It is also not known what the long-term effects associated with this treatment would be.

Gabapentin is used as an anticonvulsant and for treating migraine headaches. Recent research shows that postmenopausal women who took a daily dose of 900 mg of gabapentin had reduced hot flushes over a 12-week period. In another study women who took 2 400 mg of gabapentin had a 70 per cent reduction in hot flushes. The latter is a huge dose, which should be slowly increased from a starting dose of 400 mg. Side effects such as headaches, dizziness, disorientation and sometimes sleepiness and rashes were experienced by some of the women in these studies. The sample numbers in these trials were small and larger long-term studies are needed to determine safety and efficacy.

Vitamin E, 800 IU/day, which is often referred to as high dose, may be another option, although the clinical evidence is not definitive and the results are mixed. Because vitamin E seems to be nontoxic in low doses, is inexpensive and available without a prescription, it may be an option for women who are struggling. But results, if any, may take weeks to be felt. However, some research suggests that higher doses may cause long-term risks, and women who have heart disease, diabetes or high blood pressure should consult their doctors before taking vitamin E. Interestingly, vitamin E is present in a healthy, balanced diet and is found in almonds, hazelnuts, peanuts, peanut butter, sunflower seeds, and green vegetables like spinach and broccoli, and is used to fortify some foods. Cereals, for instance, are fortified with vitamin E.

Supplements

Plant estrogen supplements may also be helpful in reducing hot flushes. Look at the detailed information in Chapter 5 and remember that just because something is herbal doesn't mean it's harmless. Soy isoflavones and black cohosh may be most effective in this area but more research is needed to determine all the risks, benefits and appropriate doses.

Antidepressant medication

Some women who battle terribly with hot flushes and their effects cannot take hormones because of the risk or the adverse side effects. In these cases, antidepressants may work. If you remember, I wrote at the beginning of this chapter about the role of serotonin and norepinephrine in the activity of hot flushes. Research has shown that certain antidepressants seem to help reduce hot flushes. The most popular of these is *venlafaxine* (Effexor), which interacts with serotonin and norepinephrine, helping to balance their levels in the blood. It seems to be very effective and, of course, for perimenopausal women who suffer from depression, it is doubly useful.

However, as with all antidepressant medicine there are significant side effects like a dry mouth, sleeplessness and decreased appetite, so those women taking venlafaxine need to decide whether the relief they get from reduced hot flushes and less depression is worth the side effects. The decreased appetite may appeal to perimenopausal women who are overweight.

Other antidepressants that seem to work are *paroxetine* (Paxil) and *fluoxetine* (Prozac), which are serotonin re-uptake inhibitors. The latter two also have side effects, including loss of sexual desire, which is already a problem for some menopausal women, and weight gain. One of the upsides of using antidepressants to help reduce hot flushes is that the drugs begin to work within a week and it seems that very low doses are effective, which means that the side effects are not too bad.

Recent research has shown that *sertraline* (Zoloft) and *citalopram* (Ciprimal) may help reduce hot flushes in some women. However, individuality plays a part here and some women experience no relief at all with any of the antidepressants. If you decide to embark on a course of antidepressants you should do so with great care and an understanding of the risks and side effects, and you should be under the care of a competent psychiatrist who understands the biochemistry of these medicines and their possible effects on you.

Hysterectomies

My story

When I was 45, I suddenly developed the most excruciating pain during my periods. For a year before the onset of this pain I had been having incredibly heavy periods. Sometimes I thought I was bleeding to death; huge chunks of tissue or blood clots would come away and no matter how often I changed my tampon and even when I wore super-thick pads I would often wake in the night to find myself soaked. I spoke to my GP and she recommended a gynaecologist.

This suave gentleman scanned my womb and told me that I had a huge fibroid. He said it made my uterus look as though I was 12-weeks pregnant and that he felt that the only solution was to have a hysterectomy. In any case, I was in my mid-forties, had two children and was not thinking of having any more. He assured me that this was a routine procedure and most women of my age with these problems found that a hysterectomy was the answer.

He sounded very convincing, but I had always been reasonably cautious, so I spoke to my ex-gynaecologist from America, who had delivered one of my babies and knew me well. He heartily approved the diagnosis, telling me that I would feel like a new woman. One of my closest friends from America sounded very perturbed when I told her what I planned, but I was so confident that the doctor knew best and I knew so little about hormone therapy and menopause that I was sure that after the six-week recommended recovery period I would feel as good, if not better, than before.

I called my gynaecologist again, because my friend's doubts had made me anxious, and voiced my fears.

He explained the surgery and spoke to me in reasoned terms. He seemed to have all the time in the world to talk to me. I felt immeasurably reassured, booked my surgery for the week after my 46th birthday and continued quite happily with my life.

At no point during my discussions with this gynaecologist did he explain to me that I was probably perimenopausal; that heavy bleeding and clotting in perimenopause are absolutely normal; that many women's fibroids grow rapidly during this time because of estrogen surges and that as the estrogen levels out the fibroids stop growing and then shrink. He didn't say: 'Let's wait for a while. There's no immediate danger and urgency. There are no cysts on your ovaries. There are other remedies you can try.'

He didn't tell me that smaller fibroids could be removed by a laparoscopy or a hysteroscopy and larger ones by a myomectomy. He didn't say that there were hormones (progestogens, in fact) which I could take to try to stop the bleeding. He didn't say that perhaps we could try an endometrial ablation, which is a laser treatment that destroys the lining of the uterus. It is a procedure suggested for middle-aged women who don't want more children but who are battling with the exceptionally heavy periods that happen in perimenopause. At no point did he stress that a hysterectomy was major surgery and that there would be no harm in waiting a bit. In fact, the only reason to rush into having a hysterectomy is when there is a risk of cervical or endometrial cancer.

He didn't say (perhaps he didn't know) that estrogen therapy might not suit me and could have undesirable side effects, nor did he tell me that I would be plunged into premature menopause with all its attendant symptoms. He didn't tell me that hot flushes after a surgical menopause were often more sudden and severe. He didn't warn me about what could and would probably happen with sudden onset menopause – that I could gain weight, be subject to mood swings, lose my desire for sex and battle with a dry vagina. He didn't tell me that I had the option of keeping my ovaries. None of this came up. He told me blandly that he would put me on HT after the surgery and I would feel great with it. I listened and I didn't question him further. I went into surgery uninformed.

I woke up feeling deathly sick from the anaesthetic, the pain of my scar and my cut muscles. The gynaecologist arrived in his green operating gear, looking suitably handsome and exhausted. He explained that he had removed my ovaries as they were dark and had endometriosis. Once I could sit up and look around I saw that I had a patch on my thigh. This was my estrogen replacement – 7.8 mg of estradiol hemihydrate to be replaced once a week. It had taken only hours for me to become a fully menopausal woman but it would be a year before I started to feel better.

The ET did not agree with me and I had numerous reactions to it, including wild mood swings, a general feeling of insanity, pounding headaches and skin rashes. I battled with many symptoms of menopause and couldn't find the right combination of HT.

The gynaecologist, who had been so readily available pre-surgery, was impatient and abrupt with me as I questioned the treatment, and I felt that I had been utterly unprepared, and consequently disempowered and betrayed. I had not expected to feel so bereft at the loss of my womb; the psychological loss and feeling of being less of a woman was as powerful as the physiological symptoms. In the end I re-framed my situation, channelled my anger and taught myself as much as I could about menopause, constantly updating my information. Thanks to a good combination of HT and the interest in menopause that my own hysterectomy generated in me, my story has a happy ending.

If your doctor tells you that you will have a total hysterectomy this means that the uterus and part of your cervix, or your entire cervix, will be taken out. Many women who have had hysterectomies don't even know whether they have kept their cervix or not, so ask your surgeon to explain exactly what she or he intends to do in your particular case.

Some doctors retain the cervix by *laparoscopy*, which can be a good thing as some women find that they have better sex if the cervix is retained. If you are having a hysterectomy because you have advanced cancer, you may have a radical hysterectomy, which means that your womb, your cervix and part of the upper area of your vagina, as well as your ovaries, are removed.

The surgery to remove your womb can be done in two ways; through a cut in your abdomen, usually just around or on the bikini line, or through your vagina. The latter method is usually a less drastic procedure. If your doctor has recommended that your ovaries should be also be removed (an *oophorectomy*), they and your fallopian tubes will be taken out. Sometimes it is decided that if you are not yet peri- or postmenopausal and you have healthy ovaries, they will be left in. Depending on your particular case one ovary may be left in. But you should always discuss the reason for the removal of your ovaries with your doctor. If you are not menopausal you might not want your ovaries removed as this means that you will usually have a more gradual menopause, though sometimes after the womb is removed your menopause may come earlier because the blood flow to the ovaries changes.

As the medical profession becomes more knowledgeable more choices are evolving for hysterectomies, such as surgery where much of the womb can be removed by laparoscopy and the remainder through the vagina. In a different technique, the surgeon can do all the preparation for the removal of the womb by dissecting it, using the laparoscope and then pull all the bits out through the vagina. The type of hysterectomy you have depends on the method your surgeon prefers and what she or he believes will be safest for you and enable you to recover quickest.

As I wrote in Chapter 2, your ovaries make more than one of the hormones in your endocrine system, so many women who are not at risk for ovarian cancer, who do not have many or abnormal cysts or endometriosis in their ovaries, may want to think very carefully before allowing healthy ovaries to be removed. For example, it seems as though women with natural menopause continue to produce some testosterone, so the decline in this particular hormone is more gradual.

Research has also shown that those women who have an early surgical menopause may be at greater risk for heart disease because of the abrupt drop in estrogen. The issue of the removal of ovaries is very thorny indeed. There is an extremely serious question here that must be asked about your risk for ovarian cancer. Unlike many other cancers there are no clear markers or signs of ovarian cancer – it can be silent and is most often fatal, and this is why many surgeons feel that if you are perimenopausal it may be wise to remove the ovaries as a precaution. It is imperative that you take time to ask your doctor about the dangers of getting this deadly disease and elicit his/her professional opinion on whether you should keep your ovaries.

There are several reasons why your doctor may recommend a hysterectomy:

- Persistence of severely abnormal cervical cells. It is very important to monitor the cells in your cervix, which is why all women who have a cervix should have an annual Pap smear, as should women who have had a partial hysterectomy and kept their cervix, and those who have had a total hysterectomy for cancer of the cervix.

- Abnormal cells in the lining of your womb, which could lead to endometrial cancer – cancer of the lining of the womb.

- Abnormal cysts in your ovary indicating ovarian cancer.

- A prolapsed uterus (where the uterus drops down into the vagina from its normal position and may even protrude from the vagina). This can occur after childbirth and sometimes if women are seriously overweight. It can even, in some cases, be caused by chronic coughing or excessive strain when lifting heavy objects.

- Very large fibroids that are debilitating, causing pain, interfering with your urinary tract and bladder, which are too big too shrink.

- Uncontrolled heavy bleeding that cannot be stopped by other methods.

Nobody decides lightly to have major surgery that involves a general anaesthetic, yet it is amazing how many women opt for hysterectomies without the proper knowledge and preparation. It is true that many women do very well after a hysterectomy but others who have both their ovaries and their wombs removed, and find themselves in premature menopause, really battle. Many take at least a year to feel like themselves again and spend even more time after that trying to find a hormone preparation that suits them.

My sense is that if there is not a compelling health reason for having a hysterectomy, it is much easier to cope with menopause when you come to it gradually. That said, hundreds of thousands of women who have opted for this surgery are now leading happy fulfilled lives. This section is not meant to be prescriptive but to inform you about the surgery so that if and when you decide to have a hysterectomy you feel empowered and confident that in partnership with your doctor, you have made a wise decision.

Is surgery doing you a favour?

The reason I have called this chapter 'hot flushes and hysterectomies' is because hot flushes, which can vary in frequency from one a week to one an hour, are often much worse after a sudden onset menopause caused by surgery during which your womb and ovaries are removed. Sudden onset menopause can also be brought on by certain chemicals and/or some types of radiation used in the treatment of cancer.

For many years gynaecologists believed that they were doing menopausal women a favour by performing hysterectomies as a cure-all for excessive bleeding, fibroids and endometriosis. In fact, often they were plunging perfectly healthy women into premature menopause by removing their ovaries at the same time as they removed their wombs.

As you can see from my story, there are quite a few options your gynaecologist could try before you decide on a hysterectomy and the removal of both your ovaries (*bilateral oophorectomy*). My gynaecologist told me that I needed a hysterectomy because I had such a large fibroid in my uterus. He never suggested surgery simply to remove the fibroid. I had a sense that fibroids were something quite sinister; in fact they are benign growths of muscle and connective tissue in the walls of the uterus. They may grow more rapidly when your estrogen levels surge in perimenopause or may increase because of hormone therapy.

Excessive bleeding

Women in perimenopause often experience excessive bleeding because of the fluctuations of estrogen and the dropping levels of progesterone that I described in Chapters 1 and 2. A procedure that might help this condition is *endometrial ablation*, where a laser burns the lining of the womb away. Most women who have this procedure never have a period again; some have light bleeding like spotting and in a very small number of women it has no effect at all, in which case hysterectomy might be the only option.

Current thinking about endometrial ablation is that women who have this procedure may experience a false sense of relief and feel like they no longer have to worry about the lining of their wombs. It is important to note, however, that small pockets of the endometrium (lining of the womb) may be left behind after this procedure, so menopausal women who are using ET should take a progestogen as well to prevent a build up the lining in these areas.

Fibroids

As I discussed in Chapter 1, when a gynaecologist examines you a transvaginal ultrasound should be an integral part of the examination. Using this, the gynaecologist can determine the position and size of a fibroid. Once an ultrasound is done and it is recommended that your fibroid be removed, you should have an informed discussion to help you understand how the procedure will take place. There are various surgical techniques to remove fibroids. One of these is specifically directed at removing the fibroids alone and is called a *myomectomy*. It is frequently the chosen treatment for premenopausal women who want to bear more children, because it may help to preserve fertility. If you have only a few small fibroids this procedure can be done by means of a *laparoscopy*. The surgeon inserts a small instrument (a laparoscope) through the navel into the abdomen, looks at the problem and then treats the patient.

Another method is *hysteroscopy*, which is a surgical procedure that can be done on women who have a single fibroid protruding into the cavity of the womb and don't wish to have their womb removed. A small camera and appropriate surgical instruments are placed in the cervix and the fibroid is surgically removed. A *laparotomy* is another technique by which the surgeon makes a cut in the abdomen and removes the fibroid. Many women complain that they feel bloated after abdominal surgery. This is because in an abdominal laparoscopy air is blown into the abdominal cavity to improve visibility and during a laparotomy the abdominal cavity is open and not all the air that enters it during the procedure can be removed.

Finally, your doctor might suggest *embolisation* of the fibroids. This is an advanced X-ray technique where the blood supply to the fibroid is cut off, so that it shrinks.

Endometriosis

As I wrote in Chapter 1, the lining of your womb is called the endometrium and endometriosis occurs when endometrial cells grow outside the uterus instead of inside it, where they can be sloughed off during the usual end-of-the-month bleed. The endometrial cells can be found in your ovaries, your fallopian tubes and your pelvic cavity and can cause a great deal of pain. All sorts of other symptoms may be connected with endometriosis, among them constipation or diarrhoea and lower-back pain. An interesting fact about endometriosis is that there may not be any relationship between the amount of endometriosis present and the severity of the pain you are experiencing.

Your doctor can diagnose endometriosis by performing a laparoscopy. A small number of postmenopausal women may continue to experience severe pain from endometriosis. It is thought that this may be caused by the high levels of aromatase which are often present after menopause and the condition may be treated with aromatase inhibitors, which I describe in Chapter 7. Although medicines have been used to alleviate some of the symptoms of endometriosis, they will not ultimately cure the disease, and the treatment of choice is surgery.

How to handle surgery for hysterectomy

Once you have made the decision to have a hysterectomy, plan your time before and after it very carefully. You want to be able to relax when you come out of hospital, so see that you have someone who can help you, cook for you or look after you for at least six weeks when you return home. If you don't have help, enlist your friends and do some serious freezer cooking. Give yourself plenty of recovery time if your surgery is to take place before a special occasion. Things can go wrong and you may not recover as quickly as you thought you would. Many women find that their shape changes after a hysterectomy so you may want to get back into shape before a celebration.

If you have a choice, go into surgery as fit as possible. This is a great time to stop smoking once and for all. If you've always exercised you'll have an easier time. Always tell your doctor which medications and supplements you are taking and ask if you can take preparations like Traumeel or Arnica; they don't want any surprises in the operating theatre. See that you have comfy, loose-fitting garments to wear after surgery. Accept that you can't have sex for at least eight weeks after the procedure. Allow yourself time to get used to the idea of being without a womb and if you feel weepy, weep.

If you are perimenopausal be prepared for the usual symptoms and accept that you might have to tinker with various hormones before you find some that suit you. Start with very mild exercise when your doctor says you can and build up to your old regimen gradually. Remember that most women have time to get used to menopause gradually, but if you are only in early perimenopause or not yet menopausal and your ovaries have been removed, you will be plunged into menopause. If you have realistic expectations about your surgical menopause, you will deal with it much more easily.

Empowerment points

- Always get a second, or even third, opinion before you decide to have major surgery like a hysterectomy.

- Be sure that you are making properly informed choices.

- Have a baseline hormone test before you have your ovaries removed to check whether you are perimenopausal or not. If you are already menopausal or have very low levels of estrogen and have not been battling with symptoms before surgery, you may or may not need a very low dose of estradiol. Many women find that their problems start after a surgical menopause because the dose of ET they are on is just too high. Reread the HT guidelines in Chapter 4, they also apply here.

Notes

_____

_____

_____

_____

_____

_____

_____

_____

_____

7

The Heart of the Matter

Andrea was very agitated, wringing her hands, she said to me: 'I feel so afraid. I had a bout with breast cancer and though I'm now in remission, I have an absolute terror of a relapse. I live in a very health-conscious way. I eat all the right foods, I exercise and try to live sensibly.

'I am really battling with menopausal symptoms like mood swings, depression, hot flushes, night sweats, bad headaches and a pounding heart. I can't sleep and I have constant anxiety. I have no desire for sex and when I have it it's painful.

'My estradiol levels are very low but I really don't want to take hormone therapy. I would like to try something alternative to see if that will help my hot flushes. On a recent visit to my physician I found that my bad cholesterol level is high and my gynaecologist tells me that I'm more likely to die of a heart attack than of breast cancer and he wants to put me back on conjugated equine estrogens, but my oncologist is absolutely opposed to me taking HT! I am confused and scared.'

I was not surprised that Andrea was feeling anxious. She was trying to take responsibility for her health but was receiving hugely conflicting advice. Her story is pertinent both to the question of heart health and to that of cancer.

135

However, as you will find out in the next chapter, there are better prospects for a postmenopausal woman whose breast cancer is estrogen-receptor positive than one whose is not.

Research has shown that estradiol, as I explained in Chapter 2, is a steroid or growth hormone, which means it can cause breast cells which could become cancerous to increase. Very recent research has shown that women who take estrogen may be at greater risk for breast cancer, so it seems sensible not to increase the risk by taking HT. The fact that estrogen is a steroid also impacts on the issue of heart health because just as estrogen causes good cholesterol (HDL) levels to rise, it may also cause bad cholesterol (LDL) levels to rise. The WHI showed quite clearly that taking estrogen does not improve heart health; on the contrary, it might aggravate potential heart problems. So it didn't make sense that Andrea should take something that might both increase her risk of breast cancer and actually raise her already high cholesterol levels.

Facts and fables: HT and heart disease

Cardio means the heart and vascular means the veins, blood vessels and arteries. In this chapter, I use the phrase heart disease because heart and vascular diseases are interrelated.

The popular theory for most of the last century was that before their menopause women were much less vulnerable to cardiovascular disease than men. This idea led the medical profession to believe that this was because women's hearts were protected by estrogen, and when their estrogen levels fell after menopause, they were at risk. Therefore, doctors felt, it was logical to assume that if women replaced their falling levels of estrogen they would protect their heart health.

Of course, the manufacturers of hormones were delighted with this development and several large, well-designed research studies confirmed these assumptions. The best known of these was the Postmenopausal Estrogen/Progestin Interventions Trial (PEPI). When it was reported in the *Journal of the American Medical Association* (*JAMA*) in 1995, the results of the study clearly showed that postmenopausal women would benefit from a regimen of HRT because, among other things, it raised levels of HDL (good cholesterol) and lowered *fibrinogen* levels. Fibrinogen is a protein present in the blood which can cause a heart attack when its levels are raised. You may have heard your health-care practitioner referring to a *myocardial infarction*. This is simply a heart attack, which happens when parts of the heart muscle die because the blood supply to the heart has become obstructed.

In light of this type of research, women felt that much of their anxiety about HRT could be allayed and that they were taking responsibility for their health by taking either estrogen or a combination of estrogen and progestogen, and they were encouraged in this belief by their doctors. However, in 2002, as you know by now, there was trouble in paradise. The results of the Heart and Estrogen-Progestin Replacement Study (HERS), which was a well-designed, double-blind, randomised, placebo-controlled trial of 2 700 women to study the effects of HRT on heart disease, showed that after four years of taking estrogen and progestogen daily, the overall risk of heart disease was not reduced.

More problems were to come. The WHI study, which I discussed at length in Chapter 3, showed that there was an increased risk of stroke in women taking estrogen and progestogen, and that these hormones offered no benefits in relation to heart disease. The figures per 10 000 were seven more heart attacks, eight more strokes and 18 more blood clots. In 2004 the estrogen-only arm was stopped because the study showed that there was an increased risk for stroke and, as in the combined trial, there was no perceived benefit for heart disease, so it was decided that the risk of a stroke outweighed the benefits. As I wrote earlier, these results turned the medical establishment upside down. Why had they been so mistaken?

Firstly, many of the earlier trials on heart disease did not represent women fully and the information gathered was assumed instead of being based on clinical evidence. One problem was that many old-school doctors relied on obser-vation and anecdotes to guide their treatments. Another interesting fact is that a large number of the women who die of heart attacks have not shown any previous symptoms, so doctors assumed, without clinical evidence, that heart attacks in menopausal women were caused by a drop in their estrogen levels. The PEPI trial served to confirm these assumptions.

Furthermore, because doctors assumed that women didn't suffer from heart disease before their menopause, they were not carefully tested and examined for it. Finally, with more effective diagnostic techniques, such as *magnetic resonance imaging* (MRI) and scans, it became clear that the arteries of even quite young women (in their late twenties and early thirties), who were nowhere near menopause, were showing signs of the damage which precedes heart disease, indicating that estrogen was not actually protecting them to the extent that their doctors believed.

But the doctors who had spent so many years prescribing estrogen to women to prevent heart disease were not convinced. After the WHI was published, many gynaecologists criticised the trials. Their objections were that the women studied were too old and only a small proportion had significant menopausal symptoms. They failed to accept, however, that the trials enrolled more than 8 800 women aged 50 to 59, of whom more than 20 per cent reported moderate to severe vasomotor symptoms. They believed that the WHI and HERS trials failed to show that estrogen protected against heart disease because the subjects already had some kind of heart disease. So while they agreed that estrogen might be bad for those older women, they thought that if ET was started immediately after menopause it would prevent arteriosclerosis. They were determined to prove that younger women would benefit. This was called 'the timing hypothesis'.

In 2007 their thesis seemed to have been vindicated when a sub-study from the WHI, the WHI-Coronary-Artery Calcium Study (WHI-CACS), found that younger women who use ET at the onset of menopause are less likely to have calcification of their arteries (see page 142) than their contemporaries who are not taking ET. This suggests that younger, postmenopausal women on ET have a reduced risk for heart disease. Those who recommend ET as a preventative for heart disease greeted this research with delight. The International Menopause Society (IMS) issued a press release saying that the results of this study were encouraging and stated that 'women can be reassured that estrogen therapy is cardioprotective until at least 65'.

However, not everyone was convinced. Some doctors cautioned restraint and advised gynaecologists not to extrapolate too much from this data. While it is clear that short-term HT to alleviate menopausal symptoms at the onset of menopause is probably not risky, and may even help to reduce the risk of heart disease, there is **no** evidence that this initial advantage would extend to older women were they to continue to use ET.

In fact, although the coronary artery calcium scores were reduced in these younger women, there is no evidence to show the effect of estrogen on blood clots, since these events are more likely to happen in older women. Coronary artery calcium scoring is a special X-ray test, *computed tomography* (CT), which helps to check whether there is a build-up of plaque (see page 142) on the walls of the arteries of the heart (coronary arteries). This test is used to see whether or not you are at risk for heart disease, and if you are, how severe it is. Many experts believe the data in this sub-study is insufficient to prove this categorically because at the end of the estrogen-only trial, *only* the women in the younger 50-59-years age group and not the older women were measured. In spite of this, many doctors support the timing hypothesis and once again the media are picking up on these enthusiastic statements and writing things like: 'Hormone therapy actually prevents heart attacks in women who start close to menopause'.

It is dangerous to make a blanket statement like this. Heart disease may already be present in a younger menopausal woman, but may not be evident without appropriate screening. A newly menopausal woman who is overweight and has high blood pressure may already be at risk for heart disease, and giving her ET may aggravate her risk. On the other hand, her healthy contemporary who has none of these problems may benefit, especially if she has had an early surgical menopause. Once again we come back to the indisputable fact that every woman should be evaluated as in individual and her medical history and potential risk factors should be taken into consideration.

In the meantime, two ongoing studies, The Kronos Early Prevention Study (KEEPS) and the Early versus Late Intervention Trial with Estradiol (ELITE) will provide more information. The KEEPS trial is a large five-year randomised, placebo-controlled, double-blind study to determine the response of women receiving transdermal estrogen, oral estrogen (CEE) or placebos. The ELITE study will study the effect of oral estradiol with intravaginal progesterone, given to women who are less than six years into menopause, as opposed to those who have been menopausal for 10 years or more.

More research is needed to determine whether different types of estrogen, and perhaps even micronised progesterone, can play a protective role in relation to heart disease. In the meantime, it may be more sensible to look at how ageing affects the cardiovascular system and to try to understand how changes in hormone levels affect many middle-aged women, who put on weight and may develop insulin resistance as a result. These women probably exercise less as well, so all those factors may increase their risk of heart disease.

The new evidence from the WHI and the HERS trials clarified why so many women who were on HT were also taking cholesterol-lowering drugs. Instead of protecting their hearts, the 'magical' estrogen was causing an increase in both good and bad cholesterols. In addition, it seemed that oral estrogens were causing an increase in the C-reactive proteins (CRP), which as I explained in Chapter 4, are signs of inflammation and may cause heart disease when their levels are raised.

> Delia is very health conscious and was extremely worried after a recent visit to her gynaecologist, who had told her to take a hormone containing 2 mg of estradiol and 1 mg of norethisterone acetate (a progestogen) daily, because he felt it would shrink a cyst that she had in her ovary.

> 'The problem is that my GP had put me on a cholesterol-lowering drug because my cholesterol was over eight, which I told my gynae, but he didn't seem concerned. I felt very confused because I had read that recent research showed that estradiol raised the levels of both bad and good cholesterol. I was also worried because I had heard that the new dosage recommendations for HT were much, much lower than they had been previously.'

In fact, as you read in Chapter 4, a starting dose of no more than 0.25 mg to 0.50 mg of oral estradiol is recommended. I couldn't understand why a healthcare practitioner would recommend such a high dose of estrogen, given all the recent research. In perimenopausal women it might be a good idea to try an oral contraceptive, which stops ovulation and calms the activities of the ovaries, which in turn may cause the cysts to shrink, but there is no evidence that HT makes the ovaries less active. But in this case even that would have been irrelevant – Delia was clearly postmenopausal; her estrogen levels were less than 37 pmol/L and her FSH levels were high. I explained what this means in Chapter 2.

In Chapter 8 I will discuss the most conservative way to approach the problem of ovarian cysts. Delia was also concerned about her high levels of cholesterol and we know that although estrogen raises the level of the good cholesterol, it also raises the levels of the bad cholesterol and triglycerides, high levels of which are markers or warning signs of future heart disease. Finally, it would probably have been safer to give Delia her HT in the form of a patch or gel, since there seem to be lower levels of C-reactive proteins and less of a risk of clots if HT is taken through the skin.

Preventing and treating heart disease

Lifestyle is a vital factor in preventing heart disease. Ninety percent of coronary heart disease can be prevented if you live a healthy life, which is why in 2006, the American Heart Association revised its very comprehensive 2004 report and added the word 'lifestyle' to the title of the revised report, explaining that a healthy diet is not the only factor in an overall healthy lifestyle. The report incorporates and thoroughly reviews the latest available scientific evidence on preventing and treating heart disease in women. It makes practical suggestions about ways to prevent heart disease or to lower the risks and discusses and describes the most effective treatments, all based on sound clinical evidence. I have read this report and tried to summarise the recommendations in a user-friendly way. Their dietary suggestions are discussed in greater detail in Chapter 10.

Before we look at the various treatments, let's look at ways in which you can alter your lifestyle to keep your heart healthy. It should be no surprise that the number-one risk is cigarette smoking. If you still smoke, it's really time to stop! The incontrovertible fact is that toxins in cigarettes, like lead, nicotine and cadmium, poison your system, cause cancers, prevent the absorption of calcium, interfere with your hormones and lead to the hardening of the arteries. Hardening of the arteries (*arteriosclerosis*) is caused by fatty materials known as plaque being deposited or collecting on the artery walls, or by the artery wall becoming scarred or thickened. As this happens the blood flow may be interrupted, and this can get worse if blood clots (*thromboses*) form round the larger deposits of these fatty materials. When your arteries become hardened or less elastic and the blood flow to the heart is affected, you can have a stroke or suffer a heart attack.

A stroke happens when the flow of blood to the brain is interrupted, killing off or damaging brain cells in varying numbers, depending on the kind of stroke. This happens when an artery is blocked or when the wall of the artery has become weakened and bursts. In one type of stroke, blood clots or plaque form in these hardened arteries, causing a blockage by breaking away from the artery wall, travelling throughout the body and ending up in an artery in the brain, where they interfere with or stop the blood flow, causing the death of the brain cells. This is called an *embolus*. The other kind of stroke is caused by a weakened artery in the brain bursting and causing bleeding.

It is important to remember that certain hormones may increase the risk of stroke. The WHI study showed that there was an increased risk of stroke with estrogen and progestogen, as well as with estrogen alone. In 2007, results from the Estrogen and Thromboembolism Risk (ESTHER) study suggested that oral estrogen, but not transdermal estrogen, may increase the risk of thrombosis (blood clots) and that some less androgenic progestogens (see Chapter 4) and micronised progesterone may be safer than the more androgenic progestogens as far as risk of blood clots is concerned. Other studies show that women on Tamoxifen are at greater risk for stroke, clots in the lungs and a clot in the deep veins (deep-vein thrombosis).

An excellent way to prevent heart disease is to exercise for a minimum of 30 minutes a day at least five days a week, and work up a sweat. You've already read that exercise is helpful in reducing hot flushes and making menopausal women feel less symptomatic, and it's clear that it really does help to maintain good general health, keep your weight at a healthy level, and help to reduce fat levels, because you build up muscle and burn fat when you exercise. It is also known that fat women are at a higher risk for heart disease and high blood pressure.

So it follows that as well as exercising, you should have a healthy, varied diet of fruit and vegetables, good proteins, wholegrains, nuts and legumes, low- and non-fat dairy products, good fats, and drink in moderation. Your diet should severely limit saturated fats, which can cause a build-up of bad cholesterol and high triglycerides, which in turn can result in the hardening of the arteries. Being overweight can also trigger insulin resistance, which can be a precursor of diabetes, which research has shown increases the risk of heart disease. I will discuss this in detail in Chapter 10 when I look at the issues of food and weight.

Other lifestyle factors that may help to prevent heart disease are a stress-free life and the ability to deal with the kind of problems that may cause unhappiness and depression. If you are seriously depressed you should find the appropriate treatment. There are also supplements like the omega-3 fatty acids, antioxidants and folic acid which I wrote about in Chapter 5, which may help heart health. Niacin and nicotinamide have also been shown to be helpful but the jury is still out on the efficacy of all these supplements and a lot more research needs to be done before they can be recommended without reservation as being effective.

Finally, you may lead an exemplary life and still be at risk because of hereditary factors. Those genes you inherited from your parents and grandparents play a very important role. I have seen women who live like athletes but have cholesterol levels of over 10, while others can spread on the butter and munch on hamburgers and still have textbook levels!

All about cholesterol

Everybody talks about cholesterol but do you really know what role it plays in your health? Cholesterol levels are a very important marker of heart disease risk. Cholesterol is a fatty substance that is found throughout your body; in your cells, blood, tissues, brain, muscles and liver. It is present in most of the protein we eat – meat, chicken, fish and eggs – and in dairy products. Your liver produces cholesterol and also synthesises it. When we think of cholesterol we often think of it in negative terms; in fact it is essential for healthy living. It plays a vital role in cell repair, in the storage and production of energy, and as I explained in Chapter 2, all sex steroid hormones come from cholesterol. So from this point of view we need cholesterol to live. The problems occur when the levels of certain cholesterols in your bloodstream become too high.

There are a few terms that you will hear when you visit your healthcare practitioner. The first of these is *lipoproteins* (a lipoprotein consists of a molecule of fat and a molecule of protein). These are substances found in the blood that transport cholesterol. The two that we are concerned with are LDL (*low-density lipoproteins*) and HDL (*high-density lipoproteins*). The next term is *triglycerides*. All of these perform important functions in the working of your body. LDL is usually called 'bad' cholesterol because although when its levels are normal it does an essential job of carrying cholesterol away from areas where it isn't needed to areas where it can best be used, if the

144

levels of LDL become too high, it starts to stick to the walls of the blood vessels or arteries and forms deposits of the fatty material or plaque that I described earlier. This can lead to hardening of the arteries – arteriosclerosis. The job of HDL, the 'good' cholesterol, is to carry cholesterol and triglycerides to the liver, which converts them so that they can be used again in different parts of the body. If they are not needed, the liver uses the bile to get rid of unwanted cholesterol, so obviously higher levels of HDL are good because they help to protect your body from excess cholesterol.

In order to make sure that you are not at risk for heart disease your doctor will suggest that you have a lipoprotein profile, where your blood will be tested to measure your total cholesterol, HDL, LDL and triglyceride levels. This test should be done after you have fasted for 12 hours so that any foods you have eaten won't interfere with the results. The results should be within the accepted healthy levels, and if they aren't, you and your doctor will work out the necessary lifestyle changes and/or treatment. For middle-aged women the best results would read as follows:

- Total cholesterol less than five (<5)
- LDL less than three (<3)
- Triglycerides less than two (<2)
- HDL greater than one (>1)

If you have only slightly elevated levels of the first three and lowered levels of the last, your doctor may decide that if you can reach the correct levels with lifestyle changes such as losing weight, stopping smoking and increasing your exercise regimen, she or he will monitor you again and see if your test results have improved. If you have very elevated levels, or levels that are only slightly elevated but you have risk factors for heart disease such as a family history, or if you are a smoker, are overweight or drink more than two glasses of alcohol a day, your doctor will probably suggest a cholesterol-lowering drug, the most effective of which are called *statins*. These are drugs that act on a certain enzyme in the liver, causing a lowering of cholesterol in the blood. They can be taken for many years and have very few bad side effects apart from some muscle and joint pain in some cases.

High blood pressure

Other problems that might put you at risk for heart disease are high blood pressure and diabetes. I will deal with the latter in detail in the chapter on weight and weight loss, so here I will just focus on *hypertension*, which is the medical term for high blood pressure. When you have a check-up your doctor will always check your blood pressure. As your heart beats, it pumps the blood through your body and as it flows, it exerts pressure on the walls of your arteries. Your blood pressure is highest when your heart pumps out the blood and drops when the heart rests between beats. The former is called *systolic* pressure and the latter, *diastolic*. This is why you are told your blood pressure is 120 over 80 (normal for a middle-aged woman), it means the systolic pressure over the diastolic pressure. It is written 120/80. Your blood pressure usually stays more or less the same when you are awake. Certain factors – like your teenage children, fear, or illness – may cause it to rise, and it is usually lower when you sleep, which is why if you get up very quickly you may feel giddy or experience a rush of blood as the pressure normalises itself.

High blood pressure (*hypertension*) means that the top number and the bottom number are higher than normal, and doctors would classify a top number over 140 and a bottom one of over 90 as high. This means that your heart is pumping out your blood at a higher level and working harder, which can cause heart disease or, more commonly, stroke. As you get older your blood pressure tends to rise, which is why so many older women are on medication for high blood pressure. Several things, including your diet – too much salt and too many fatty foods – water retention, being overweight, certain hormones and illnesses can affect your blood pressure. Stress and tension can also cause high blood pressure because agitation causes your heart to beat faster. There are several different types of medication which can help to lower your blood pressure and your doctor may prescribe some or all of the following: *diuretics*, which help to prevent water retention; *ACE inhibitors*, which help to bring your blood pressure down; and *beta blockers*, which help to regulate your heartbeat by calming your body's responses.

Many cardiologists will recommend a scan of your carotid arteries, which are the major arteries on either side of your neck, running from your heart into your brain. If the walls of these arteries are clear and free from plaque, the fatty material that builds up if you have arteriosclerosis, then even if your cholesterol levels are raised, you are not at such high risk for heart disease.

Medicines to prevent heart disease

Other medicines your doctor may prescribe to prevent heart disease are drugs called *anticoagulants*, which are used to prevent clotting in the blood. People often mistakenly think that they make your blood thinner. If you are at risk for heart disease, your doctor and cardiologist may recommend that you take an aspirin or half an aspirin daily, but you should not embark on this course without the knowledge, recommendation and agreement of your healthcare practitioner. Just because you can buy aspirin over the counter doesn't mean it's harmless; there may be many side effects, including internal bleeding and stomach upsets, as well as kidney failure. If pure aspirin upsets your stomach, coated aspirins are also available.

New risks for heart disease

Your cholesterol levels and your lifestyle are not the only markers that may indicate to your healthcare practitioner that you are at risk for heart disease. Advances in research are revealing new risks. You've already read in Chapter 4 that taking oral estrogen raises the levels of *C-reactive protein* (*CRP*). This protein is produced by the liver only when you are experiencing severe inflammation, injury or disease. It is part of the normal immune response to problems in your body. Research has shown that although CRP levels may be raised when you have a heart attack, it is not clear what role it plays in heart disease; whether it is just a marker of the disease or whether raised levels may be a risk factor in heart disease. However, there is a growing body of evidence that it may be a risk factor.

Another marker seems to be high levels of *homocysteine*, which is an amino acid that helps to make protein and build and maintain tissues. In Chapter 5 I discussed various antioxidant supplements that are thought to lower homocysteine levels. The reason we want to lower these levels is that recent research seems to show a strong link between high levels of homocysteine and the risk of stroke and heart disease. It seems that high levels result in a build-up of bad cholesterol in the arteries, causing hardening. High levels combined with smoking and high blood pressure make your risk of heart disease even greater.

A further problem may be high levels of something called *fibrinogen*. Fibrinogen helps the blood to clot, which is absolutely vital for survival, but when the levels of fibrinogen in the blood become too high, the clotting mechanism can become a danger and cause clots to form in your arteries. As is the case with C-reactive protein, the presence of fibrinogen may indicate inflammation in the walls of your damaged arteries, which is why high levels in your blood may act as a warning flag for heart disease. Lifestyle and certain hormones can cause your fibrinogen levels to rise, but guess what the number one cause is – smoking! I know I am repeating myself but the evidence is too compelling not to keep mentioning the huge risk that smoking poses to your health.

Earlier I wrote about lipoproteins. A new lipoprotein, called *lipoprotein(a)* or *Lp(a)* has made its appearance. It seems to be formed when a particular protein in the body attaches itself to a molecule of LDL. The bad news is that when LDL carries this specific protein, it appears to interfere with your body's ability to dissolve blood clots, and when this happens you are at increased risk for stroke because of the interrupted blood flow.

Because these are such new discoveries it is not clear what will be effective against raised levels, but it seems certain that a healthy lifestyle and giving up smoking, drinking moderately and exercising, as well as taking cholesterol-lowering drugs should help keep these risk factors at bay.

Empowerment points

- You should always be treated as an individual. All the personal risk factors, such as your lifestyle and family history, whether you smoke or are overweight, plus any others, should be taken into consideration and carefully discussed.

- If you're a smoker, stop smoking immediately.

- Be aware of the risks involved in heart disease and take control of your life.

- Women who are having heart attacks don't often complain of chest pain; they are more likely to report pain in their necks, the middle of their backs or their jaws. They often describe palpitations, a feeling of indigestion, shortness of breath and often nausea, which may be combined with vomiting.

- If you're anxious about taking a particular medication don't be afraid to question your practitioner or get a second opinion. You might not want to take a risk that your practitioner deems acceptable.

- Until there is more evidence, HT should not be used to prevent cardiovascular disease when there are unambiguous studies which show that there are other drugs, like statins, that really work.

Notes

_____

_____

_____

_____

_____

8

The C Word: Cancers in
Menopausal Women

Andrea's story, told in Chapter 7, graphically illustrates the fact that the issues of heart disease and cancer are vital to middle-aged women. Both diseases are tied up with the question of whether peri- and postmenopausal women should take HT. Since middle-aged women are more vulnerable to certain types of cancer, I think it is important to give a laywoman's perspective on these illnesses. This will not be an in-depth discussion, but it will give you some general information that will empower you.

Most of us are terribly afraid of cancer, even more so than of heart disease, which is strange since research has shown that cardiovascular disease kills far more women than breast cancer does, but fear is irrational. Even as I write these words, I feel anxious and hesitant about writing about cancer. I am almost superstitious. Why go into this? Why mess with it? The spectre of cancer is so terrifying. We have friends who have died of it and know others who are battling with treatment. We may also know some who are in remission. However, if we can try to conquer these fears and give ourselves the chance to understand the dynamics of cancer and heart disease, how to lower our risks, especially if we are vulnerable, and to be aware of the risks, we can increase our chances of living to a healthy and happy old age. As we age the risk factor increases, so it's very important to understand how cancers occur so we can live in a way that will help to prevent them, or at least, decrease the risk.

There are, of course, hundreds of different types of cancers, but the ones that I write about are those that seem to be associated with women in menopause: breast cancers, endometrial cancer, vulvar cancer and ovarian cancer. In fact, these are all very complicated diseases – the subject of breast cancer deserves a book all on its own. My object here is to give a general overview to help you understand a little more about these cancers, to be aware of the risks and to see that there are treatment options available. There are really good associations out there and the 21st century allows women to be much more enlightened, to understand the nature of their cancer and how they can participate in their treatment and recovery. The bulk of the information is about breast cancer because it is the most widely researched and the most common cancer that attacks middle-aged women. There are excellent websites and information centres with toll-free lines available (some of these are listed with the references at the end of the book).

As is evident in this book, I am not keen on too many diagrams but I think that in order to help you conquer the fear of breast cancer and to arm yourself with knowledge, I will use a couple of diagrams to show where breast cancers usually begin and where they travel. Breasts are of major psychological and physical significance for most women. They are the symbols of beauty and femininity, the sign that we have changed from girl to woman and then to mother, as we nourish our children from our breasts. The image of a woman cradling her baby at her breast is as old as humanity. This is why when our breasts are cancerous or removed we feel so bereft and why breast cancer has so many psychological implications.

Our breasts are specifically designed to make milk. They are made up of different tissues – fatty and connective – and groups of tiny milk-producing glands. They are divided into sections called *lobes*, which contain even smaller lobes, known as *lobules*. It is in these lobules that milk glands are found. When we breastfeed the breast milk flows out of the breast through tubes (*ducts*) to our nipples.

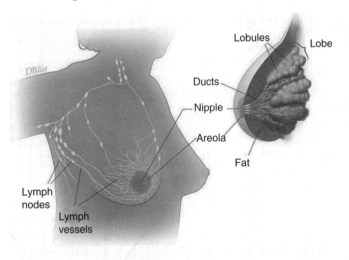

The parts of the breast and the lymph nodes and lymph vessels near the breast

Source: 'General Information about Breast Cancer'. National Cancer Institute. US National Institutes of Health www.cancer.gov

As you can see in the diagram the breast also has tiny vessels, which are very similar to veins. These vessels are called *lymph vessels* because they belong to the *lymphatic system* and carry a clear fluid that cleans the tissues throughout the body. The role of the lymphatic system is to guard our body from infection, and to help in this function there are little areas called lymph nodes throughout the body, including in the armpits, neck area, near the collarbone and in the groin and chest, where lymph fluid collects. These *lymph nodes* collect materials like bacteria and cancerous cells that are harmful to the body and prevent them from entering the bloodstream. So when a lot of harmful material is gathered in the nodes they can become swollen and painful, a sign of infection or that something is wrong, which is why your doctor feels for swollen lymph glands when you complain of feeling ill. But be aware that a malignant node is generally painless.

The cells that make up the tissues in our bodies are constantly growing and dividing as new cells are needed, but sometimes the way in which the cells form new cells goes awry and there is spate of new cell growth when new cells are not needed because the old cells haven't died. This mass of cells in the tissue becomes a lump or growth (*tumour*) and this is what can be felt or detected by means of a screening. At different times during your cycle your breasts may feel lumpy because of the rise and fall in your hormone levels. Some women only have lumpy breasts at certain times of the month and others always seem to have lumpy breasts, which shows you that not all lumps are dangerous or malignant. These non-threatening lumps are called *benign* and generally only one out of ten breast lumps is malignant. The most common cause for a breast lump in most menopausal women is a cyst. The lumps you should worry about are the ones that are diagnosed as malignant. These little masses of cells may start out very small indeed, so small that they cannot be felt in a breast examination, which is why healthcare practitioners, especially those involved in dealing with cancers, believe in a screening process called *mammography*, which helps them to identify and deal with the cancer in its earliest stages.

Mammograms and ultrasounds: screening for breast cancers

'That's it!' said Leigh triumphantly. 'I never need another mammogram, thank goodness. It was a horrible experience.'

'Why not?' I asked in amazement.

'I've just been for my annual check-up and my gynaecologist says she can pick up any changes in my breasts with her yearly examination and she also gave me information which showed that radiologists couldn't claim scientifically that there was a better survival rate for women who had regular mammograms than those who didn't!'

I was dumbfounded. I knew immediately what she was talking about. In medical research there is an independent non-profit organisation called the Cochrane Collaboration that reviews the available research on different healthcare interventions and then reports its findings so the healthcare practitioners can see whether the research is valid or not. In 2001 a Cochrane review stated that the research that was currently available did not show that there was a survival benefit if there was mass screening of women and that furthermore the available evidence did not show that women with breast cancer lived longer if they had been screened. It suggested that those who recommended screening and those who wanted to be screened should consider these findings carefully.

All hell broke loose among those who felt that the review was incorrect, because many of the studies and the statistics they had reviewed were faulty, so that it created a misleading impression about the efficacy of screening for breast cancer. As I explained in Chapter 3, it is all too easy for doctors to take what they want from a report and sell it to their patients as the truth. It is true that mammograms may be done by inadequately trained radiographers, and that there can be misdiagnoses which cause tremendous anxiety when a woman is told there is a problem when there isn't and, in some cases, death, when someone is told she is fine when she is not. But all this tells us is that we should understand that a tool, however effective, can be misused.

Believers in mammography responded to this review in depth, stating that they understood that no study is perfect but that many of the criticisms cited in the review were incorrect and that in fact there had been careful control of the statistics, which they believed to be valid in spite of their drawbacks. They said that in general the research showed that mammograms are effective in reducing deaths from breast cancer.

In 2004 researchers from the American Cancer Society, reviewing the randomised trials of over 40 years, concluded that the trials generally showed that mammograms substantially reduce death from breast cancer and that while there are still problems like false positives, which means that a lump is diagnosed as cancerous when it is benign, or false negatives, which is when a patient is told she is in the clear when she is not, the 20 per cent reduction shown overall is very statistically significant in both absolute and relative terms. In January 2005 another Cochrane review examined randomised controlled trials conducted with a follow-up time of nearly 20 years and came to the conclusion that regular physical examinations and yearly mammograms are very effective in detecting recurrences of cancer and in reducing the mortality rate of breast cancer survivors.

This sounds pretty convincing in statistical and medical terms, but how can we make sense of it? Let's imagine that you have a small cancerous lump in your breast that is less than 1cm in size. It is called a *ductal carcinoma in situ* (DCIS), meaning a cancer in a specific part of the breast duct that has not invaded the surrounding duct. These cancerous cells are confined to the inside of the ducts and because they have not become invasive, which means that they have broken through the wall of the breast ducts to affect other breast tissue, there is no risk of the cancer cells spreading. This is why DCIS is sometimes known as a pre-cancer.

DCIS cannot usually be felt as a breast lump or other breast change, and so most cases are found by routine screening with mammograms. If this DCIS is detected by screening and appropriately treated, the recovery rate is excellent because it has not spread. In fact research has shown that recovery may be over 95 per cent, because steps can be taken to prevent it developing into invasive breast cancer and treatment for DCIS is usually very successful. However, if the DCIS is not detected and therefore not treated, approximately between a quarter and half of all these areas of DCIS will develop into invasive breast cancer. And the chances of survival can be 40 per cent less!

As cancers grow they become more aggressive and start to invade the surrounding areas, which in the case of the breast, would probably be the lymph nodes, and then the blood-stream. This movement, when a group of cancer cells starts to travel and damages other organs or tissues or forms other secondary growths is called *metastasis*.

From my personal perspective, I would suggest you have a mammogram once a year after you turn 40 if you are taking HT. Since the first edition of this book was published, there is new research showing that women in the 40- to 49-year-old age group should be screened based on their individual assessments, their own individual preferences and their cancer risk, which I will discuss later. All women over 50 should, if they can, have an annual mammogram. Breasts of postmenopausal women are less dense which means that their mammograms are more effective. But obviously, if you already have become menopausal in your forties, you may be a better candidate for a mammogram than 50-year-old woman who is still having regular periods. It goes back to the fact that all women should be treated as individuals.

If you have very dense breasts, you should expect to have an ultrasound as well. If you are very anxious because you are at high risk it is a good idea to have an annual mammogram and then an ultrasound every six months. Research has shown that for women who are at very high risk for breast cancer, *magnetic resonance imaging* (MRI), when performed in venues specialising in breast cancer screening, is much more sensitive than mammography, though, like all techniques, it has its drawbacks and is, of course, very expensive.

However, an annual MRI may be recommended for women who have a BRCA altered gene, those women who have not been tested but who have a first line relative that has a BRCA-positive cancer, and who have had a three or more false negative biopsies. Use of this diagnostic tool has expanded and MRI is now also used in certain specific cases after a woman has been diagnosed for breast cancer to determine the extent of the disease and as guidance for both biopsies and the localisation of the cancer. It can also be used to evaluate if the treatment recommended is being effective.

The dreaded mammogram

Mammograms strike fear into the hearts of many women. Some women have had one and found it so uncomfortable that they swear they will never have another; others have been put off by gruesome descriptions of mammograms being like having your breast slammed in the freezer door or lying on a cold concrete floor while your breast is squished between two weights. Still others are worried about the amount of radiation they might be exposed to when they have their annual mammogram.

The truth is a well-performed mammogram is no more than slightly uncomfortable. You will be taken into a private room and told to undress from your waist up. Here your breasts will be positioned on a plastic shelf. You will need to stand in two different positions, your breasts will be sandwiched, but not in any way that should hurt – if it is unbearably painful ask the radiographer to stop. If you know your breasts are very tender, take a painkiller before you embark on the process.

Try not to have a mammogram just before your period when your breasts may be very full and tender. Some women find it comforting to take a close female friend or relative with them and others may want to be with their partners or husbands. My view is that whatever makes you feel most at home should be the rule. Here's a tip: I have found that if you stand on tip-toe so that you let your breasts lift on to the little plastic ledge of the mammography machine it feels much more comfortable. It is a bit undignified but most of us have felt far worse during gynaecological examinations and if you are really uncomfortable you should find a centre that specialises in breast screening. Firstly because experts will probably interpret the results better and secondly because the woman who does your examination will probably make you feel more at ease.

If you are worried about exposure to radiation it will probably help you to remember that you are exposed to far greater levels when you sit in front of your computer or shop at a mall.

Since the first edition of this book was published, digital mammography has become more common. This kind of mammography uses the same technique as film screen mammography, but the image is recorded directly into a computer. The image can then be enlarged or highlighted. If there is a suspicious area, your radiologist will then use the computer to take a closer look. If digital mammography is used your radiologist may read your mammogram with the help of computer-aided detection (CAD) programs, and can then transmit your mammogram to your doctor via e-mail.

Once the procedure is over you will be asked to wait while the radiologist looks at the pictures of your breasts. If all looks clear, she or he will probably tell you to get dressed and will then spend a little time with you, telling you that all is well and suggesting when your next visit should be. Usually, after you have had children, your breast tissue changes – this is called an *involuted* breast, which means that it has sort of collapsed inward, so the fatty tissue is not too dense. If you have very dense tissue because you are hormonal or on HT, or because you have had a breast implant or reconstruction and the image doesn't look clear, or the radiologist sees something that looks out of place, she or he will suggest you come along to another room where an ultrasound machine is set up. Your breasts will be scanned to see the area of concern more clearly. There may be a tiny lump or there may be small areas of calcium that are clumped together which might also be a sign of cancer.

The scan doesn't hurt at all, I promise you. You lie on a bed next to a screen and the radiologist spreads a gel over your breasts and moves an ultrasound probe, a flat object, with light pressure over your breasts while watching the screen to see more clearly what's going on. To you, it will look like the map of the moon, to the expert it will give a clear indication of whether there's something to worry about. The only problem is that if the radiologist hasn't explained why you are there, you may feel a bit panicked. Stay calm. Often the scan is just routine, to make absolutely sure that any shadowy areas that are shown in the mammogram are no more than more dense bits of tissue.

The problems begin when the doctor sees that there is indeed an abnormal mass. But remember that most suspicious findings are not cancerous; perhaps only one in five or even fewer will be problematic. A needle biopsy will usually be performed. This should be done by a specialist radiologist in a specialist radiological suite, using either a mammogram or ultrasound for guidance. An oncologist friend says that doing a free-hand biopsy is like sticking your hand into the haystack and trying to find the needle.

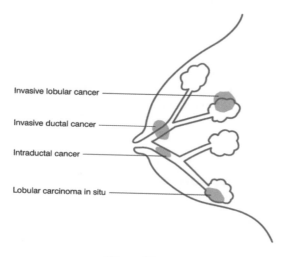

Sites of breast cancer

By kind permission of Dr Carol-Ann Benn

There are several ways to determine if the lump is malignant. The specialist will use the ultrasound and a needle to take a sample of tissue and the cells, which will be sent to a pathology laboratory to see if they are harmful. There are two types of needle biopsies. The *fine needle biopsy* is most effective in collecting cells from cysts and lymph nodes and can also be used for solid masses. A *core needle biopsy* is generally performed on a breast lump to collect both tissue and cells. The needle used for this procedure is slightly thicker but neither procedure, in the hands of an expert, should be too painful. If it is unbearably painful, there is something wrong – and not with you! The specialist may also suggest another form of biopsy where either a bit of the lump or the entire lump is removed so that the pathologists can examine the tissue carefully. This is done only if the material collected from the core biopsy or fine needle biopsy comes back as inconclusive, doesn't have typical characteristics, or doesn't fit with the clinical findings of the specialist. A biopsy can also be performed if the suspicious area is in a place that is hard for a needle to reach. From the pathological point of view, if you have cancer, your samples should be checked to see if the cells respond positively or negatively to estrogen and progesterone, because this will affect your treatment options.

I am not saying that once you have an annual mammogram you can abdicate your responsibility to yourself and your health. Living well is one of the first lines of defence, as is an understanding of the possible risk factors in your particular situation. It would also be sensible to know how to examine your own breasts once a month.

How to examine your own breasts

Decide when you want to examine your breasts and make it the same time each month. Remember that breast tissue reacts to hormone changes in your body so your breasts could feel a little lumpy or tender just before or during your period, or if you are on HT, or are perimenopausal and experiencing the wide fluctuations of estrogen levels that I discussed in Chapter 1.

Some women like to examine their breasts in the shower, others in the bath, or while lying in bed. It's up to you. Probably the best way is to get your doctor to give you a thorough clinical breast examination. Then feel over your breasts yourself so you know how they feel after they have been given the all-clear. This will help you to be more confident when doing a self-breast exam that something feels different; a harder lump, or one that wasn't there before.

Be alert for *any* change sin your breasts. A change can be an important warning sign. Look at your breasts in a mirror, hold each one in your hand and look down at it to see if you can detect any changes in shape (I'm not talking here about weight gain or loss). Are there any strange rashes or dimpling? Has your nipple changed and moved inwards or is the skin round the nipple tender or inflamed, itchy or painful? Is the skin crusty or an angry red? Is there any fluid or discharge coming out of your nipple? Raise your arms and check again that everything still looks the same.

Now get into the bath or shower, or lie down, and gently move the first three fingers, held flat and together, in a circular motion over your entire breast from the top to the bottom and from over your cleavage to under your armpits, exerting a gentle pressure and feeling deep into the breast tissue. Use the right hand to examine the left breast and vice versa. Ideally you should do this examination both standing and lying down. Having said all that, I must admit that I am useless at breast exams. I immediately think that a rib is a sinister lump and I can never remember what my breast felt like from one month to the next. If this is the case with you as well, get your GP to examine your breasts thoroughly. But even if you are uncomfortable examining yourself, you must be alert to any of the changes in your breasts that I have mentioned above.

Risk factors

The first thing to be aware of here is that 50 per cent of women who get breast cancer have no obvious risk factors at all, which is my opportunity to say that no woman should ever, ever blame herself for getting breast cancer. Plenty of healthy women, living as well as possible, get breast cancer. If you are at a high risk because of your family history, you can take responsibility for your health and see that you are monitored and screened regularly. There are steps you can take to lower your risk profile and live as healthily as possible. However, blaming yourself and immersing yourself in guilt can only impede your recovery. Everyone is going to have risk factors for some illness or another.

One of the strongest risks of breast cancer, which I will explain later, is your age. Your genetic make-up will determine whether you suffer from certain illnesses like diabetes, cardiovascular disease or cancer. In your make-up there is a trigger that will determine what will happen to you and it may happen no matter how healthily or unhealthily you live. In any case, as we get older and live longer, we are at greater risk for some kind of cancer or another as the cells in our bodies age. I am appalled at those alternative medicine writers and practitioners who put this kind of burden on women with cancer. You are who you are, and ultimately your genetic make-up may be the culprit, not you. Of course relaxation techniques and appropriate living can improve your immune system and your chances of recovery, but the burden of recovery should not be placed on you alone. Work in partnership with your surgeon, oncologist and counsellor. Allow yourself to work through the grief, rage and fear, and don't hide those feelings. You have not wished cancer upon yourself!

This is also probably the place to mention alternative and complementary cures. If you have read Chapter 5 you already know my bias, but 'natural' cures may be devastating for cancer patients in terms of the false hope, the cost and the often harmful effects, and because they promise to work and don't, which could deprive the cancer patient of valuable time and exposure to conventional medicines which have been shown to work.

The same rules apply to alternative cures as to conventional treatment. What is the evidence that they work? What are the interests of those involved and what are their medical qualifications? I accept that many people have had horrific experiences with conventional doctors but I have heard equally horrific stories about complementary healers. Be aware and don't allow despair to make you gullible. Also, don't forget the power of the placebo effect that I discussed on page 101. Those who offer these 'cures' should allow the most thorough scrutiny possible. Anecdotal evidence can never replace sound scientific evidence. If supplements make you feel better, take them. Just remember to discuss what you're taking with your oncologist – any potent natural medicine can cause serious side effects or interfere with some of the conventional treatments you are taking. I recommend that you look at the articles on complementary and alternative cancer cures on www.quackwatch.com, my favourite site for logical, balanced comment on this subject.

Now to the factors that may increase your risk of getting breast cancer (remember even if you have one or more of these risks you may never get it at all).

Age

Age is the strongest risk factor for breast cancer. Like most cancers, the risk of developing breast cancer increases as women get older. Nearly 80 per cent of breast cancers occur in women older than 50. This happens because there are changes in your breast cells which can cause cancer, and obviously the longer we live, the more time there is for this to happen. This is why I recommended earlier that women over 50 have annual mammograms. You can't stop ageing but you can have regular screenings.

Family history of breast cancer

BRCA1 and BRCA2

This is number one on the list. About 10 per cent of breast and ovarian cancers are inherited, which means that they are caused by an altered gene that has been passed on from parent to child. Remember you do not *actually* inherit cancer but you may inherit a higher risk of getting it.

Family history of breast cancer refers to any first-line relative – your mother, sister, daughter or father – who may have had it. Information about this is especially important if these relatives had breast cancer before they were 40, this is called early breast cancer. You should also mention if any of your second-line family members on either your father's or mother's side, such as a paternal or maternal grandmother, or aunt, or even first cousins had breast cancer.

Information about your family history of breast cancer becomes even more important if there are three relatives on the *same* side who have had or have breast cancer. If you have had a bout with cancer, such as endometrial cancer, you may also be at high risk for breast cancer. *Genetic make-up* is therefore a risk factor. The reason for members of one family being susceptible to breast cancer may be in their genes.

There is a lot of talk and confusion surrounding two genes called *BRCA1* and *BRCA2*. Every person has these genes and normally they play an import role in preventing breast and ovarian cancers. But sometimes a change may occur in these genes and they do not work as they should in controlling the growth of the cells. Instead they allow the cells to grow at an abnormal rate which may lead to caner. We inherit two copies of each and every gene – one from our mother and one from our father. So if either one of your parents carry an altered BRCA1 or BRCA2 gene, you have a 50 per cent chance of also having this altered gene. This does not mean that you are definitely going to get breast cancer but it does mean that it increases your possibility of developing breast cancer. Certain groups of people have been found to be more likely to carry these altered genes, for example people of Ashkenazi Jewish descent and members of Afrikaner families. Other population groups have also been found to be more likely to carry these altered genes.

Thanks to ongoing medical research there is a test available which can determine whether you are a carrier of one of these altered genes. But it is very important to understand that unlike a mammogram or other screening tests, this test is specifically for people who are thought to be at high risk for breast or ovarian cancer.

Anyone considering this test should first meet with a qualified specialist and do a thorough evaluation of their family history to be sure that this genetic testing is the right path to take. People can determine whether they carry an altered BRCA gene that may be responsible for the cancers in their family, and if they do carry an altered gene they can develop a strategy with their doctors and discuss the options that are available to decrease their cancer risk, as well as ensuring that they have ongoing monitoring which will help detect the cancer early, when the prognosis may be better.

A downside is that no screening or testing is infallible and some people become terribly anxious when they realise that they carry an altered gene which increases their risk of cancer, and they may act impulsively without considering all the available options. Remember that scientists are continuing to discover new genetic markers for breast cancer, so if you know that you have these factors your doctor will help you decide what you want to do.

Although HER2 is NOT a risk factor for cancer because the genetic abnormality is *in* the tumor and *not* in the person, I have placed the information here because many women ask me about it and I want to use this opportunity to discuss receptors, particularly estrogen receptors, which are relevant for women with breast cancer. In order to understand HER2 cancer, you need to know something about receptors and growth hormones.

Firstly, it is important to understand that the life cycle of each one of the millions of cells in our body is programmed to behave in a specific way but sometimes this process can be changed by various factors, one of which I will explain below. In the development of cancer a key factor is a change in the growth rate of the cell. Now let's go back to receptors. In Chapter 1, I explained that receptors are special groups of cells that are present in the organs and tissues, and respond to messages from the different hormones in your body. In fact your doctor will tell you about these receptors when they explain your breast cancer pathology report. There are receptors for the female hormones, estrogen and progesterone, present in your breast cells. These cells respond to messages from these hormones. Estrogen or progesterone will 'tell' the receptors to increase normal breast cell growth, where for example, it can make the cell repair or reproduce itself, or they can cause abnormal breast cell growth. Remember that each of these receptors only responds to their own specific protein or chemical, like the right key opening the right lock. Some of these chemicals I mentioned above are called growth factors and they attach to these receptors and stimulate cells to grow.

The HER2 gene is responsible for making HER2 protein. HER2 is one of the proteins found on the surface of certain cells. So we could say that HER2 is a receptor for a *particular* growth factor called *human epidermal growth factor*, which occurs naturally in the body.

Usually the HER2 protein plays an important role in normal cell growth and development. It transmits signals directing cell growth from the outside of the cell to the nucleus inside the cell. Sometimes, however, there is a genetic alteration in the HER2 gene that causes human epidermal growth factor to attach itself to HER2 receptors on breast cancer cells and stimulates the breast cancer cells to divide and grow. The problem starts because some breast cancer cells have a lot more HER2 receptors than others. When this happens, the tumour is described as being HER2 positive. It is thought that about one in five women with breast cancer will have HER2-positive tumours. This excess of HER2 is due to an altered gene, which can occur in many types of cancers, not only breast cancer. It is very important to understand that this altered HER2 gene is only present in the breast cancer cells, not in the rest of the cells in the body, and cannot be passed on to other family members.

The problem with HER2-positive breast cancers is that they tend to grow more quickly than other cancers, so you may have heard the specialist talking about your cancer being more 'aggressive'. When this happens, tests can be done to find out whether you have HER2-positive breast cancer. Usually the specialist oncologist will have a sample of cancer tissue from previous biopsies or your surgery. Testing may also have been done for HER2 in your initial surgery.

If you test positive for HER2, a drug called *trastuzumab* (Herceptin) has been developed and can be effective against this type of cancer. Recent research also suggests that Herceptin may help women with early breast cancer to help reduce the risk of the cancer coming back or recurring. It is currently known that chemotherapy and/or hormonal therapy can reduce this risk. A number of research trials looked at giving Herceptin as a treatment at the same time a woman received chemotherapy, to see if this further reduced the risk of cancer recurring. The results of these trials were very promising; the cancer came back in fewer women who had Herceptin combined with chemotherapy, compared with women who only had chemotherapy. There are side effects which may include fever and chills, weakness, nausea, vomiting, coughing, diarrhoea, and headaches. Usually these side effects lessen after the first dose. As I will discuss later in the section on treatment, chemotherapy and/or hormonal therapy can reduce this risk of beast cancer returning and as you can see, research has shown that Herceptin in combination with chemotherapy may help reduce the risk of the cancer recurring.

You may remember reading about several cases in different countries where women took their medical aids to court to ensure that this particular treatment, which is very expensive, would be paid for by their medical aids and they won. Your own specialist will advise you of the best treatment.

The hormone connection

It seems clear that there is a strong causal relationship between estrogen and breast cancer, so a long exposure (more than five years) to estrogen and high doses of estrogen are listed as potential risk factors. Therefore, the following are risk factors:

- Early menarche: meaning that you got your first period at an unusually young age, so your body has been exposed to estrogen for longer than normal.

- The longer exposure to estrogen also applies to late menopause.

- Long-term hormone therapy speaks for itself. If you're putting estrogen into your body you are increasing your exposure to it. This also applies to high doses of estrogen therapy (ET). The jury is still out concerning the length of time a woman may safely use ET but it seems as though a period of less than five years does not increase the risk. But ET may increase the growth of breast cells, breast density and breast pain, and it is thought that estrogen progesterone therapy may make the interpretations of mammograms more difficult.

- A late first pregnancy is also a risk factor because in the first place, you've had long-term exposure to estrogen, then during your pregnancy you have large amounts of estrogen coursing through your system at an age when you are starting to be at higher risk anyway.

- If you've never had a baby you could be at higher risk. This almost seems contradictory, but it relates to the hormone prolactin that is involved in pregnancy and the production of milk, which inhibits the production of estrogen. The interruption of estrogen production in a woman's life for a significant amount of time is thought to be protective.

- Dense breast tissue is also related to hormones. This is a risk factor because if your breast tissue is dense, it is more difficult to spot any abnormalities either during a clinical examination or a mammogram and many women who are on HT have much denser breast tissue. Interestingly, women who have had cosmetic plastic surgery of the breast, such as breast enlargement with implants or breast reduction, do not have increased risk of breast cancer, though mammograms need to be done more carefully on these women.

- I call the other risk factors the lifestyle risks. These include being extremely overweight after menopause. This is a risk because the enzyme aromatase, which is in the fatty tissues, can produce excess estrogen. Obviously your diet plays a part here since an unhealthy diet can lead to excess weight and part of an unhealthy diet is eating too many hydrogenated fats, which have been shown to put you at risk. It is important to eat well. Choose a diet that is low in saturated fats (fried food and red meat) and high in vegetables and fruits. Broccoli, cabbage, Brussels sprouts, kale and cauliflower are especially rich in a substance known as Indole-3-carbinol, which has been shown to be a major anti-cancer agent. A good rule of thumb is to make sure that your daily diet includes something red, something yellow, something orange and something green from the fruit and vegetable families. Lack of exercise contributes to excess weight and general unhealthiness, so this is a logical risk factor. Research has shown that drinking more than two glasses of alcohol a day is also very risky. The reason for this is that alcohol may increase the levels of estrogen in your blood or interfere with the way it is broken down and used effectively. If your liver doesn't do its job properly because of excess alcohol, it may not be able to get rid of harmful substances that may cause cancer.

The problem is that while you can take responsibility for your daily breast health, most cancers are so tiny when they start out that even an expert can't detect them with a physical examination. We know from research that it is better for us to treat cancers as early as possible, before they become aggressive or invasive. In fact, it's just common sense that a smaller tumour would probably be easier to treat, which is why I believe in regular screening.

Strategies for dealing with breast cancer

Julie, who was in her forties, found out over the phone that she had cancer. She was told that she would be having surgery the next morning and would meet her surgeon for the first time in the pre-op ward of the hospital. When she ventured a protest she was told brusquely that it was her breast or her life! Within 24 hours she suffered both the trauma of learning she had cancer and a radical mastectomy (where the whole breast is removed as well as some pectoral muscles, the chest muscle that moves the arm).

For a year following the surgery she was in a deep depression, her balance had been altered, she felt ugly and she had had no counselling to help her deal with her trauma. Whenever she told the oncologist how down she felt, her feelings were brushed aside. 'You're alive,' she was told. 'What more do you want?' She was left with an underlying unresolved anger and felt depressed and guilty and ashamed that she wasn't more grateful to her 'saviour'.

Julie had every right to feel ill-used. A year after the surgery she visited another oncologist and a surgeon who took the time and trouble to explain the process of breast reconstruction and performed the surgery that reconstructed Julie's breast. The surgeon dealt with her angst and despair, listened to her without judging her and helped her to find professional counselling. It is now five years since her bout with breast cancer and though Julie is aware of the risks, she is living well and happily.

I have included this story because I passionately believe that all women with cancer should be treated with dignity and respect; their partners and families should be involved; they should be entitled to clear and unambiguous explanations of their disease; they should have the right to question their doctors as much as they want; and they should never be made to feel ignorant or helpless. They should also always be given the opportunity to get a second opinion on treatment decisions. A sympathetic atmosphere and appropriate counselling should be an integral part of the treatment and no woman should be bullied or rushed into a hasty decision about a mastectomy or surgery. By the time the cancer is diagnosed it has been around for a while and it is far better to be allowed to make a careful and informed decision than to feel helpless, angry and patronised. Being treated with respect will help you to take control and be a partner with your specialist in fighting your cancer.

When you get the bad news make an appointment to see your oncologist or cancer specialist. Make a list of questions. This applies to all medical consultations. I always tell my clients to keep a piece of paper and pen handy before an appointment and to write down anything that comes into their minds about their problem, no matter how trivial they might think it is. When you are shocked and emotional you won't be able to think clearly and if you write down whatever comes to mind during the time before the appointment with your specialist, you will be able to address issues that you might otherwise forget or suppress during the consultation. Ask about anything and everything. It is your body and your life, and you have the right to question your doctor. Never ever feel embarrassed or anxious about wasting his or her time. If you aren't satisfied with an answer or don't understand something, that's fine, ask for clarification. The doctor's job is not to be judgemental about your perceived level of intelligence; it is to help you heal as quickly as possible.

Take your partner or husband with you to the consultation. I think that the support of your family and friends is vital at this time. You set the boundaries and don't be afraid to ask for exactly what you want. I think children handle trauma such as a mother's illness better when the information they are given is straightforward and there are no hushed whispers and mystery surrounding the problem. Uncertainty is terribly frightening for a child.

Treatment options

Depending on the type of cancer you have and how advanced it is, there are different treatment options. Usually you will have some kind of surgery to remove the lump and the infected area. You should discuss the type of surgery with your specialist surgeon and the choice will probably depend on the size and position of the lump, the size of your breast, and what you hope for from the surgery. This is a good time for your surgeon to refer you to a plastic surgeon to discuss your options for reconstructive surgery. Many surgeons now work in conjunction with a plastic surgeon since research has shown that for many women immediate reconstruction seems to lessen the trauma of breast mastectomy or lumpectomy.

During surgery for breast cancer it is common to leave a clear margin of 1 cm around the lump. At the same time the surgeon may surgically remove some of the sentinel lymph node under the arm on the side of the breast that has the cancer to ascertain whether the infection has spread. The sentinel node is the first node into which the duct in which the cancer is found drains. Treatment is and should be tailored to the needs of each individual. Cancer treatment should not be of the 'cookie cutter' variety. In the first place, treatment may differ depending on whether you are peri- or postmenopausal. So if a friend has had breast cancer and her treatment was different from yours, don't panic; your treatment will be the most effective for your particular cancer or your own circumstances.

Radiation therapy, which is when the cancerous area is blasted with X-rays, may be suggested after the surgery to make sure that all the cancer cells are killed. Many of you may have heard the word *adjuvant* therapy – it simply means after surgery. If your doctor talks about *neoadjuvant*, it means before surgery. Sometimes a woman may have radiation therapy or chemotherapy before the surgery if she has a very large and aggressive tumour, to help shrink it and keep the cancer localised. In other cases she may first be given one of the two medications I write about below before her operation.

After surgery some women will be given chemotherapy, which is a chemical treatment given in either pill or injection form, that travels through the bloodstream and kills the cancer cells in the body. The course usually takes several months and some women have miserable side effects, but once again, your individual biochemistry will dictate this.

If you have an estrogen- and/or progestogen-positive tumour, which means that exposure to one or both of these hormones causes the cells in the tumour to grow, as I explained above a logical step would be either to suppress your estrogen or block the estrogen receptors throughout your body. This can be done surgically with a total hysterectomy and oophorectomy, where your womb and your ovaries are removed (see Chapter 6), or by giving you hormone treatment. This is not the HT that I have talked about throughout this book but a sort of 'anti'-hormone treatment or hormone blockade that is called *adjuvant endocrine therapy*. It stops your own internal estrogen from reaching the estrogen receptors or stops your body from making estradiol. So women on this treatment may take Tamoxifen as well as chemotherapy, or may not have chemotherapy at all and just take Tamoxifen or an aromatase inhibitor, which blocks the enzyme aromatase from converting the androgens in your body to estrogens. It is thought that cancers develop in places where the activity of this enzyme is highest, like the breast.

As I explained in Chapter 4, Tamoxifen is a selective estrogen receptor modulator or SERM. This means it has an estrogen effect in certain areas of your body that will benefit you, and block unwanted estrogen effects in other parts of your body, so that the amount of active estrogen is not increased. Another hormonal treatment is the use of *aromatase inhibitors* (AIs). Two of these, *Letrozole* (Femara) or *Anastrazole* (Arimidex), work by blocking an enzyme, aromatase (see Chapter 2), which is responsible for making small amounts of estrogen in postmenopausal women. The AI hampers the production of estrogen and actually reduces the total amount of estrogen in a woman's body so that less estrogen can reach the breast cancer cells. But aromatase inhibitors cannot prevent premenopausal women's ovaries from making estrogen, so they are usually used in postmenopausal women.

Another hormone blocking treatment is *luteinising hormone-releasing hormone analogue* (LHRHa), such as *Goserelin* (Zoladex), which suppresses the LH (see Chapter 2 to remind yourself about LH) from your pituitary, which means that the production of estrogen from your ovaries is greatly reduced. LHRHas are now being tested as adjuvant therapies in addition to Tamoxifen or an AI in premenopausal women.

The bad news is that while these treatments are dealing with your cancer they may also be causing some very nasty side effects. You can understand why: Tamoxifen blocks certain estrogenic effects; chemotherapy can induce menopause-type symptoms; and the removal of your ovaries will plunge you into menopause, causing all the symptoms of dropping estrogen levels that I discussed in Chapter 1. This is why Tamoxifen is usually prescribed for no longer than five years, since long-term treatment with it may put you at risk for blood clots, endocrine cancer and sometimes the formation of cataracts. On the upside it may prevent bone loss and may have a beneficial effect on your cholesterol levels.

Unlike Tamoxifen, Anastrazole and Letrozole don't cause cancer of the womb and seldom, if ever, cause blood clots. But they can increase a woman's fracture risk because they remove almost all estrogen from a postmenopausal woman's body. Women using an aromatase inhibitor should discuss this risk with their doctors and have a bone density test to see whether they should also be taking a medication to strengthen their bones. There may also be certain side effects with aromatase inhibitors, such as joint pain and muscle aches. Research is still under way to determine the length of time women should be taking this treatment.

Researchers are constantly searching for new options and at the moment one of these third-generation SERMs, *Arzoxifene*, a new SERM is in Phase 2 trials (See Chapter 9) and is being explored as a potential agent to reduce the risk of, or delay, the development or recurrence of cancer This drug seems to have strong breast anti-estrogen activity and an absence of uterine agonist activity, which means that it does not lead to thickening of the lining of the womb as can happen with Tamoxifen. Another new treatment option is *Fulvestrant* (Faslodex), which also acts on the estrogen receptors (ERs) but it doesn't just block the action of estrogen on the estrogen receptors, it eliminates this action and may be a good treatment option in the future for those women whose breast cancers have progressed or recurred after treatment with Tamoxifen, Anastrazole or Letrozole. Fulvestrant is given as a monthly injection and side effects include hot flushes, mild nausea, and fatigue

Breast reconstruction

One of the biggest issues for most women who are told that they must have surgery is the removal or mutilation of a breast or both breasts. Luckily, plastic surgery has made such huge advances that many women who have had surgery for breast cancer can have their breasts reconstructed. Reconstructive surgery means plastic surgery to restore or preserve the shape of the breast. In the past, surgeons and oncologists would recommend that women wait until after the completion of all their treatments before having their breast reconstruction, but today plastic surgery techniques are so advanced that *immediate reconstruction*, which means reconstruction is started at the same time as the breast surgery to remove the cancer, may be best for most women. This is called *onco-reconstructive surgery*.

There are several reasons for this. From a surgical perspective most plastic surgeons agree that the *aesthetic* result, the way the breast will look, is generally better when the surgery is done at the time of the mastectomy or lumpectomy. At one time reconstruction was only offered to women who had mastectomies; now, even if you've only had a small part of your breast removed, plastic surgery is available to restore balance and symmetry between the two breasts.

Sybil was in her late eighties when she was diagnosed with breast cancer, but she did not want the life-saving mastectomy procedure. When her surgeon asked her why not, she replied that she had been told she was too old to expect breast reconstruction. She had had a long and happy marriage and, as a deeply religious woman, she believed that when she died she would be reunited with her beloved husband. She explained to the surgeon that her husband had loved and admired her body, especially her breasts, which had been part of the very good sexual relationship they had enjoyed. She did not want to meet him again without one of her breasts.

The surgeon reassured her and said that she always worked with a plastic surgeon and they would make sure that she had a breast reconstruction at the time of her mastectomy without increasing the length of the operation. Sybil came through the treatment well and was very pleased with her 'new' breast. She lived a happy and cancer-free life for the next five years, and died peacefully in her sleep at the age of 94.

Research has shown that there is a real psychological benefit in beginning the reconstructive process at the same time as the initial surgery. For some patients it is life-affirming at a very frightening time. Some women have found that after a consultation with their plastic surgeon they choose to have the kind of breasts they've always wanted and decide to have a breast reduction or breast enhancement after their lumpectomy or mastectomy.

So here is rule number one: When you have your first consultation with your surgeon you should ensure that you are referred to a plastic surgeon for an evaluation and a thorough discussion of your options in breast reconstruction. Many surgeons work in conjunction with a plastic surgeon and are very comfortable with this type of working relationship. There are those surgeons who believe, as Julie's surgeon did, that their job is to chop out the cancer and save your life, but since it is likely that you will still be alive 10, 15 or many more years after your initial surgery, others believe that in addition to treating your cancer you should also be offered a good quality of life. It seems clear that women who have breast reconstruction generally have a better self-image than those who don't. Breast removal without reconstructive surgery often adversely affects your self-esteem, your femininity, your sensuality and your sexuality. Not all women choose to have reconstruction but all women should be equipped with enough information to make an informed decision.

You and your surgeons will decide when to do the reconstruction. Most surgeons will opt for immediate reconstruction if it is safe and feasible, because there is less scar tissue, which makes the plastic surgery easier, and the psychological benefits are enormous.

Once you've decided to have reconstruction, there is a very important factor which you must internalise and which should be discussed with your plastic surgeon to avoid any future disappointment. The most gifted surgeon in the world will never be able to perfectly replace the breast you're about to lose, even if she or he uses the best techniques available.

The upside of reconstructive surgery is that it is a safe option that allows you to look and feel better and to wear the clothes you want to wear – you may eventually find that you can wear revealing, sexy evening dresses and bathing costumes unselfconsciously, and that you feel more sensual and sexually at ease. A reconstructed breast is more convenient and comfortable than an external prosthesis, which is a specially designed unit that resembles a breast, which you put into your empty bra cup. The bare scar left if the breast is not reconstructed may serve as a psychologically disturbing daily reminder of what you have been through.

There are two main methods of reconstruction. In *implant reconstruction* implants are placed under the chest muscle. In *flap reconstruction* the plastic surgeon uses your own body skin, muscle and fat from your tummy or elsewhere to reconstruct your breast. The two flaps that are most commonly used are the *latissimus flap*, taken from your back, which is a relatively small operation, and the *TRAM flap*, which uses the lower abdomen as the donor site (for skin, fat and muscle).

The TRAM flap is the more popular option, though it requires more intensive surgery, so it is best used for healthy patients who can tolerate longer time in surgery and an extended recovery period. The use of implants may mean an easier recovery and is also a popular choice. Many surgeons think that when your own tissue is used, the reconstructed breast looks better and feels more realistic than a breast with an implant, but the complications of the flap reconstruction outlined above persuade some women, particularly very athletic and/or thin women, or those with careers on the line, to opt for the implant. Some surgeons think that if possible, women who are going to be treated with radiation should have flap reconstructions, because the materials that make up the breast prosthesis do not radiate well.

There are no simple rules and the best reconstruction option for each patient should be carefully considered. The reality is that if you feel good about yourself then whatever you've chosen is the right choice for you.

The downside of an implant is that it often requires two smaller operations after the initial surgery. A temporary implant, known as a tissue expander, will be put into your breast and will be gradually inflated in the surgeon's office until the size of the reconstructed breast matches that of the other breast. At a later date this tissue expander will be replaced, in a brief outpatient procedure, with a permanent implant.

Finally, if your nipple and areola have been removed, they can be reconstructed under local anaesthetic about three months after the reconstruction. Some women say they can't be bothered about replacing the nipple, but many find they are much happier when their breast looks complete.

Other cancers

There are other types of cancers that affect women and I will cover these briefly, just to keep you informed and to enable you to recognise some of the warning signs and to know what questions you should ask your doctor and what questions she or he should be asking you.

Paget's disease

Many women don't know that Paget's disease is also a type of breast cancer. It usually shows up as an irritation of the nipple, which looks like some kind of skin problem because the area is inflamed, red, crusty and may sometimes ooze, so dermatologists and other doctors may mistake it for some kind of common skin dermatitis and prescribe a cream to soothe it. Be alert. Paget's disease means that there is cancer in the milk ducts of the breast which has spread to the nipple.

Vaginal cancer

Many peri- and postmenopausal women suffer from itchy and dry vaginas caused by low levels of estrogen. If you have this problem and the condition is not helped by the application of topical estrogen or an estrogen ring, you need to make sure that there is nothing untoward going on by making an appointment for a thorough vaginal examination and the accompanying screens, because vaginal cancer may occur in middle age.

Cervical cancer

Your cervix is the lower part of your womb that connects to your vagina. The best way to detect cervical cancer is by having a Pap smear done once a year. In this procedure some of the cells of your cervix are scraped off painlessly and sent to a laboratory to be checked. Some cervical cells can look abnormal but are not cancerous or pre-cancerous. If there are abnormal cells, your cervix can be checked by a procedure known as a *colposcopy*, during which the cervix is examined with a high-powered magnifying lens and a light that are inserted into your vagina.

Please note that even if you no longer have a cervix because your womb and cervix were removed after a Pap smear revealed abnormalities, you *must* still have an annual Pap smear to check for something doctors call 'skip lesions'. These are unusual but it is wise to be cautious, so if you have had a hysterectomy for reasons other than an abnormal Pap smear, and are in a long-term, monogamous relationship, most experts suggest that you have a vault smear every ten years, just to make sure all is well.

Women are at risk for cervical cancers if they *smoke*, have had *many sexual partners*, or have a *partner who has had many sexual relationships*. This is because they are at greater risk of catching a sexually transmitted disease like the *human papilloma virus* (HPV), which research has shown to be strongly associated with cervical cancer and cancer of the vulva. Vulva is the term for all the external genital parts that lead into your vagina. HPV is one of the strongest factors implicated in the risk of getting cervical cancer. Many women have HPV and while doctors believe that women with cervical cancer must have been infected by this virus, it is very important to understand that *not* all HPVs cause cancers. HPVs are a group of more than 100 types of viruses called papilloma viruses because some of them can also cause warts, or papillomas, which are benign tumours.

However certain 'high-risk' types of HPV can cause cancer of the cervix. These types include HPV16 and 18. About two thirds of all cervical cancers are caused by HPV16 and 18. Currently there is no cure or treatment for the HPV infection but the infection can disappear without treatment because a woman's immune system will have successfully fought the virus. The good news is that there are now two vaccines available: *Gardasil*, which protects against HPV6, 11, 16 and 18, and *Cervarix*, which protects against HPV16 and 18.

Apart from ensuring that you have a Pap smear once a year, you should be aware of the following signs which might indicate cervical cancer: painful intercourse, bleeding after sex and pain while urinating (though these could be attributed to a dry vagina from an estrogen deficiency), lower-back pain, abnormal bleeding, or an unusual discharge from your vagina. If you are very sexually active and at a high risk for carrying HPV, some doctors will test for it when in combination with the Pap smear.

Once you have been diagnosed with cervical cancer, spend some time with your oncologist discussing your treatment options. The colposcopy that I described above will have alerted your doctor to anything abnormal; the biopsy that follows it will have taken a section of the tissues and cells so that they can be examined by a pathologist to confirm your doctor's diagnosis. If the lesions are malignant your doctor will recommend a hysterectomy, which may have to be an extended hysterectomy, in which the womb, the top of the vagina and the surrounding lymph glands are removed. Your doctor may call this a Wertheim's hysterectomy. If a woman's reproductive years are over, an oophorectomy will also be performed (see Chapter 6). The surgery may be followed by the appropriate cancer treatment – radiation or chemotherapy. Research has found that radiation therapy can be very effective.

Endometrial cancer

The endometrium is the lining of your womb (see Chapter 1). It is a well-documented fact that endometrial cancer, cancer of the lining of the womb, is usually associated with *unopposed estrogen* or *excessive levels of estrogen*, where the lining of the womb builds up because you are on an HT regimen of estrogen only and do not have the monthly bleed associated with progesterone (see Chapter 1).

Even if you are on continuous, combined HT, don't be lulled into thinking that you are not at risk. An imbalance in the estrogen and progestin you are taking can still cause the lining of your womb to become too thick. If you still have your womb, you should have an annual vaginal ultrasound examination to evaluate the lining of your womb.

It is interesting that the risk of endometrial cancer increases with the number of years you have been on estrogen-only therapy. You remain at risk for several years after you have discontinued the hormone therapy. So today it is standard practice, if you still have a womb, to take a progestogen along with estrogen. Research has shown that taking the two together, which is called *continuous combined* therapy, may be safer than taking them *sequentially*, which means taking the estrogen first for a couple of weeks followed by the progesterone. A progesterone-releasing intrauterine device inserted into your uterus is another option because this can be very effective in preventing a build-up of the lining of your womb. In Chapter 4 I wrote that if you are taking HT and you have a womb you must be monitored regularly. The same applies to women who have kept their wombs and are taking Tamoxifen – studies show that these women are at a greater risk for endometrial cancer.

Monitoring for endometrial cancer

All women who have kept their wombs, especially those on HT, should have an annual gynaecological examination. You should also have yourself checked if you are experiencing unusual bleeding, if you have problems when you urinate, if sex is very painful, or if you have pain in your pelvis. If you are not on HT you may have *vaginal atrophy*, which is the drying up of your vagina, and which may account for some of your symptoms. The pelvic examination will reveal this. Your gynaecologist should examine your pelvis to see if your uterus has become abnormally enlarged. She or he should then, as a matter of course, do a transvaginal ultrasound. This scan will show if there are any abnormal features in your uterus.

During the ultrasound examination your doctor will see if the lining of your womb is thicker than the normally accepted range and will measure it. The doctor will then decide whether further investigation is needed and will take a sample of the lining by inserting a *pipette*, which is a thin, flexible tube, into your womb and removing a small amount of the lining. This sample will be sent to the lab, where a pathologist will examine it to see if there are pre-cancerous or cancerous cells.

Some doctors may prefer to do a D&C (dilation and curettage; a surgical procedure performed under general anaesthetic, where the neck of the womb is stretched – dilation – and a surgical instrument is used to remove the lining and contents of the womb – curettage), but this is more invasive and you would need an anaesthetic.

But there are some doctors who are now qualified to do an outpatient hysteroscopy (Chapter 6) which will allow you to recover more quickly since you don't need a general anaesthetic. This is probably a more controlled and accurate way of obtaining tissue for evaluation from suspicious areas. Note that if you are taking Tamoxifen you should have the lining of your womb screened every six months. If you have bleeding, your doctor should take a sample of the lining and may do this using a hysterescopic-directed biopsy, either as an outpatient procedure or under general anaesthetic

If your cells are shown to be pre-cancerous or cancerous your doctor or specialist will discuss the different treatment options with you. If the cells are pre-cancerous but you don't show any risk factors – you are not on unopposed estrogen, you are not overweight, you don't smoke or drink to excess, or have high blood pressure or diabetes – your doctor may monitor you within three months, or may prescribe a high-dose progestogen.

If the cells are cancerous the treatment follows much the same route as treatment for cervical cancer. Surgery is per-formed after careful clinical evaluation of the stage that the cancer has reached. This will determine the extent of the operation. Samples of tissue from the organs that have been removed will be checked for cancerous cells. After surgery, depending on what you and your oncologist have decided, you will have the appropriate cancer treatment.

Ovarian cancer

These words strike dread into the hearts of most women and their doctors. The reason is that the survival rate of women with ovarian cancer is poor. It is a deadly and silent cancer, and is often only detected when it is quite far advanced. Because your ovaries contain reproductive tissue the cells are programmed to grow, but when this programming alters, abnormally fast growth of cells and tissues takes place. These little growths may be benign, which means that they stay in one place in the ovary and don't move into the surrounding areas, but in some cases the growths are cancerous and start to invade the neighbouring tissue.

Many of you may have been told by your gynaecologists during an examination that you have an *ovarian cyst* (a sac filled with fluid). You may want to look back at Delia's story in Chapter 7. The rule is that all ovarian cysts in postmenopausal women should be investigated. If they are benign, there is no problem. It is only when the cysts are malignant that doctors worry.

The most common reason for ovarian cysts is that a little egg-containing follicle in the ovary, which I described in Chapter 1, grows bigger and doesn't burst – sometimes it releases the egg, sometimes it doesn't. In the normal course this little follicular cyst will shrivel up, but sometimes it just remains. If the cysts are benign the best treatment is conservative. In other words, your doctor will keep an eye on them with regularly scheduled vaginal ultrasound examinations.

There are other little cysts in the ovary called *endometriotic cysts*, which are filled with blood and can become very painful, but they are not necessarily dangerous. When these are noticed on an ultrasound scan your doctor will make an informed decision about how to deal with them. Some specialists will do a blood test called a *CA-125* that screens for cancer. This test shows a certain substance, present in cancerous cells, that has been released into the blood. However, some doctors are wary of a result that shows raised levels of CA-125 because other conditions, such as gastrointestinal cancer, can also cause this elevation.

Ovarian cysts are not usually cause for alarm unless they are increasing rapidly or have certain abnormal features which show up on an ultrasound. If you tend to get them you may find that once your ovaries stop their reproductive function after menopause you may no longer be troubled with them. If you are perimenopausal and battle with painful ovarian cysts, many doctors prescribe an oral contraceptive, which stops you ovulating, so that your ovaries 'quieten down'.

The strongest risk factor for ovarian cancer is those women with a family history (mother, sister or daughter) of the disease. Second-tier relatives like aunts and grandmothers also constitute a risk but it is not as high. Some women who have a genetic mutation in their BRCA1 and BRCA2 genes and are susceptible to breast cancer may also be at risk for ovarian cancer. It is thought that women who have never had children may be at greater risk for ovarian cancer than those who have. Your risk for ovarian cancer increases with age. However, it is now thought that long-term users of the low-dose oral contraceptive (more than 10 years) may be protected from ovarian cancer because this pill stops ovulation. But don't forget though, that there may be an increased risk of breast cancer among long-term oral contraceptive users, so we need more research to clarify this.

Sometimes ovarian cancers may be misdiagnosed, so be aware of certain symptoms such as swelling and bloating, which may occur as the tumour grows in the ovary. A woman may feel nauseous or suffer other symptoms that are usually associated with indigestion, like gas and bloating, and a general feeling of being too full, which often results in a loss of appetite. She may also suffer from diarrhoea or constipation.

Be alert for ongoing symptoms of indigestion that aren't cured with the appropriate medicine. A gynaecologist friend remarked that he remembered an old professor at medical school telling the class of the many times he had seen 'ovarian cancers drowning in a sea of antacids'!

A biopsy should *never* be done on the ovary of a menopausal women. The most effective way for your doctor to determine if the growth is cancerous is to do a laparotomy, a procedure I wrote about in Chapter 5. The incision in this surgery should not be a bikini cut but a proper up-and-down cut. At the time of this procedure the surgeon will determine whether there is a malignancy. Once this is identified, specific surgery is performed, usually a total hysterectomy, which includes the womb, fallopian tubes and ovaries.

The apron of fat which hangs from the large bowel is also removed (*omentectomy*) and any other tumours greater than 1cm or those that can be felt during the surgery, which may mean removing some of the bowel. The surgeon will send all the removed tissue plus the fluid that was in the cavity (*washings*) for diagnosis and staging. Staging is a process to see how far the cancer has spread, especially if it is not obvious to the surgeon during the surgery. Staging is very important because it helps the surgeon and the oncologist to decide on the correct form of follow-up treatment, depending on the extent and type of cancer. If an expert does not do this type of surgery then any cancer that has spread outside the ovary may be missed and not properly treated.

Some gynaecologists who don't have the ability to perform this meticulous routine or the knowledge to diagnose this type of cancer, want to be conservative and try not do this extensive surgery, but it is very dangerous and the patient may then require repeat surgery and/or additional therapy.

I mentioned that if you are diagnosed with breast cancer you should consider your options carefully. If you have been diagnosed with ovarian cancer, my sense is that speed is of the essence; usually because by the time it is diagnosed it will be quite far advanced. Ovarian cancer patients usually have chemotherapy after surgery, but because there are different types of ovarian cancer your oncologist will decide on the most effective course of treatment and will inform you whether radiation therapy would be beneficial in your particular case.

Empowerment points

- Don't rush into surgery without considering all the options and getting a second opinion.

- Make a comprehensive list of questions before your consultation. Some people get flustered or anxious when facing their doctors. Take someone with you to make notes, or use a tape recorder. It is impossible to assimilate all the information you will be given when you are in a highly emotional state.

- Live as healthily as possible but don't ever blame yourself if you get cancer.

- Be sure to have an annual gynaecological examination. An annual mammogram is a must if you have specific, individual reasons, are older than 50, or are on HT. For peace of mind, if you are at high risk for breast cancer, arrange to have an ultrasound every six months in addition to your annual examination.

- Work in partnership with your oncologist to get the best out of your treatment. If something worries you or you don't understand some point of information, don't be afraid to ask over and over again until you are satisfied that you understand what's going on.

- Once you are diagnosed, get good counselling. Having a safe place to let off steam, scream, weep and shout will help you deal with those overwhelming feelings.

Notes

_____

_____

_____

_____

_____

_____

_____

_____

_____

_____

_____

_____

_____

_____

_____

_____

9

The Bare Bones: Menopause and Osteoporosis

Nina is a pretty, vivacious woman in her late fifties; small boned and petite, she glows with health. She started having very irregular periods when she was 40. When she told her gynaecologist, at the time, he didn't seem worried.

'He told me that it was normal and when I went back to him at 42 because my periods had stopped altogether, he told me once again that it was normal. I trusted him so I did nothing about it.'

The next time she saw him he did some hormone tests. 'He told me that I had no estrogen in my body whatsoever but that since I was so young he felt it was only the onset of menopause.'

Once again he did nothing, and she stayed with his practice for the next five years. Then she started hearing her friends discussing their menopausal symptoms. Many of them were going to the same gynaecologist, a different one from the one she consulted. 'They raved about him and, because they seemed to know so much about menopause, I felt I should be seeing the doctor from whom they had learnt everything.

'I changed doctors but I didn't really like his practice; the waiting room was overcrowded, he never spent quality time with me and when I saw him, he kept interrupting my appointment to talk to other patients on his constantly ringing phone. It was like being part of a factory assembly line. To be fair, he did tell me to have a bone density test which had never been suggested to me before. I had the scan and then thought nothing more about it.

'Five months later I ran into some friends who were talking about their bone density scans and I realised I hadn't heard anything about my results, but thought this was probably because my bones were normal. I never imagined there could be a problem because I felt so well, but I thought I'd better phone my doctor and ask.'

Nina called the doctor's receptionist, who took the file through to the doctor. 'He obviously had someone with him. I heard the receptionist give him my file. When he was talking to me he used my name all the time, which made me very uncomfortable because I knew he had a patient with him. I asked for my bone scan results. I heard him riffling through papers, then he suddenly said: "Oh my God! You've got very bad osteoporosis in both your hip and spine. You must go onto to a bisphosphonate immediately!"

'"What's osteoporosis?" I asked him – I'd never heard of the condition. He explained briefly and irritably. I was really upset and asked him why no one had come back to me with my results, which were obviously serious, in the five months that had passed since I had my test.

He said impatiently: "This is a huge practice; my nurses can't waste their time phoning everyone with their results." I thought he had a point as far as cases where the results were normal were concerned, but if results came back which showed that something was seriously wrong, I felt it was his responsibility to inform his patients. I ended up at a specialist bone clinic. Today I take Fosamax once a week and my bones aren't bad at all.'

It is clear that Nina was treated very badly. Her first doctor didn't explain to her that a woman's periods become erratic in perimenopause or test her hormone levels. Even when she told him that her periods had stopped completely he still didn't test any levels and, in addition, gave her wrong information based on his assumption that because she was young she was not yet in full menopause.

When her next doctor eventually had her hormone levels tested and saw that the estrogen levels were very low, he never explained about the different levels of estrogen. To say that she had 'no estrogen whatsoever in her body', is as you know from Chapter 1, absolute nonsense. He never suggested that she have a mammogram or a bone density scan. He didn't ask her if she was taking calcium, which is standard procedure for a middle-aged peri- or postmenopausal woman.

Although he advised her to have a bone density scan, her doctor didn't even bother to look at the test results or inform her that she had bad osteoporosis. He also took no responsibility for his negligence, which could have had serious consequences if Nina's condition had been left untreated. He violated patient/doctor confidentiality by naming her and discussing her condition in front of another person who may have known her.

The worst part of Nina's story is that so many years elapsed while she was losing bone density, so she never treated the problem with calcium, hormones or bisphosphonates (drugs that slow bone loss). I think the doctors *assumed* that because she was young, did not drink or smoke, and exercised regularly, that she was not at risk. Remember, osteoporosis is a silent disease and the *only* way to determine whether there is a problem is to do a bone density scan.

Osteoporosis is a hot topic in menopause. Some practitioners refer to it as bone fragility. It has become very controversial because until recently, the gold standard treatment for peri- and postmenopausal women with osteoporosis was estrogen replacement therapy but the WHI study challenged this thinking and ideas changed. The study showed that women who were taking HT had an overall 24 per cent reduced risk for total fractures but that the other problems – increased risk of stroke, heart disease and breast cancer – did not seem worth the gain in bone density. Furthermore, other research shows that a couple of years after a woman stops taking estrogen the improvement in bone density is lost.

Books about osteoporosis seem to follow the same trend as many books about menopause. They are very dense and there are pages and pages of scientific information about osteoclasts and osteoblasts. As I researched this chapter I realised that osteoporosis is a 'dry' subject but you do need some technical information in order to understand it properly. Once again, knowledge is power. Once you have grasped the facts you will be empowered and able to take charge of your health in this area, so persevere, even if you have to read some of what follows a couple of times.

The human skeleton is made up of bone, which develops in babyhood and carries on growing until we reach our peak bone mass in our mid-twenties. The phrase 'bone mass' refers to bone density, which is the quantity of bone in a certain area. Imagine two pieces of Emmenthal cheese exactly the same size. The one has large holes and only a little cheese, the other has small holes and a lot of cheese. The latter is denser than the former.

When bones are at peak density, they are at their optimal strength. Bones are made up of a protein called *collagen*, which provides the framework of the bone, and a mineral substance called *calcium phosphate*, which adds strength to the bone and makes the framework harder. We have two types of bones: *trabecular*, which are spongy and softer, and *cortical*, which are very hard. Trabecular bone is found at the ends of long bones and in the spine, while the cortical bone on the outside makes up the shaft of the bones. This combination of hard and soft materials makes bones more flexible and stress resistant.

Because bone is made up of these tissues, it doesn't remain static when we reach peak bone density in our twenties. Throughout our lives, the bone tissue is breaking down and then being built up again. Interestingly, the body ensures that the bone material is distributed in areas that are under

The structure of bone

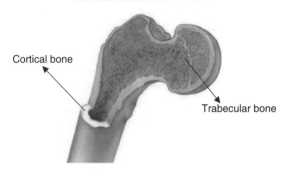

Cross section of bone

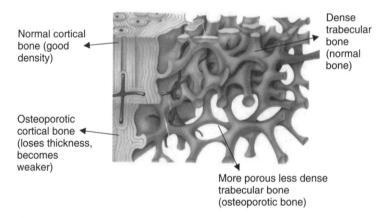

Normal cortical bone (good density)

Dense trabecular bone (normal bone)

Osteoporotic cortical bone (loses thickness, becomes weaker)

More porous less dense trabecular bone (osteoporotic bone)

Diagram showing normal bone and osteoporotic bone

Based on drawings from a poster produced by Hologic, SA Scientific

the greatest stress. As we get older, in areas where there has been a lot of wear and tear, and that need to be repaired or strengthened, the older bone material is replaced with new bone material. Obviously the old bone can't just stay there so the body breaks down the old bone tissue and ensures that it is removed by cells in the bone known as *osteoclasts*.

During this process, which is known as *resorption*, calcium and phosphorus are released into the blood. Once this has occurred the new bone material replaces the old material, using other bone cells known as *osteoblasts*. This process is called *formation*, and the two actions together are called *bone remodelling*. The greatest amount of bone turnover takes place in the trabecular bone, which as I wrote above, is mainly in the vertebrae of the spine and in the ends of the long bones like the femur, which fits into your hip joint.

The osteoclasts break down the old bone tissue, then the osteoblasts take over, building the new bone tissue before it is absorbed into this new layer of collagen and bone minerals, where it becomes an *osteocyte*. It is actually the osteocytes, embedded in the bone, that send out the messages to the body that a specific area needs, for one reason or another – stress, damage or wear and tear – to be remodelled. Osteoclasts and osteoblasts have another very important job; they regulate the supply of calcium in the body.

As I wrote in Chapter 5, calcium maintains the cell structure and is a mineral that is essential for bone formation, cardiovascular, nerve and muscle functioning. It is also very important in metabolising food, so too little calcium may mean that you put on weight. Because it is such an integral part of a healthy body's functioning, calcium needs to be maintained, not only in the bones but also in the blood. A calcium imbalance, too much (*hypercalcemia*) or too little (*hypocalcemia*), can lead to a wide variety of symptoms. Too much induces a feeling of exhaustion, weight gain, high blood pressure, dehydration, depression, an irregular heartbeat and, in extreme cases, coma. Too little results in muscle cramps, irregular heartbeat, low blood pressure and sometimes seizures.

Resorption and the process of remodelling, which continues throughout the life of the body, is controlled (once again) by the hormones, in particular *parathyroid hormone* (PTH), which regulates calcium and phosphorus in the blood, and estrogen, testosterone and *calcitonin*, which influence the activity of the osteoclasts, the cells that break down bone material.

This is probably the best point at which to write a bit about the vital role that estrogen plays in maintaining women's bone density and the reason why, in the peri- and postmenopausal years, we lose bone so quickly. While we are young, healthy, reproductive adults with normal circulating levels of estrogen, the places in our body where bone is remodelled (the remodelling sites) are controlled by estradiol.

As I wrote above, estrogen influences the activity of the osteoclasts, whose job it is to break down bone material. Because the estrogen limits their activities, we don't lose bone in the normal course of events, but as we become peri- and postmenopausal and our estrogen levels fluctuate and drop, this carefully regulated activity of bone resorption speeds up. The osteoclasts at sites all over the body begin to get overactive, breaking down more bone material and releasing more calcium and phosphate into the blood. The body can't deal with too much calcium phosphate because there isn't enough calcium and vitamin D naturally in our bodies to replace the minerals we are losing. Because we are losing more bone material than we are replacing, our bones become fragile and our risk of fracture is greatly increased. This is why doctors may recommend that women who have an early surgical menopause, causing a sudden drop in their levels of estrogen, should consider taking estrogen therapy. Research has shown that premature menopause often leads to rapid bone loss and a higher risk of osteoporosis and fractures.

Osteoporosis is a condition in which bones may fracture with very little force and sometimes no force at all. It is one of the major contributory causes of death in elderly women and a powerful reason for the diminished quality of life of women who suffer hip or vertebral fractures and/or multiple fractures as a result of this silent disease. Women who have osteoporosis die at an earlier age than those without it and suffer enormous pain and distress as a result of their crumbling bones. If you are going to live a long and healthy life you need to be extremely aware of the risks for this disease and try to prevent it if you can.

As I mentioned, if you are fortunate enough to have peak bone density, you have a much lower risk of fracture, but as we age, both bone density and bone strength decline. When bone loss occurs, it affects the bone density, which in turn affects the strength of the bones. Because we lose bone density and strength as we get older, we need to be able to predict whether we are at risk for fracture and take steps to reduce this risk.

Bone mineral density and bone strength

There are four ways of looking at bone mineral density (BMD) and bone strength. These are: bone mineral density (the amount of bone material packed into a certain volume of bone); the micro-architecture (the three-dimensional structure of the bone – the way the different types of bone are laid down to form the bone.

If you look at a section of bone under a microscope, you can get a sense of whether the structure is sound or not); the mineralisation of the bone (when bone tissue or material is broken down, releasing calcium and phosphate); and the bone-remodelling rate (the rate of resorption and formation of the bone material).

Bone density contributes to bone strength so we need to determine it by means of a bone scan called *dual energy X-ray absorptiometry* (DEXA), which measures the bone density of two different types of bones – those in the lumbar spine, which is made up of the five vertebrae in the lower back, and those in the total hip and the femoral neck of the hip, which is where most hip fractures take place. The femur is the long bone in the upper part of the leg. The bone has a head and shaft, which fit into each other at the femoral neck like a ball into a socket.

DEXA scan

This test can be known as the DXA or the DEXA scan. For this test you will be asked to lie on a bed and a special X-ray machine will take measurements of your bones. Be reassured, the radiation level of this machine is extremely low. This test produces a T-score, which shows how the measurement of your bone density differs from the normal peak bone density of a young, healthy adult. Your bone density is normal if your T-score is –1 to +1. You have *osteopenia* if your score is less than –1 (< –1) and more than –2.5 (> –2.5). If you have osteopenia you are more likely to be at risk for fractures than if your bone density was normal. If you have osteoporosis your score will read –2.5 or less than –2.5(< –2.5).

A good rule of thumb is to have a bone scan when you become perimenopausal or as near to that time as possible (your symptoms will tell you that you are perimenopausal or, if you don't have any symptoms, you can have the scan in your late forties). If your bones are healthy you should have your next scan about two years into your menopause, because by then you may have much lower levels of estrogen. After that it will be up to your specialist to advise you how often you should have a scan, which she or he will judge according to your results.

But remember, if you have a surgical or chemical menopause, stop your hormone therapy, or develop a thyroid problem you should have a bone scan within the year to check that all is well. It is important to ensure that the healthcare practitioner who reads your DEXA results has been properly trained to interpret these readings. Beware those who tell you that they can determine your bone density by performing a heel scan, which is called *peripheral site measurement* in medical terminology. This scan is usually done with smaller, much less accurate machines on your heel bone and is often administered by people who are not trained in this area, such as pharmacists. This is not a validated tool to measure fracture risk. Bone density tends to vary from one part of the body to another so this measurement is not as accurate as a measurement taken at the hip or spine, since changes in your heel may happen long after they have occurred in your spine.

Because the DEXA is only two-dimensional it can't show the actual structure of the bone, but it is theoretically possible to examine the structure of bone with an ultrasound scan to determine its quality as well as its density. This can only be done for diagnostic purposes since the ultrasound can't be reproduced. Your doctor may measure the breakdown of bone in your body by doing a blood test and a urine analysis.

This is a bone turnover test. Bone turnover reflects what is happening in bone at a moment in time – if bone turnover markers are elevated, this suggests that bone loss is occurring. These elevated bone markers are an independent way to prevent fracture risk.

A pathologist should also be able to measure the calcium, phosphate, PTH and vitamin D in your blood and the levels of creatinine and calcium in your urine. These tests are done to exclude other causes of bone loss which may require correction. These levels are markers, much like cholesterol levels in monitoring for heart disease, which tell the specialist about the activity of your bones and whether you are at increased risk for fractures.

Risk factors for osteoporosis

Although the assessment of bone mass plays an extremely important part in diagnosing osteoporosis, it is very important to understand that like most other conditions, there are multiple risk factors which can cause osteoporosis. Knowledge of all these risks plays an important role in the diagnosis and treatment of osteoporosis. In fact the World Health Organisation (WHO) together with the International Osteoporosis Foundation (IOF) is working with several other interested bodies to develop an easy-to-use fracture risk assessment tool for doctors to use with patients, since the DEXA scan may not be readily available to all people. If you are one of the lucky ones who can have a DEXA scan, the accuracy of the diagnosis made by your doctor can be improved if she or he also takes your other risk factors into consideration.

Indeed, without assessing other risk factors, up to 75 per cent of those who need treatment for osteoporosis, may be missed! I have listed these risk factors and explained why they may put you at risk. As with heart disease and cancer, family history and genetic make-up play a large part in determining whether you are at risk. Small-boned women, like Nina, and Caucasian women may be at greater risk.

It is thought that more than 50 per cent of women are at risk for osteoporosis because they have first-line relatives like a mother or sister with the disease. So if you know your mother has battled with osteoporosis you need to be more alert and live the kind of life that will lessen this risk.

Remember, as with most of the conditions I have written about in this book, lifestyle plays an important role in your level of risk for osteoporosis. Heading the list is, of course, smoking. Not only do the toxins in cigarettes block the absorption of calcium, but smokers have lower estrogen levels, which contributes to overactive osteoclasts. Smokers often have an earlier menopause than non-smokers and research has shown that they have an 80 per cent increased risk of fractures. Women who are heavy drinkers are also at risk for osteoporosis, which is logical because they often eat poorly and have low body mass, while excessive alcohol interferes with their body's absorption of calcium and vitamin D. Because estrogen plays such an important role in controlling bone metabolism, anything that interferes with your estrogen levels, like excessive drinking, will affect your fracture risk.

In fact, anything that lowers your estrogen level can put you at risk. So *surgical menopause* and/or early menopause, which was Nina's problem; not having your period (*amenorrhoea*) for a number of reasons such as chronic stress; *not ovulating*; and *high prolactin levels*, which as you recall inhibit estrogen production, are all risk factors. If you are extremely thin, you are also at risk. Anything that contributes to *low body weight*, like excessive dieting, eating disorders or fanatical exercising, will also put you at risk for this disease, since the absence of fatty tissue will affect your estrogen levels (see Chapter 1). As you age you are at greater risk for osteoporosis. You are also at risk if you *never exercise* because, as you will read, appropriate exercise is actually bone strengthening. If you go back and look at all these risk factors it is encouraging to see how many of them are under your control, which means that even if you are at risk for osteoporosis you can change your lifestyle to reduce your risk of fracture.

Certain medicines like anti-epileptic medication, long-term cortisone treatment, drugs that thin your blood, thyroid medication, aromatase inhibitors (which I discuss in Chapter

7) and chemotherapy may also put you at increased risk for fractures. It is important to know that there are several illnesses which put women at risk for osteoporosis. These include kidney and liver disease, thyroid disease, bone cancer and rheumatoid arthritis. In fact, anything that because of inflammation and infection causes a high level of C-reactive protein or homocysteine in the blood can put you at risk for osteoporosis. In medical language, these two markers of the immune system, which you read about in Chapters 4 and 5, are called *cytokines* and affect the process of bone material breakdown. Your doctor should be aware of all these risks when she or he takes your medical history.

Reducing your risk for osteoporosis

There are some easily achievable ways of lowering your risk for osteoporosis. You have already realised the importance of living and eating sensibly, but there are other things you can do to look after yourself. Firstly, if you smoke – stop. If your alcohol intake is excessive, stop drinking or if you are disciplined, reduce it. As I have written, too much alcohol can increase your hot flushes and put you at risk for cancer. Complete abstinence may not be necessary but, as you will read in Chapter 10, it's just sensible for peri- and postmenopausal women to be temperate if they drink.

Exercise is essential if you want to lower your fracture risk and here the kind of exercise you choose is very important. Your bones are living organisms composed of cells and tissue. The cells in the bone 'talk' to each other about how much stress is being put on the bone, so that they can respond to this stress by building new bone. If the appropriate amount of stress is exerted, new bone will be built, so any exercise that puts stress on the bone is beneficial to bone strength. However, there is a downside. If too much stress is put on the bone and the body responds by breaking down and trying to build the new bone, the bone builders may not be able to cope, so you will find yourself with a stress fracture, which occurs as a result of too much exercise or too much pressure on a certain area, like the pounding action on the ankle bone when marathon runners run too long and too hard.

It is interesting to note that astronauts who spend significant time in space lose bone density because of the weightlessness of space. Because of the zero gravity, there is no stress on the bones to encourage the formation of new bone, but the body continues its work of breaking down the bone materials. Astronauts who have been tested have lost some bone in their spines and quite a bit more in their hip areas.

Before you embark on an exercise programme, especially if you haven't exercised before, you should check with your doctor that it's okay to go ahead. Be moderate. Take it gradually and work up to your desired regimen. Probably the most effective type of exercise for peri- and postmenopausal women is walking. A large body of research has shown that it is beneficial for not only the weight-bearing bones but for the skeleton as well. Women who walk regularly for a minimum of 30 minutes at least four times a week will have better and stronger bones than those who don't.

I have always recommended that peri- and postmenopausal women walk weighted. Walking is an excellent way of increasing the metabolism, but you may also need to increase the stress on your bones as you walk. I think that unless you have excellent posture, carrying small hand weights when you walk may make you either lopsided or round-shouldered and, in any case, it is better to let your arms swing freely. A better option is a waistcoat like a sleeveless fishing jacket with pockets to which you can gradually add small diving weights. A diving belt to which you can add weights is also a good idea. Start with very low weights, about 2 kg, and gradually, by adding another kilogram each week, work up to 15 per cent of your body weight. If you weigh 60 kg, you should eventually be carrying an extra 9 kg.

I believe that exercise should be varied, like your diet, because apart from the boredom factor, I think that it is important that you exercise all parts of your body for optimum results. Resistance or weight training twice a week is another kind of exercise that ensures that all the muscles in your body are strengthened, which in turn, is beneficial for your bones because apart from anything else, you may fall less often as your muscles become stronger. Join a reputable gym with good trainers or find yourself a well-recommended personal trainer and check his or her qualifications carefully. Get an expert to design your weight training programme and be suspicious if there are too many repetitions, more than 10 to 15 is too many. The initial weights should be set low so that you don't strain yourself. Don't be overambitious. You can add more weight gradually but never so much that you hurt yourself or have to lift the weights in an inappropriate manner. There are right and wrong ways to lift weights and your trainer or instructor should be able to show you the correct way. Go slowly, it takes time to build your muscle and nothing worth doing well comes quickly or easily. Don't forget to cool down once you have finished.

Another important type of exercise is something that increases your flexibility and balance. Fracture risks are increased when women become older and fall more often because they lose their balance. Either Pilates or yoga would be an excellent addition to your exercise regimen, and both of them, if correctly taught, are ideal for middle-aged women. I do Pilates and find that it has helped my posture and balance by 'centring' my body. This type of exercise uses a technique called core stabilisation, where the muscles that support your spine and upper body are strengthened with the use of special machines and carefully designed exercises. It is a gentle but thorough form of exercise and helps improve your posture, co-ordination, balance and flexibility. Yoga also increases your suppleness and flexibility through a series of floor exercises that don't jar your joints. Both types of exercise stress the importance of breathing correctly, balancing, focusing your mind and using carefully controlled movements.

Many peri- and post-menopausal women complain about joint pain and resort to glucosamine and chondroitin supplements to help relieve the problem. Glucosamine and chondroitin are natural substances found in and around the cells of cartilage. Together they help protect the cartilage. It seems that glucosamine may play an anti-inflammatory role, while chondroitin is thought to keep the cartilage strong and resilient (see Chapter 5).The results of a recent long-term study, Glucosamine/chondroitin Arthritis Intervention Trial (GAIT), under the aegis of the National Institute of Health

(NIH), showed that these supplements did not provide relief from osteoarthritis pain to all the participants in the trial, but a much smaller subgroup study (see page 42) showed that those who had moderate to severe pain experienced significant relief, which means that further research is needed to confirm these findings

Supplements and osteoporosis

In a perfect world healthy eating is the best way to obtain calcium because of all the essential vitamins and minerals that are found in high-calcium foods. Research has shown that dairy products are the best sources of calcium. Four cups of dairy products, such as milk, yoghurt and cottage cheese would give you about 1 000 mg of elemental calcium and the good news is that it makes no difference whether they are whole, low-fat or fat-free dairy products. More calcium is required in old age – 1 500 mg/day.

However, you will recall that in Chapter 5 I wrote that most peri- and postmenopausal women don't get enough calcium in their diets and must supplement this. So if you're not eating enough calcium-rich foods – milk and milk products, especially cheese; sardines with bones; dark leafy greens like kale and broccoli; sesame seeds; oranges and soybean products – you should take between 1 200 and 1 500 mg of *elemental* calcium daily and no more! Calcium carbonate seems to contain the most elemental calcium and is better absorbed with food, but you can take calcium citrate if you prefer it, either with meals or on an empty stomach. Just see that it contains enough elemental calcium – the actual basic calcium that is available in the tablets.

There are all sorts of calcium products in the marketplace but research indicates that calcium carbonate and calcium citrate are the most effective types. Studies show that you should not take more than 500 mg at a time because it won't be properly absorbed. Read the label on the brand you are taking and work out how to split the dose. If the calcium is a good brand it will tell you whether to take it with or without food. This is important, but I know how stressed women can get, so it is probably okay to take it when it suits you, rather than not take it at all. Try to have at least one dose with food if that is recommended.

Make *absolutely* sure that any calcium you take is combined with an adequate amount of vitamin D, which is essential for calcium absorption because it helps your body to use this vital mineral most effectively. There has been some very important research recently which has shown that in healthy women, levels of vitamin D (25 OH vitamin D) should be between 36 and 40 ng/mL. Many postmeno-pausal women's levels of vitamin D are too low and some-times your healthcare practitioner will decide to do a test to determine whether your levels of this essential nutrient have dropped below 30 ng/mL. The recommended dose of vitamin D is now 800 IU daily. You need hours of sun exposure to make enough vitamin D, and overexposure to the sun is ageing and dangerous. It is much simpler to make sure that whatever supplements you are taking contain enough of this vitamin.

In Chapter 5 I mentioned that soy isoflavones might have a protective effect on bone. A growing body of research agrees with this and there is ongoing research to determine whether isoflavones help maintain or build bone density. Some good trials have shown that soy isoflavones are effective in main-taining the bone mineral content in women who are in late menopause, but other research shows that they do not pro-tect women in early menopause against bone loss. It's your call. Talk it over with your doctor. If you have decided to take soy for menopausal symptoms, as well as a preventive treatment for osteoporosis, you must be monitored either by having a DEXA scan with an appropriate follow-up time, or a urine analysis which will allow your healthcare provider to see whether you are losing calcium and creatinine.

Treatments for osteoporosis

The next section is quite technical, but I truly believe that all women should understand how the medication they are taking works, and what their choices are. There are very effective and powerful agents available to prevent the breakdown of bone material. These can be *anti-resorptive*, which stops bone resorption activity; *anabolic*, which means a medication that stimulates the formation of bone; or *dual-acting*, which does a bit of both.

The first category includes bisphosphonates, SERMS (see Chapter 4), estrogen and calcitonin. Before I write about these different treatments, it is important to understand something about bone biology that recently came to light. Research found that there was a connection between the osteoblasts and the osteoclasts; whatever you do to the one happens to the other. This connection is known as 'coupling'. This is relevant because of the way medication prescribed for osteoporosis works and will make sense later in this chapter when I describe newly available medications.

I have already discussed estrogen and it is clear that even a very small amount (0.014 mg) of additional estrogen possibly protects the bones. Bone loss will accelerate when you stop HT, so have yourself assessed and if necessary, ask your doctor to prescribe an alternate medication for bone protection. The risks of HT may outweigh its benefits, so if you don't have menopause symptoms, don't take HT to prevent osteoporosis.

This is probably a good place to mention tibolone. As you saw in Chapter 4, this product has a combination of weak estrogenic, androgenic and progestogenic effects on your body and is often recommended for women with osteoporosis because it has been shown to increase bone mineral density. There are worries about tibolone and its associated risks with heart disease, so there will need to be more research before doctors can say with certainty that the benefits outweigh the risks. Because studies have highlighted the risk associated with long-term HT, it seems more sensible to look at other medication if you need treatment for osteoporosis.

Bisphosphonates

The bisphosphonate category contains two well-known medicines, *alendronate* and *risedronate*. You might recognise them by their trade names, Fosamax and Actonel. Bisphosphonates suppress the activity of the osteoclasts so that the breaking down of bone is limited. These medications can be taken daily or weekly, depending on your particular case. Most women who are on them don't seem to suffer from bad side effects, though some complain of stomach upsets, others of aching joints, or both.

At the time of writing there is a new bisphosphonate under trial called *zoledronate*. This is given *intravenously* (an injection into the vein), in fact it is called an intravenous infusion, and after three years of the ongoing Horizon-PFT trial, the data on the efficacy and safety of zoledronate is very promising. If these results continue, zoledronate will be considered as a first-line treatment for osteoporosis. One of the upsides of this treatment is that it will only be given at 12-month intervals, which would eliminate much of the discomfort associated with daily or weekly doses of bisphosphonate. As far as dosage of bisphosphonates is concerned, the length of time for which you will need to take the medication will depend on your own individual case.

Anabolic agents

Teriparatide (Forteo), which is based on parathyroid hormone (PTH), which regulates the amounts of calcium and phosphate in your blood, is an anabolic agent. It is given as a daily injection *subcutaneously* (under the skin). Studies have shown a real increase in the bone mass of the women using it. Side effects of this product are rare, but include nausea, muscle cramps and headaches.

I have already written about SERMs in the chapters on hormones and cancers. SERMs are hormones that have a beneficial estrogen effect on certain areas of your body, blocking unwanted estrogen effects in other parts of your body so that the amount of active estrogen is not increased. The best-known SERMs are Tamoxifen and the second-generation SERM Raloxifene. These SERMs have an estrogenic effect on your bones, controlling the activity of the osteoclasts, which are the cells responsible for breaking down bone material.

In general, Tamoxifen would be used primarily to prevent osteoporosis but some doctors use Raloxifene (Evista) because it increases bone mineral density in the spine in women with osteoporosis, and although there are side effects such as muscle cramps, increased risk of blood clots and sometimes hot flushes, some women who aren't happy taking bisphosphonates do very well on it. Raloxifene also lowers the levels of bad cholesterol (LDL). Currently Raloxifene is a second-line treatment, after bisphosphonates, which are still the gold standard, but further research is needed to understand all its risks and benefits.

Two new third-generation SERMs, *lasofoxifene* and *basedoxifene*, are now in phase-three trials. (A short digression here to explain what these different trials mean: All medicines passed by a regulatory body, as I discussed in Chapter 3, have to have undergone extensive testing to make sure that the benefits of the drug outweigh the risks, so a drug looks very promising if it reaches Phase 3 trials. These trials are both expanded controlled and uncontrolled trials, and are conducted after Phase 2 trials have obtained evidence. This suggests that a drug will be effective at an optimally selected dose. Phase 3 trials gather additional information about the safety of the drug to evaluate the overall benefits and risks, and provide adequate information for physician labelling. Phase 3 trials usually include between several hundred and several thousand volunteers.) These third-generation SERMs could help to treat women with breast cancer who enter early menopause due to chemotherapy and are, as I explained earlier, at high risk for premature bone loss. Lasofoxifene appears to decreases bone loss, has favourable effects on blood cholesterol levels and may also prevent the growth of certain breast cancer cells. Basedoxifene acetate is promising as a treatment for osteoporosis, and may have fewer adverse effects on the lining of the womb and less vasomotor effects than those SERMs that are currently used in clinical practice. The jury is still out and more controlled clinical trial data is needed to confirm these results.

Calcitonin, which I discussed earlier in this chapter, is a hormone produced by the thyroid. As a medicine, its job is to control the activities of the osteoclasts and prevent overactivity. Its trade name is Miacalcic or Miacalcin and it is given as a nasal spray, which means that among its side effects, which are fairly mild, there may be some nasal irritation. Studies have shown that it is effective in reducing fractures of the spine but not hip fractures, so that although it does reduce bone resorption it is not a first-line treatment like the bisphosphonates.

New treatments for osteoporosis

In the first edition of this book, some of the medications that I wrote about were still undergoing trials to ensure their efficacy and safety. Today, several have been approved as effective treatments for postmenopausal osteoporosis. One of those is *strontium ranelate* (Protos). It works in a very different way from the two medications I mentioned earlier. Anti-resorptive agents (bisphosphonates) reduce fracture risk by slowing down the breakdown of bone by the osteoclasts (resorption), *but* because of 'coupling', which I mentioned earlier, they also slow down the formation of the bone by the osteoblasts.

On the other hand, anabolic agents like Teriparatide increase the formation of bone but also increase the breakdown of the bone. Strontium ranelate was found to have a different effect. It works by 'uncoupling' this process of bone remodelling so that in a dual action, it simultaneously helps to decrease the breakdown of bone while increasing the process of bone formation. Instead of just strengthening one part of the bone (see diagram of the structure of bone) because of its ability to 'uncouple', it improves the structure of trabecular bone and stimulates the formation of cortical bone.

Finally there is also some interesting work under way which looks at the effects on bone of growth hormone (GH) and insulin-like growth factor hormone. GH works in conjunction with the parathyroid hormone, which plays such an important role in bone formation. But I must beg you not to mess around with the GH that is offered to you by complementary healthcare practitioners. The interactions of these hormones in our bodies are extremely complicated and they may result in bad side effects when used in ignorance.

Empowerment points

- Living well is a good way to help protect yourself against osteoporosis: eat sensibly and exercise at least five times a week.

- Osteoporosis is a silent disease and only proper screening will show whether you are at risk for it.

- Know your risk factors for osteoporosis. If you do, you can eliminate any that are within your control and protect yourself against those that aren't, like a family history, a particular medication or illness.

- Take adequate calcium and vitamin D.

Notes

_____

_____

_____

_____

_____

_____

_____

_____

_____

_____

_____

_____

_____

10

Food Is My Drug of Choice: Weight and Diet in Menopause

The workshop had been over for a while but I noticed that Tessa and Stephanie were still deep in conversation. They were discussing diets: the most popular subject among many middle-aged women.

Tessa must have been very pretty when she was younger; her eyes sparkle and her hair shines, but she is very overweight; as she heaved herself up she was breathing heavily and though the room was not particularly warm, there was a fine sheen of moisture on her skin. Stephanie was reasonably slim, though some unwanted kilos had obviously settled themselves on her hips. Although she and Tessa were the same age, she moved lightly and easily and seemed full of energy.

'I don't know why you're complaining, you look great!' Tessa exclaimed. Stephanie shook her head. 'I don't mean to sound like I'm looking for compliments but since I've started menopause, I don't know what's wrong with me. I've never had a problem with weight but suddenly I've picked up four kilos. I have always exercised and I haven't started eating more or anything but it's really hard to lose. It doesn't matter what I do, it keeps coming back. I'm fed up!'

'You don't know how lucky you are. I think I've been dieting all my life,' said Tessa. 'There isn't a diet I haven't tried. I've always thought there must be something wrong with me. Yesterday I saw a new nutritionist and she said I may have something called met ... meta ...?'

'Metabolic Syndrome?' I interrupted.

'That's right,' Tessa responded. 'She says that is why I'm not losing weight, but she's told me there's a medicine that will fix it and help me to lose weight as well. I can't wait.'

'That's funny,' said Stephanie, 'my GP was also telling me about it but he said that he thought I was insulin resistant. He took some blood and said he would see if my insulin levels were up and would then give me this great medication. I think it's called Glucophage.'

I thought, as I listened to them, that one of the most difficult aspects of menopause is weight gain. Because it is such a loaded topic there is a lot of confusion around it. Tessa's nutritionist was quite wrong when she said that Tessa couldn't lose weight if she had metabolic syndrome – a change in lifestyle, diet and exercise is far better than taking a drug.

How often, while watching the Oscars, have we stared in horror as a star of decades past who we once idolised lumbers on stage to receive an award, beautifully coiffed and made up, but fat. What has happened to the object of all that teenage envy? I used to be shocked when I saw them, but I know better now. It is a fact of life that when you become peri- or postmenopausal you will put on some weight. The most important thing is to find out how to remain reasonably slim, while at the same time living happily and well.

My aim in this chapter is not to bombard you with scientific information that will confuse you, or to give you advice that you find unpalatable and hard to follow. In any case, every woman is different and has her own way of handling things, so the cookie-cutter approach won't work here any more than it does with any of the other problems of menopause. I won't give you any diets to follow; what I will do is explain basic biochemistry relating to weight and hormones, information that you have probably been given during your peri- and postmenopausal years and that may have confused you.

I will also share some suggestions that may work for you. As you read this chapter, many of the isolated facts that you have learnt in the preceding chapters come together. You've read that being fat puts you at risk for various illnesses and increases menopausal symptoms; that exercise is beneficial in protecting your body and helping you to lose weight; and that eating correctly optimises your health, so you will understand why being an appropriate weight for your age in peri- and postmenopause is essential if you are going to live to a happy and healthy old age.

There are several things to notice about Tessa and Stephanie's conversation. Stephanie complains that since she has become menopausal she has put on weight, which she is battling to lose. Like most women, unless you are unusual, you will put on a couple of kilos during and after menopause. There may be several reasons for this. As your hormone levels begin to change in menopause they affect the way your body fat is distributed so that it moves away from your legs and arms and seems to settle around your stomach and thighs. This would account for the phrase 'middle-aged spread', which strikes fear into so many hearts. In addition to causing discomfort – that awful tight waistband and the resulting red ring – increased waist circumference, as you will read below, has some serious health implications for middle-aged women.

The theory is that the body knows that its levels of estrogen are dropping and, as I explained in Chapter 2, estrogen is produced both in your ovaries, which are now slowing down, and in your fatty tissues. In an effort to conserve estrogen, your body may want to retain or even encourage more fat storage, so it seems that the metabolism slows and the fat is redistributed to the areas where it produces the most estrogen – waist, bottom, hips and thighs!

Quite apart from that, when you age your metabolism slows as certain hormone levels drop, your thyroid is not as efficient and you become less active. The sad fact is that you can't continue to live as you did when you were 20. Once your doctor has ruled out any hormonal imbalances or illnesses, you are going to have to change your lifestyle if you don't want to get too fat. A very large study done over a period of four-and-a-half years showed that women who made an effort to change their lifestyles did not gain weight, in fact, some actually lost it. A control group of women who had not been on a low-fat, calorie-reduced diet with increased physical activity gained an average of 2.5 kg. These results clearly show that you don't have to get fat after menopause. You can stay reasonably slim or maintain your weight.

The first point is that there is no quick or magical way to keep your weight down when you are peri- or postmenopausal. Stephanie hadn't actually started eating more, but her metabolism had begun to slow down and her body had redistributed fat, adding it to her hips, stomach and thighs. This redistribution of her fat mass began to compromise her muscle mass. Since she was already exercising, Stephanie needed to look at the amount she was eating and to cut down on quantity because her slower metabolism couldn't deal with the amount of calories she was consuming. It is thought that in order to lose weight peri- and postmenopausal women should cut out 3 000 to 4 000 kilojoules a day (for those of you who are old-fashioned and prefer to think in calories, that's about 700 to 950; 1 calorie = 4.2 kilojoules).

Stephanie also needed to reassess the type of food she was eating. If you have always been slim in spite of the fact that your favourite snack is four slices of chocolate cake washed down with a fizzy drink and you never exercise seriously, it's hard to face the reality of ageing and the changes it brings. As you will read below, certain changes will take place in your body when you start to gain weight that make it even harder to lose it. The fact that Stephanie had always exercised was in her favour and if she is careful, it seems unlikely that apart from those few kilos about which she is sensitive, she will put on more weight.

When I married I weighed 52 kg. I can't believe I ever fitted into my wedding dress and I have kept just one glamorous outfit as a bittersweet memory. Menopause, too little exercise and too much of the 'wrong' foods have taken their toll. Often clients bring photos of themselves when they come to talk about menopause and I sympathise, but the reality is we are no longer 18 and our bodies are changing inexorably as we get older. So instead of mourning the changes, we need to learn to deal with them.

There are certain health implications of gaining too much weight in middle age – breast cancer, heart disease, diabetes and high blood pressure – but apart from those, I think it's important to feel good about yourself, to be able to exercise without puffing and panting, to feel not only light-hearted but light-footed and to be happy in the knowledge that you really are looking after yourself, so that your menopausal years are happy and healthy.

Before I discuss various diet options and the kind of exercise programme that may suit you, I would like to get the serious stuff about weight gain out of the way. In the past 10 years or so, a new catchphrase has come into play: insulin resistance. The moment Stephanie mentioned to her doctor that she couldn't lose the weight she had gained he immediately suggested that she was insulin resistant. I meet many menopausal women who blame their weight gain on their insulin resistance, but the fact is, it is not the insulin resistance that made you fat in the first place, it is the weight you gained that caused you to become insulin resistant. Here's why: As I wrote in Chapter 2, insulin is a hormone secreted by the pancreas. Insulin plays an extremely important role in maintaining the steady levels of glucose in your body's cells by regulating the process whereby the sugars and to a lesser extent, the fats and proteins you eat, are properly broken down and used to make new tissue.

This may be a good place to explain how your body digests food and breaks it down into various components. The major component is glucose, the sugar that is vital for energy production in the cells. Insulin ensures that the broken-down foods are used as *efficiently* as possible and that the food energy that is not needed is properly stored and released when it is needed. It also controls the way fat is stored in the body. However, all sorts of problems can be triggered by raised insulin levels and many women who gain weight in midlife may start to experience these.

When you are overweight, eat the wrong foods and/or don't exercise, your insulin doesn't work as well as it should. This is insulin resistance. It means that although there is enough insulin available in your system, the cells it regulates do not respond to it. If the relevant cells don't respond to insulin they cannot metabolise the glucose. So, because glucose isn't being used and stored properly, after a while, and this can take years, it begins to build up in the blood, which can eventually cause diabetes.

Remember that your body is a very complex and delicate machine. In Chapter 1 I described how the pituitary pumps higher and higher levels of follicle stimulating hormone (FSH) when the ovaries don't respond to normal amounts of FSH. The same principle applies with insulin. When the cells in your body; in your muscles, tissues and liver, don't respond to insulin, the pancreas goes into overdrive and pumps out more insulin, which is still not properly used because of the insulin resistance, which after a number of years, may further raise your glucose levels. This is why you will be asked to have a fasting blood glucose test, and some-times a glucose tolerance test to check your levels, if your doctor suspects you have either insulin resistance or type 2 diabetes. As with cholesterol tests, you fast before the test so that the results are as accurate as possible.

Once you understand how your body becomes insulin resis-tant, it is not terribly difficult to correct the problem, as long as you remember that insulin resistance does not initially cause weight gain, it is a direct result of being overweight. So, don't let your doctor tell you that you are fat because you are insulin resistant – you are insulin resistant because you are fat! The reason for the confusion is that if you are fat because you are insulin resistant it can be much harder to lose weight.

Simply, if you have become insulin resistant because you have gained too much weight, you need to get back into shape and lose the weight that is causing the problem. Basically, one of insulin's jobs is to promote the proper use and storage of fat and to ensure that it is effectively used (burnt) by the muscles to release energy. In a very complex process, when you become fat, the excess fat interferes with the way the muscles metabolise fat. If you are insulin resistant you need to do something about it. There is no reason for you to take medication at this point but you must bring your weight down and start to exercise. The *best* and most effective medicine for insulin resistance is the correct amount of exercise and weight loss. Research has shown that exercise increases your body's response to insulin; it improves insulin sensitivity

If you ignore the diagnosis of insulin resistance and continue with your old lifestyle, eating too much, drinking heavily, not exercising, the symptom of insulin resistance could lead to *type 2 diabetes*. This is different from ordinary diabetes, where your pancreas doesn't make enough insulin to metabolise the glucose in your body. In type 2 diabetes, your pancreas keeps making higher and higher amounts of insulin but when it 'sees' that this doesn't help, it becomes exhausted and stops producing the appropriate insulin.

If type 2 diabetes is not treated, you could be at risk for all sorts of serious illnesses including heart disease, damage to your eyes and kidney disease. Another danger of insulin resistance is *metabolic syndrome* (now more commonly known as *insulin resistance syndrome*). Metabolic comes from the word metabolism, which is the way your body breaks down or synthesises food to keep it functioning. Syndrome is the medical term for a disease that can be diagnosed because you have a number of symptoms that characterise it. The symptoms of this syndrome are diabetes or insulin resistance and the resulting glucose intolerance (which simply means that your body is metabolising glucose incorrectly), plus two or more of the following symptoms: increased waist circumference (greater than 80 cm), high blood pressure, obesity, high levels of triglycerides and low levels of good cholesterol (HDL), and raised levels of our old friend C-reactive protein (see Chapters 4, 7 and 8). There are women, however, who may be neither obese nor have an increased waist circumference but who still suffer from insulin resistance syndrome. The biggest issue in relation to this syndrome is that if you have it, you are at serious risk for cardiovascular disease.

This may all sound very frightening but the good news is that insulin resistance can be reversed and type 2 diabetes can be well managed. Some excellent research has shown that you can improve with medication like glucophage, which increases insulin sensitivity throughout your body, OR you can get with the programme by losing weight and exercising properly. There is some excellent research out there that shows that by seriously modifying their lifestyles women with metabolic syndrome actually reduce their chances of getting diabetes, and here's the really interesting part, the group that was on medication did less well than the group that dieted and exercised. Tessa told Stephanie that she had been diagnosed with metabolic syndrome and it is clear that the 'medicine' her doctor was prescribing would help her, but she also needed to put in the effort to lose weight and to exercise.

Having said all that, I think it's time to get back to reality, which is that most of us will put on a couple of kilograms at menopause but if we look after ourselves our weight will remain more or less stable. This is nothing to worry about. When medical literature talks about women with increased waist circumference, they are talking about women whose waists measure more than 90 cm and whose body mass index (BMI) is higher than 30.

BMI shows a healthcare professional whether you are underweight, just right, overweight or obese. The way to work it out is like this: Calculate your mass (frequently referred to as 'weight') in kilograms and divide it by your height in metres squared. The equation looks like this:

$$\frac{\text{mass in kilograms}}{(\text{height in metres})^2}$$

For example, if you weigh 60 kg and your height is 1.65 m, the calculation would be 60 divided by 2.72 (which is 1.65 squared), giving an answer of 22, which means your body weight is normal. Here is a table to guide you:

Body Mass Index	What the numbers mean
Below 18.5	Underweight
18.5 – 24.9	Normal
25.0 – 29.9	Overweight
30 and above	Obese

Diets

If you are like most women, you will have tried an amazing number of diets in your lifetime. Who can forget the Grape-fruit Diet, the Drinking Man's Diet or the Scarsdale Diet; which of us hasn't been to Weigh-Less or WeightWatchers or SureSlim? Today, flavours of the month include the X Diet, the Cabbage Soup Diet, the Zone, the Atkins Diet and the South Beach Diet. As with everything in our world, there is a plethora of choice. Basically diets fall into two broad categories: low carbohydrate, high protein or low fat, high carbohydrate. I will describe the basics of both and you can make your choice based on the information, selecting the one that will best encourage a long-term healthy lifestyle.

Carbohydrates are compounds made up of sugars, starches, cellulose and gums. They are an extremely important source of energy and play a vital role in fat production in our diets. *Simple carbohydrates* are things like cane sugar, beet sugar and fructose. Lactose, which comes from milk, is also a simple carbohydrate. Your body absorbs simple carbohydrates (apart from fructose) very quickly, which is why if you eat a sweet or drink a sugary drink when you feel in need of a boost you suddenly feel better. The big problem is that you will quickly need another sugar 'fix' because this energy high doesn't last very long. *Complex carbohydrates* – bread, potatoes, pasta and rice, as well as wholegrains – are com-posed mainly of starches. Other complex carbohydrates, for instance vegetables and fruits, are composed of starch and dietary fibre. The good news about complex carbohydrates is that they take longer to absorb and the glucose reaction to them is not as rapid and doesn't end as fast, so you feel more satisfied and don't feel hungry quite as quickly again.

Very low carbohydrate, high protein

This category is best represented by the Atkins Diet. It comprises a very low carbohydrate load, where only 25 per cent of the diet is carbohydrates and 75 per cent is protein and fats.

The diet works on the theory that when you don't eat a lot of carbohydrates your insulin levels will be reduced, which will encourage your body first to burn its stored carbohydrates and then, when they are depleted, to use the energy stored in fat cells and to burn fat for energy. The process where your body burns fat without carbohydrates is called *ketosis*. Your body may also lose essential stores of water when you diet this way. The problem is that you may be eating more protein and fat than is good for you and not enough grains and fruits, which are complex carbohydrates that are highly recommended for protection against various cancers and that contain essential antioxidants which may guard against raised levels of C-reactive protein and homocysteine.

People who are on an extreme form of this type of diet have bad breath and often feel queasy or giddy and have very bad headaches. Although weight loss is quick and effective, if you decide to take this route you need to have your cholesterol levels monitored because you are probably eating more saturated fats than are good for you. As with most extreme diets there is hot debate about the efficacy and safety of the Atkins Diet. What has emerged is that although the diet is effective, at the end of a year people on more traditional, moderately low carbohydrate diets, had lost more weight or stuck to their diet better, which is probably no surprise to most of us who find ourselves becoming bored and fed-up after a lengthy period on any one diet.

Another problem is that very high protein levels can be associated with the loss of essential minerals and calcium from your bones, putting you at greater risk for osteoporosis. Also, some carbohydrates like vegetables, fruits, wholegrains and legumes, are really good for your health and contain important vitamins, minerals and fibre. Extra protein just won't fill the gap left by excluding them. So, though the Atkins Diet does recommend a variety of leafy, green vegetables, some experts think that the selection isn't varied enough to compensate for the variety of complex carbohydrates missing from the diet.

High carbohydrate, low fat

The Pritikin Diet, an example of this type of diet, assumes that 63 per cent of your food intake will be carbohydrates, 20 per cent fats and 17 per cent proteins. The theory is that by increasing your intake of carbohydrates your body will speed up the mechanism whereby it metabolises carbohydrates so the excess carbohydrates will not be stored as fat. Proponents of the high carbohydrate diet believe that your body will know that you have had enough carbohydrates and won't demand as many.

The other advantage of a high carbohydrate, low fat diet is that you limit your fat intake, but there are downsides. The first is that our bodies need appropriate amounts of fat to function properly – hormones, cell functions, brains, central nervous systems, skin and tissues all benefit from the correct amounts and types of fat. The other problem with high carbohydrate diets is that people may think any carbohydrate, like white bread, marshmallows and cakes, will be fine, instead of better carbohydrates like fruits, vegetables and wholegrains.

Also, if you are consuming huge amounts of carbohydrates your body is programmed to react by pumping out higher quantities of insulin and glucose, and I have already discussed how these high levels can lead to heart disease. Finally, spiking glucose plays havoc with your appetite and leaves you feeling hungry instead of comfortably satisfied after a meal.

Here's a little tip: if you are offered a 'low-fat' drink look at the ingredients carefully. Something is making it taste better and something is needed to take up the space left by the fat that has been removed; it may be sugar, which will add to your calorie intake.

The moderate carbohydrate diet

This is probably the most sensible diet for perimenopausal and menopausal women. It includes a moderate amount of carbohydrates, about 45 per cent, about 35 per cent proteins and 20 per cent of mainly healthy fats like olive oil and avocado. After years of yo-yo dieting it seems to me that the main 'trick' to losing weight and maintaining the weight loss is a lifestyle change, which is ultimately more effective than a diet that helps you lose weight quickly but is not sustainable. I have also found that if I lose weight too quickly, I regain it quickly.

Many middle-aged women diet for special occasions, because they need the motivation to look good, but if they do succeed, 10 to one the weight will be back within months of the wedding, or the 21st, that special birthday celebration or exotic trip. My advice, from bitter experience, is to change the way you eat on a daily basis. If you eat a varied diet that has the right amount of healthy carbohydrates, fats and protein there is always room for some of the luxury foods, like a glass of wine, or a chocolate, or a luscious dessert.

All the research that I have done has given a clear message: portion control and reduced calories. So wave goodbye to a diet that says eat only four pieces of chocolate cake a day. You will lose weight because you will have restricted your food intake, but ultimately it won't be sustainable because you will die of boredom and because the calories in a piece of chocolate cake are actually quite high because of the fat content.

Fats

Your body needs fat to function optimally. There are 'good' and 'bad' fats, and there are different fats. The three main kinds of fats are saturated fats, which include animal fats, dairy fats, and coconut and palm oil. The fats in avocado, olive oil, canola oil and peanut oil are known as monounsaturated fats and the vegetable oils like corn and sunflower oil as well as fish oils, flaxseed oils, sesame and walnut oil, are called polyunsaturated fats. In small quantities polyunsaturated fats are fine for us, it's only when the vegetable oils have been heated at a very high heat followed by bubbling hydrogen through it (which is the way margarine is made) that they become the very unhealthy hydrogenated fat or trans fats. Beware of these. They have a very bad effect on your bad cholesterol (LDL).

Animal fats have small amounts of trans fats, which is why dieticians recommend low-fat milk and lean red meat. A bit of butter now and then doesn't hurt anyone, just watch the quantities and don't slather it onto your toast (a pity, because there are few things as delicious as hot buttered toast, though if you're into lifestyle change the toast had better be made from rye bread!). Essential fatty acids like the omega-3 and omega-6 fatty acids are all quite healthy and, in some cases, flaxseed and fish oil for instance, are beneficial in small to moderate quantities and it's fine to add olive oil to your diet. However, rather than just adding these supplements, eat enough fatty fish, which is particularly good for you. You should eat this at least three to four times a week because it is very rich in omega-3 fatty acids and has been shown to help reduce your risk of heart disease. Remember to remove the skin before you eat it to reduce the risk of contaminating agents such as mercury, which are now polluting our seas. You know enough to stay away from deep-fried foods and foods like cakes and biscuits, ice-cream and hamburgers, sausages, salami and bacon, which are rich in fat. The problem is that they taste great, but we know that they are harmful and not doing our middle-aged metabolism any favours.

Stick to lots of fruit and vegetables; fish, especially fatty fish like salmon, but really any fish; wholegrains and rye bread or a rye bagel, if you need some toast or bread; and see that your food is poached, grilled, steamed or boiled, or if you roast anything keep the oil to a minimum.

Foods that make sense

Like most peri- and postmenopausal women you are probably a walking encyclopaedia of the foods that are good for you, but here's a quick overview to jog your memory or to confirm that you've been right all along.

Protein

Lean meat, fish (eat a lot of this; its benefits are amazing); chicken without the skin (though I always eat the wing and I'm not stopping now. Don't be fanatical, if you want a bit of skin now and then, it's not going to kill you); legumes; soy products; and low-fat dairy products.

Vegetables and fruits

Each of these has its own special benefits. Go easy on the potatoes and bananas, but see that you have at least five or more servings of a variety of vegetables and fruits a day. Chose those that are strongly coloured like spinach, carrots, berries and tomatoes because these contain more micronutrients. Fruit juice is not as healthy as whole fruit because the fibre content is lower and it is not as filling.

Healthy fats

Fish oils, avocado, nuts, olive oil, canola oil and flaxseed oil.

Wholegrains

These are grains like wholewheat, barley, oats, cracked wheat, whole cornmeal and brown rice that have not been refined, so much of the goodness in them, like the fibre and the germ of the grain, is retained.

Dark chocolate

In *moderation* this is good for you! Research has shown that it can increase HDL levels and improve endothelial (the cells that line the blood vessels) function in healthy adults.

Stay away from:

Processed foods; greasy foods; fast foods; highly refined foods; cakes; rich desserts; carbonated, sugary drinks; sweet milky drinks; sweet alcoholic after-dinner drinks; alcohol in general; sweets and milk chocolate – though everything in moderation, so eat what you want occasionally but in small amounts.

As far as alcohol is concerned, women should not have more than one drink a day – 250 ml of wine or about 100 ml of spirits like vodka. A glass of wine or a tot of spirits contains roughly the same amount of alcohol. If you are at a party, dilute your wine with sparkling mineral water, have plenty of water and don't mix your alcoholic beverages with sugary cold drinks. Cocktails may taste wonderful but they are very high in calories.

Exercise and weight

Throughout this book I have stressed the benefits of exercise in protecting you against chronic diseases including heart disease, type 2 diabetes, high blood pressure, cancers, osteoporosis and depression. The good news is that middle-aged women who exercise do much, much better on the weight front than those who are sedentary. Literally hundreds of pieces of research have shown that no matter how fat you are physical exercise is great for your health and vital if you want to lose or maintain weight. Women who exercise have smaller waists, which mean they are at lower risk for insulin resistance and type 2 diabetes, and have lower levels of bad cholesterol. Regular exercise also helps to maintain your weight loss.

What is important is the amount of exercise you do. A gentle stroll round the garden or the mall does not constitute serious exercise. The current recommendation is 30 minutes at least five times a week; enough to *work up a sweat*. But if you are trying to lose weight it will obviously be helpful to increase your daily physical activity to 60 minutes.

You need to make a commitment to an exercise regimen and stick to it, which means that you should apply some careful time management. Women often tell me that they are too busy to exercise. But if you cut back on the time you spend sitting at the computer, watching television or other unnecessary sedentary activities, you will find that you there is plenty of time to exercise. Try to walk whenever possible; park further away; take the stairs rather than the escalator or the lift; spend time in your garden.

When I wrote about osteoporosis I recommended walking weighted, resistance training and Pilates or yoga as forms of exercise that will contribute to maintaining your bones. New research indicates that you should include some kind of resistance training at least twice weekly. When you decide to make exercise part of your lifestyle you shouldn't stick to one type only. Apart from the boredom factor, you need to challenge your body. The moment you reach a comfort zone, the benefits of exercise are not as great. You need to work on all aspects: cardiovascular, muscle tone, flexibility, suppleness and good posture. This doesn't mean that you have to go overboard and become an exercise fanatic. In fact, if you over-exercise, apart from the injuries you could inflict on your body, if you're too lean you could be depleting your already low levels of oestrogen and you also won't look great. Every middle-aged woman needs a bit of fat to plump out her skin.

Find an expert and work out an exercise regimen that will fit in with your lifestyle and really work for you. Decide when you have adequate time to exercise, see whether you can be flexible and whether you have the discipline to go it alone day in and day out.

If you are like me, you would rather be lying on your bed with a novel and a bar of chocolate than working up a sweat, so exercise with a trainer or work out and walk with a friend. It's less easy to skive off that way. There is a lot of choice available. Some women do well with personal trainers, others like to work out at a gym with a pre-designed programme, still others prefer to walk and exercise with a friend or their partners. As long as you have a varied programme that encompasses some aerobic work, some resistance training and some flexibility and stretching, you are doing the right thing. The bad news is that you must exercise five days a week. The good news is that all exercise programmes say that you must rest your body, so you can enjoy your days off. In any case the benefits of exercise are wonderful. Exercise is a great safeguard against depression and stress. Many of us have found that when we feel down, food is our first comfort stop, but studies have shown that if you exercise you are less likely to be depressed and to turn to food to cheer yourself up.

Eating for comfort

Some time ago I had a bad year. I felt depressed and that my life was out of control. But there was one area I convinced myself that I was in charge: eating. Whenever I had that empty, sinking feeling, I went to the fridge or cupboard and tried to make myself feel better.

I say I tried because for a few moments it worked, but moments later I would feel more depressed than ever. The brief high that the comfort food had given me wore off very quickly and I found myself in that cycle of eating that starts with something savoury, say a packet of chips, then goes on to a chocolate, then a fizzy drink, then a piece of chicken, followed by something else. I was guilty but defiant, and tired all the time because I felt too down and listless to exercise, and when I didn't exercise I felt even more angry and depressed.

At night I would lie in bed and touch the roll of fat round my hips and remember how none of my clothes fitted me any more and how I didn't want to look at myself naked and feel really miserable, but the next day, in spite of the stern lecture I had given myself, I would be back at it again. Food had become my drug of choice.

Many middle-aged women will know what I'm talking about. Food can become as much of an addiction as alcohol and drugs. The problem is that you need to eat in order to live, which is why, when you decide to lose weight and keep it off you need a serious lifestyle change. It's very clear that eating something with lots of refined sugar (a simple carbo-hydrate) does give us that quick boost, but it's not sustained and we probably find ourselves craving some more choco-late or cake or whatever is at hand to get that energy back. Insulin levels go higher, digested meal blood sugar goes a bit higher than it should, then it drops quickly and we need an energy boost.

It is a medical fact that the feel-good neurotransmitter sero-tonin that I wrote about in Chapter 4 regulates not only mood and sleepiness (which is why we often feel sluggish after a meal high in carbohydrates) but our appetite and desire to eat. It's a very complex biochemical procedure that works like this: when insulin is produced, most of the amino acids in the blood drop and only *tryptophan*, which is one of the things that triggers the production of serotonin, reaches the brain (see Chapter 4).

So, if you eat a meal that has a lot of carbohydrates in it and the tryptophan levels are higher than the other amino acids, the raised level of tryptophan triggers a greater production of serotonin. The other side of this coin is that foods rich in protein seem to inhibit serotonin production, which is why many women on very restricted diets, or diets very low in carbohydrates and very rich in proteins, may feel down and depressed or moody and start craving Chelsea buns. It's also well known that certain carbohydrates seem to increase serotonin levels more quickly than others, especially simple carbohydrates, so it's quite logical that our brains, knowing that our serotonin levels are low, would encourage us to pick up a bun, or something else that is starchy, to help us feel better.

The food fix is different for different individuals because our biochemistry is different. I'm sure you've heard women talking among themselves about the different foods that make them feel better when they're down. Many middle-aged women battle with depression, as I will explain in Chapter 11, but going on an eating binge isn't the answer – talking to a therapist to help you over your rocky patch may help. But many feelings, not only depression, may trigger a compulsion to overeat. Don't act out your feelings by raiding the fridge. Ask yourself what you are feeling when you start eating compulsively, crave something sweet or eat throughout the day. Don't try to submerge your feelings of anxiety, fear or anger with food. Ask yourself what you are feeling when you make for the fridge. For example, if you are anxious, acknowledge that feeling and just sit with it for a while.

Some women find it helpful to write about their feelings, others discover that when they deal with them by seeing a therapist or working through them in a group, their need to overeat disappears. The age of perimenopause can be a time of many conflicting emotions and feelings, and it is important to recognise and deal with them constructively. Some women, who during this time have become obsessed with food, their weight and dieting, find that joining Overeaters Anonymous (OA) helps. This is a gentle, non-threatening way to deal with food and weight issues. You can access your nearest branch through the Internet.

Some women find that taking antidepressants during the perimenopausal period helps them, while others discover that eating correctly and exercising is the answer. Once again, it depends on your individual context. I found that eating sensibly actually stopped the sugar cravings because my glucose levels were balanced rather than spiking, and when I was eating properly and exercising, I no longer felt out of control. You can get back on track with a proper lifestyle programme, but the slippery path to overeating and not exercising is steep.

Many women have found that it is very helpful to go to a dietician when they have decided to re-examine their lifestyles and eat healthily. A sensible, sympathetic ear really works in this area because you can check your weight and often find out why something is or isn't working. You can get a meal plan that will be individually tailored to your food likes and dislikes. It's pointless going on a diet that includes most of the foods you hate. You may lose weight in the beginning but you will soon give up.

Studies have shown that women who are monitored in a one-on-one programme maintain weight loss better than those who do it alone. You will probably begin your weight loss programme by seeing your dietician once a week and, as you lose the weight and get the hang of sensible eating, your visits will be fewer, but still regular. Some women who have kept their weight down for more than five years go biannually and always have the option of increasing the number of appointments if they are worried about their weight. Others find it works to go to group weigh-ins and lose weight and keep it off that way, but if you can afford it, I think that the individual attention really helps.

Empowerment points

Now that you've had a little reality check, let's look at how you can manage your weight in menopause and still enjoy your life. The rules below are what I have learnt over the years as I have struggled to lose my middle-aged spread.

- There is no such thing as a painless way to lose weight. By this I mean that there will be some things you will have to give up, like second helpings and fast food (or at least not eat it more than three times a year). If you decide to try one of the hundreds of diet pills that are on the market, be careful. They usually don't work, so you'll have wasted your money and when they do work they can often have serious side effects. (Ephedra for example, which was much touted as being able to speed up your metabolism, was found to be dangerous, ineffective and has now been removed from the shelves of most reputable health food stores and pharmacies.) As you read in Chapter 5, you need to be very careful about the medical claims and the effects of the supplements you take.

- Stay away from fad diets. They may work well at first but the weight you lose quickly may be mostly water and lean muscle mass instead of fat; you'll gain it back, perhaps even more than before, and it will be harder to lose. Lose weight on a sensible meal plan at a sensible rate: not more than two to four kilograms a month.

- No second helpings. This really works. Look at your slim friends. At a dinner party they seldom have a second helping or they take a tiny bit to start and may have a minuscule second taste.

- Watch your portions. Look at a fat woman helping herself to food at a buffet. The chances are her plate is laden. Most research concludes that in the matter of losing weight and maintaining it, it doesn't matter what the diet is, once the portions and calories are restricted, people lose weight.

- Watch your calories. It's no good having small portions of high calorie food. Well, it's better than having large portions of high calorie food, but it's not sensible. That's why dieticians often suggest that rather than ordering a huge plate of pasta with a rich cheesy sauce you have a big green salad with your meal. It takes up space, it's healthy and it's low in calories. My suggestion is that when you eat a salad you dress it with something tasty and interesting. Feeling deprived and bored when you eat is the quickest route I know to a trip to the sweet cupboard.

- If you know you're going to a dinner party or will to be eating dinner at a special restaurant, pace yourself during the day. Certain slim women, who seem to eat huge quantities at night, often leave out lunch or breakfast. Obviously this isn't the healthiest way to do things, but it gives you a bit of room to manoeuvre.

- Some women do better when they eat every couple of hours. So you may have breakfast at 8am, a snack at 10am, lunch at 1pm, a snack at 4pm and dinner at 7pm, with a snack at about 9pm. If the food you eat is sensible, you will keep balanced levels of insulin and won't have uncontrollable food cravings.

- Learn to know what true hunger feels like. Don't eat out of habit, boredom or for comfort and don't wait until you're ravenous before you eat. When I was overeating I felt hungry, or at least in need of food, all the time. I had forgotten what proper hunger felt like and only remembered it when I started to eat properly and felt satisfied for the periods between meals.

- Vary your diet. As I have emphasised, to lose or maintain weight requires a lifestyle change and there's no point in dieting frantically for two weeks for a special occasion and then putting it all back on. It's too depressing. There really are plenty of choices out there. You don't have to sit glumly over an endless array of cottage cheese and plain lettuce. Ask your dietician to help you find a way to include the foods you like in a meal plan. You'll be surprised at how many things you can eat and still lose weight.

- Find someone to monitor you. It's sensible when you start your new lifestyle regimen to get help from a professional who can help you through the bad bits and explain why you aren't losing weight when you could have sworn that you had stuck to your meal plan. Professionals understand how your metabolism works and can give you lots of helpful hints. Research has clearly shown that women who had support when they were on diet and then went onto a weight maintenance programme did much better than those who had to go it alone.

- Don't eat out of depression or boredom and don't eat to suppress your feelings. There's a moment of triumph and defiance, and then reality bites. Learn to recognise when you are anxious or angry and develop mechanisms to deal with those feelings. OA is very helpful in enabling you to recognise why you are eating compulsively.

- Watch the amount of alcohol you consume. There's no problem with a glass or two of wine, but it can play havoc with the levels of glucose in your blood, which can make you very hungry. Also, when you drink too much your willpower falters.

- Don't fall into despair if you've pigged out. And don't make it an excuse to go on a binge. Say to yourself: 'I ate exactly what I wanted last night. It was delicious and I enjoyed every mouthful. It made no difference and today I'll resume my eating plan.' Don't beat yourself up and don't justify feelings of guilt and depression about what you perceive as overeating in retrospect by saying: 'I've messed up so there's no point in going on with my meal plan and my exercise.' Take everything one day, or even one meal, at a time.

- Treat yourself occasionally and do it guilt-free. There's no reason not to have the hot-buttered toast (as long as it's rye toast!) or the piece of cheesecake or the Christmas pudding. Just don't go mad, and watch your portions. If you're eating mindfully and savouring your food it's amazing how a little goes a long way.

- Exercise for at least 30 minutes five times a week. See that you have a varied exercise programme and always work up a sweat.

- Ensure that you drink enough, but not too much, water. Six to eight glasses a day will stop that hungry feeling you may get when you're dehydrated. Those women who drink more than two litres of water a day may have mineral imbalances and often have urinary tract infections and urinary problems, a situation that doesn't help women who already have vaginal dryness and urinary incontinence.

- You are not a 'bad girl' when your diet goes awry or you diverge from your meal plan. What you've done may not be great for your health, but that's it. Take the emotion out of eating once and for all. When you eat well and exercise you're being kind to and looking after yourself. A middle-aged woman doesn't need to be bullied and bossed about her weight or judged on it. It's no one's business but your own. Do it for your health's sake and the rest will follow.

- Some women are very disciplined in their eating habits from Monday to Friday and then eat more or less what they want at the weekend. Others are generally disciplined all week but eat luxury foods and have a drink or two when the need arises: a dinner party, a meal at a restaurant, or a special occasion. It depends on what suits you best.

- TAKE CONTROL. What you eat should NEVER control you. Don't give your power away to a bar of chocolate or a piece of cake!

Notes

_____

_____

_____

_____

_____

_____

_____

_____

_____

_____

_____

_____

_____

_____

_____

_____

_____

_____

_____

_____

11

Heart, Mind and Body: A Menopause Miscellany

View 1

Alexandra sipped her coffee reflectively. 'It's the dreaded pole in the back in the middle of the night,' she said. 'I don't know if other menopausal women feel like me, but sex has become a bore. I mean he hasn't talked to me all day except to ask if I've collected the package from the post office. During dinner he's exhausted and afterwards he slumps in front of the TV with a whisky in his hand and drops off to sleep. He falls into bed still without saying a word; he snores loudly and suddenly in the middle of the night he grabs me. I couldn't feel less like sex by that time.'

View 2

'How do I feel about sex?' Sue grins. 'I love it. I'm in my mid-fifties and he's quite a bit younger but he makes me feel great. I love his energy and, to be frank, his body. We talk for hours in bed and laugh a lot. He makes me feel beautiful.'

View 3

'I used to really enjoy sex,' says Connie. 'We've been married a long time and now that the kids are gone, we don't have to worry about someone bursting into the bedroom at the wrong time. I love my husband and I feel like sex, but it's so painful that I don't even let myself get excited any more. John's become anxious about even touching me. It's become a huge worry. I've also been very depressed during this last year, worse than I can ever remember apart from a bad period of postnatal depression after our third child was born.'

View 4

'After my hysterectomy, I was really worried about our sex life,' says Vicki. 'My gynaecologist removed my cervix as well as my womb and for a while I didn't feel like going near my husband because I felt so different. Perhaps it was in my mind. I don't know, but after a while my hormones were sorted out, I started using the estradiol-releasing ring so my vagina didn't feel sore any more and sex isn't bad at all. I still have an orgasm and I'm not sure if I could tell you whether it feels different or not. In any case I've always felt that Dave liked sex more than I did, he still thinks I'm sexy and wants to make love nearly every night. I decided that if we just made love and I didn't make a big thing about it, it would become easier – like a pleasant habit. In fact it's fine. He's really happy with our sex life and so am I.'

I have called this chapter 'Heart, mind and body' because I think they are all connected in healthy, functioning peri- and postmenopausal women. Sexuality in midlife is dependent on many different things – psychological, physical and social. Since all these aspects of our lives are intertwined and since they affect us particularly during the peri- and postmenopausal years, I will discuss all of them in greater or lesser detail. They are intrinsic to the way we feel about ourselves, how we relate to our sex lives, our psyche and the way we look during menopause.

One of the biggest issues for menopausal women is sex. In Chapters 2 and 4 I mentioned that many perimenopausal women suffer from a low level or even a lack of sexual desire, and I wrote that this might be the result of lowered levels of testosterone, but I also wrote that I had a lot of thoughts on the subject. I don't think that the only solution to women's lowered libido is to slap on the testosterone. Women are very complex and there may be myriad reasons why they don't have the same level of sexual desire and energy that they had when they were young.

Each of the women I quote above has a different take on her sex life. Alexandra's husband is a farmer who gets up early and is exhausted at night. He doesn't bother to talk to her any more; she feels that he doesn't even see her, and for him sex has become a mechanical exercise. While Alexandra doesn't find sex painful, like many menopausal women she's lost interest, and with good reason! She feels like a whore and there is no intimacy in their relationship. If Alexandra were confronted with a loving man who appreciated her, she might be surprised at how sexy she felt.

Sue is lucky; after a painful divorce she found someone who thinks she's gorgeous and has the energy and stamina to make sex fun. He's made her change her mindset and she has no sense that she shouldn't be enjoying sex in middle age.

Connie is suffering from painful intercourse – *dyspaurenia*. It's very common in menopause when estrogen levels drop and a woman's vagina becomes dryer because the cells lining the vagina have less estrogen. She is also suffering from depression, which is also very common in peri- and postmenopausal women, and is well known for putting a damper on sexual desire.

Unlike Connie, Vicky has dealt with the changes in her body and seems to have moved on to a new and rewarding sexual period in her life. Her hysterectomy didn't seem to affect her ability to have an orgasm and though she doesn't describe sex as an earth-shattering experience, it is pleasant and comfortable.

Physical changes that may affect your sex life

Lower levels of hormones, especially testosterone

A lot of research has focused on whether women enjoy sex less after menopause or hysterectomy. The interesting thing is that for many years it was thought that when your hormone levels, especially your androgen levels (see Chapter 2), dropped, you lost the desire. But as I have written repeatedly, women are complicated and although some women did very well with added testosterone or a combination of estrogen and progesterone, others found that the HT made no difference at all. As I indicated in Chapter 4, women who have had a natural menopause continue to produce amounts of testosterone similar to those they produced prior to menopause, so low libido cannot necessarily be blamed on lower levels of testosterone.

The *methyltestosterone* implant may have had a good effect, but the studies did not clarify how much of the increased sexual desire was the result of the placebo effect, the idea that sex would be more appealing if there was additional testosterone – women's minds play a big role in their sexuality. Another problem with the implant is that it probably gave women more testosterone than their sensitive adrenal cascades could deal with and many found themselves with all sorts of unwanted side effects like aggressiveness, greasy skin, unwanted facial hair, adult acne and weight gain. They also had raised levels of bad cholesterol.

Newer research has shown that women battling with lowered sexual desire after a surgical menopause had improved sex lives when using a testosterone patch which gave them a daily dose of 300 mcg of testosterone, in conjunction with transdermal ET. As I discussed in Chapter 4, it may be better to take a hormone through your skin because it seems to create fewer side effects, but there are women who just don't respond to this patch. Although many doctors feel that the treatment option may be the way forward for those women who suffer from low libido.

Some women swear by DHEA and there is ongoing research to establish the efficacy and safety of this hormone, which I have written about in Chapters 2 and 4. If you decide you want to try DHEA only take it if you are under the care of an experienced endocrinologist or a doctor who really knows about it. Certain medications that middle-aged women may have to take such as beta-blockers, antidepressants and corticosteroids can also cause low levels of libido. It's very important to ask your doctor about the possible side effects when you start taking a new medicine.

Very sensitive, tender breasts

Many women going through perimenopause, or who are on HT, suddenly experience very tender and sensitive breasts. Being sensitive in this case doesn't mean that you become more sexually aroused, it means you can't bear to have your breasts touched, which can be a big problem for a man who finds touching his partner's breasts exciting and for the woman involved, who has always enjoyed this aspect of her sexuality and now finds herself shying away.

Tender breasts can probably be blamed on fluctuating levels of estrogen, though sometimes progesterone can cause your breast tissue to retain water, which can also make the breasts oversensitive. Sometime balancing your hormone levels with HT can solve this problem, but as with most menopausal symptoms, this one will usually resolve itself. Your best bet is to be frank with your partner and find another part of your body that can be touched and that will give you pleasure, not pain.

Dry vagina

When you are a young, reproductive woman, or even when you are older but not yet menopausal, your vagina is probably well lubricated and looks, on examination, plump and luscious. As you embark on perimenopause and your estrogen levels start to drop, the endothelial cells that line the vagina become thinner and less estrogenated. This is called *vaginal atrophy*.

A gynaecologist can see at once if this is happening, because the walls of your vagina will look pale and dry. These endothelial cells also line your urinary tract so when they lose estrogen you may suffer burning during urination, urinary tract infections, urinary incontinence, stress incontinence and vaginal itchiness. (Remember to check that the reason for all these symptoms is your dry vaginal and urinary tissue, and not anything else more serious, as I explained in Chapter 7. It never hurts to be sure.)

Obviously, if you aren't properly lubricated and your vagina is dry, sexual intercourse will be painful. Many menopausal women find that even though they are aroused, it hurts when they are penetrated and during the sexual act. This pain may induce them to fear sex and become uptight and worried, which further inhibits sexual arousal. Most women know that even in the days when their vaginas weren't dry a lack of sexual desire or the feeling of suddenly being turned off prevented them becoming moist and ready for sex, so when they are menopausal the situation becomes fraught with pitfalls.

Luckily the cure for a dry vagina is relatively simple. There are several different vaginal estrogen creams and products that can help to alter the state of your vagina. Most of them have very low levels of estrogen and work excellently. This type of estrogen is effective locally and because, as I explained in Chapter 4, only very small amounts enter your system, you aren't exposed to any risk. If you decide to use conjugated equine estrogens (CEE) you may find that the effects are not just local, and the lining of your womb may thicken. It's a question of finding the solution that suits you best.

Vicki chose the estradiol-releasing ring, but there are estrogen creams, vaginal pessaries and tablets that also work well. Women who are on HT find that they don't usually need an estrogen cream, but the problem is that of all the menopause symptoms, the one that continues when the others subside is the dry vagina. It's not going to improve when your hormones settle down after perimenopause. If you don't want to use a topical vaginal estrogen some practitioners suggest a silicone-based vaginal gel before sex. Water-based lubricants also work well and may not be as irritating, but they can dry up while you're making love, so you need to find the type that suits you and your partner best. To increase intimacy, ask your partner to help you apply the gel. Interestingly, some research has shown that postmenopausal women who have regular sex have a slower rate of vaginal atrophy or dryness than women who are not sexually active, so if you don't have regular sex, think about getting a vibrator.

If you are experiencing painful sex, I would urge you to find a solution. The psychological element is very strong here. If you don't deal with this problem it can become a vicious circle, which may be difficult to break.

Lack of sensation during sex

The bad news is that many women who are well into middle age no longer have the tight, supple vaginas they had in their youth: babies and life have taken their toll. It helps to remember that the vagina is a 'potential' space. This means that the walls of the uterus fold in on themselves and there is no space there, but when something like a tampon or a penis is inserted, or a baby is born, it opens to provide the space needed. Over the years, the tissue and muscles have stretched; the vagina is no longer as elastic as it was when you were younger. During sex these muscles may not be able to tense as they once did. The problem is that many women may not find sex painful but may have no sensation when they make love.

Some of these women believe that a vaginal reconstruction will be the answer. However, don't follow this route blindly; this surgery is usually performed when there is bad tearing or scarring. For those middle-aged women who have problems when the womb drops into the vagina or the bladder falls down, a hysterectomy would be the surgery of choice.

If you don't have any of those problems, the best way to deal with this is to change your position when you make love, so that you are able to feel your partner's penis.

There are no set rules for this; you'll just have to experiment a bit. Another problem that could compound the situation is that many men no longer have the firm, long-lasting erections they had in their youth. I mention this because it takes two to tango and many middle-aged women blame themselves when sex is no longer as good as it used to be. As you get older, it may take longer to feel pleasurable sensations or build up to a climax than it used to, so you need patience and sometimes a sense of humour; but laugh with each other.

Middle-aged men can suffer from all kinds of potency problems for a variety of reasons – lowered testosterone levels, high blood pressure and other medical problems, stress, performance anxiety and prostate cancer, as well as some of the medications prescribed for these. Prostate cancer in particular can have huge implications for the lives of middle-aged couples, especially in the area of sexual dysfunction. If your partner is battling, talk to an expert. There's no shame in this and there are many ways to deal with the problem or get around it. If you are embarrassed to discuss sex with your partner and explore all your options, this too can become a vicious circle. The same applies to asking for what gives you pleasure and saying what doesn't. Many sexual issues can be resolved with frank and open discussions and mutual respect.

Hysterectomy

Like Vicki, some women may battle after they've had a hysterectomy. Women may be profoundly attached to their wombs and there may be psychological issues around their own feelings of diminished femininity and a sense of loss. But if they deal with these, the problems are usually short-lived. Most women find that they are functioning quite well six months after their hysterectomy, though for some it may take up to a year to get back to normal.

There has been much discussion about whether the removal of the cervix affects sexual functioning or not. I've done my own anecdotal research and it seems that most women find that they still have orgasms after a hysterectomy, though whether they are the same type or not is open to discussion. That said, some women say that their orgasms feel different, especially if stimulation of their cervix was important to their sexual response. These are women who get pleasure from cervical stimulation, which means that for these women the loss of their cervix may make their orgasms less intense. During sex the uterus contracts, so women who found these contractions pleasurable and noticeable, especially during their orgasms, will no longer feel these after a hysterectomy and will notice a difference in the depth and intensity of their orgasms. Generally, women will still feel the pleasurable vaginal contractions. The good news is that most women experience a clitoral orgasm and since in a normal hysterectomy the clitoris remains, most women find that they can still have a very satisfactory orgasm.

There are two different kinds of orgasm, the *external* orgasm, achieved through stimulation of your clitoris, and the *internal* orgasm – when your G-spot and the area round it are stimulated. We've all heard about the G-spot, which is the region situated in a woman's genital area behind her pubic bone. This area surrounds the urethra. Tiny glands called Skene's glands are found here in the upper wall of the vagina and the lower end of the urethra. The name G-spot is given to the area where the Skene's glands are found. These little glands are like prostate glands in men. Their size differs from one woman to another, and they may not even be present in some women. The theory is that the G-spot is extremely sensitive and if this area is stimulated women can climax. So certain women who have very tiny Skene's glands, or none at all, may not experience an internal orgasm. Other women who still have their cervix experience orgasms when the cervix is stimulated or when there is pressure on the anterior wall of their vagina, or both. Because a woman's orgasm is highly individual, women can have orgasms that combine all three sensations. What this information tells you is not to despair when you have a total hysterectomy, you can still achieve great sexual pleasure.

Sleep deprivation

No woman who is feeling exhausted from lack of sleep is going to feel sexy. The only thing she can think of when she gets into bed is whether she is going to fall asleep and if she does for how long the sleep will last. Insomnia is very common in peri- and postmenopausal women. It comes in many forms.

Some women find they no longer experience a deep uninterrupted sleep, but that their nights are disturbed, either because they are battling with night sweats and wake several times drenched to the skin, or they have troubled dreams, or they sleep so lightly that the slightest sound wakes them. Other women fell into a deep sleep but wake unusually early, with a panicky feeling or a pounding heart; still others struggle to fall asleep or are wide awake after only an hour.

Fluctuating hormonal levels are not the only problems that deprive women of sleep; depression, anxiety and stress can also affect sleep patterns. Another issue is the loud levels of snoring that may emanate from your ageing partner. Something can be done about this and he should consult a specialist. Many women who start to take antidepressants (SSRIs) during the perimenopausal stage find that they sleep better. Having a glass of warm milk may encourage sleepiness because the milk contains lactose, a carbohydrate that may affect the serotonin pathways (see Chapter 10).

You may also want to ask your doctor for one of the newer, safer and less addictive sleeping pills to get you back into the habit of uninterrupted sleep. Often insomnia is a self-fulfilling prophecy because you are so worried about not falling asleep that you work yourself up into such a frenzy and then there's no way you'll be able to sleep. Certain supplements, such as melatonin, have been recommended for the problem. It is thought to be safe in small doses, but more research needs to be done to determine its efficacy and long-term safety. If you want to try it, consult your doctor first. Calcium and magnesium are thought to help promote sleepiness, but once again, the jury is out until more data is in.

Regular exercise can be helpful in promoting sleep, as can eating sensibly and not too heavily at night. Remember not to drink too much: alcohol may help put you to sleep, but you will wake dehydrated and with a pounding headache, and the other risks of alcohol aren't worth it. Research suggests that for the sake of our health we should sleep for between seven and eight hours a night, though not longer, so you should get to bed at a decent hour at least a couple of nights a week.

Exhaustion can lead to raised cortisol levels, an impaired immune system, anxiety, poor cognitive functioning and depression, which are risk factors for other illnesses like heart disease. There are all sorts of behavioural suggestions like not reading or watching television in bed, creating a calm environment and a darkened room, but I think that each woman knows what suits her best at bedtime. I for one can't fall asleep unless I read for a while. We probably need a bit less sleep as we get older, so don't stress if you are waking up earlier, as long as you wake feeling rested and alert – your body will tell you whether you are getting enough sleep or not. Don't panic if you have one or two sleepless nights, but find help if the situation persists.

Body appearance (you AND your partner)

'The problem,' says Amy, 'is that I hate the way I look. My boobs hang, my hips are wide and my skin is mottled and not smooth any more. I've got a double chin and no matter how much I exercise, I just don't feel firm. I don't feel sexy, in fact, when I look at myself I'm "turned off", although the weird thing is that Rob tells me I'm gorgeous and he loves my body and he is always eager to make love.'

Amy is blonde and extremely pretty and although she's no longer slim, she glows with vitality and is beautifully groomed. From what she has just told me, her husband agrees with this assessment, but she can't accept her middle-aged self. Many of us hold in our minds a picture of ourselves at 18 and it's very hard to accept that gravity and life have altered us. We are going to continue to age, no matter how much time and energy we put into preserving ourselves, and one day we're going to be old. This is a fact of life. It doesn't mean that we can't be sexy and attractive in midlife because we are no longer young and firm.

Take Sue and her younger lover: 'I love the way I feel,' she says. 'I work out and my body is as good as it's going to get, but that's okay because I feel healthy and good about myself. I like looking good, but I've accepted that I can't wear things like tight midriff tops. So I buy clothes that suit me and get vicarious pleasure from shopping for my daughter. It may sound like a rationalisation, but I don't think the faces of young girls are as interesting as the faces of my friends. Those lines add character; they tell a story of lives well lived, full of happiness and sorrow and laughter.'

I agree with Sue. I was very inspired by a book by Janet Juska called *A round-heeled woman*. Aged 66, she decides she's tired of being celibate and advertises in the *New York Review of Books*: 'BEFORE I TURN 67 – next March – I would like to have lots of sex with a man I like. If you want to talk first Trollope works for me. NYR Box 10307.' I opened the book with some trepidation, I thought it might contain gratuitous sex and I wasn't sure what I would find. In fact I was blown away by her courageous and endearing story. It contains a hopeful message for all older women who think their sexy days are over. It also says to single women that there's nothing wrong with wanting a physical relationship and letting the world know it.

We have to stop buying into the mindset foisted on us by the media; that young is better. There is nothing more attractive than a good-looking, middle-aged woman who is happy with herself and her life. When a woman feels good about herself, it's amazing how few people judge her physical appearance. And while we're lamenting our lost looks, let's spare a thought for our partners. Their bodies are no longer firm, a beer belly is often the first thing we come into contact with in bed at night, they have more hair on their chests than on their heads, their skins have reacted to years of sun and weather, and their bodies no longer look the way they did some 30 years ago, when a glance from them made us go weak at the knees.

Their appearance may be what's turning us off, but most men don't spend an inordinate amount of time worrying about that. They have absolute confidence that we will still find them sexy and attractive, and that we couldn't ask for more than to make love with them every night. At worst, if your man is not the Adonis he once was, you can close your eyes and fantasise.

Sex should be a shared experience, but as I wrote above, as we get older the satisfying sensations take longer to happen. This means that you need to pay attention to foreplay and to try to rekindle the intimacy of your first sexual experiences together. In our busy lives we may need to schedule time for sex; anticipation can be exciting. So try to create a romantic environment that will make this a special time for both you and your partner. You may find that you are not as energetic as you once were and are too tired for sex at night, but there's nothing wrong with weekend afternoons. Take the phone off the hook, be glad that you don't have to worry about the children bursting in and enjoy yourselves!

Your menopausal skin

Exercise and a sensible lifestyle should help you maintain a reasonable body and good health, but there's no doubt that the skin is a major indicator of age. We've all looked into the mirror and seen the fine lines, wrinkles, sunspots, uneven pigmentation and the larger pores that are signs of an ageing skin. If you have worshipped the sun all your life it's bad luck, because nothing, except perhaps smoking, is more ageing.

However, regardless of how much sun damage you've already inflicted on your skin, you should never go out without a sunscreen. I believe that to try to minimise the age spots, you should wear a sunscreen on your hands as well. Look at the hand that is nearest the window when you drive to see why. If sun spots get too bad, they can be burnt off.

Before I describe the products and treatments that are available to help our ageing skins, a quick word about skin cancer. We all have little moles all over our bodies, some of us more than others, but you should go to a dermatologist for a yearly check-up to monitor any moles that may have changed. You are at risk for skin cancer if you have a *family history* of it, are *fair-skinned*, have *red* or *fair hair*, and have had many *years of sun exposure* or any *unusual moles*. Skin cancer can appear anywhere on your body, but it is usually found in those areas that have had the highest exposure to the sun.

Melanoma is the deadliest skin cancer and it can occur anywhere on the body. When found early, before it penetrates deeply into the skin, melanoma is completely curable, so it is important to have it diagnosed early. Be alert for a mole that suddenly changes colour, gets darker or bigger, or seems to be composed of more than one colour. If a mole is itchy, inflamed, or painful, if the skin is broken and it bleeds, you should alert your doctor. Red areas that bleed easily in sun-exposed skin should also be checked because this might indicate a cancer known as *basal* or *squamous cell carcinoma*. While rarely fatal, these cancers can grow rapidly and become severely disfiguring.

If something on your skin looks suspicious, the dermatologist or surgeon will do a biopsy (see Chapter 8) to remove as much of it as possible and send this section of cells and tissues to the laboratory to see if it's cancerous. Many doctors like to get two opinions when a melanoma is found because it is difficult to diagnose. If the diagnosis is positive the specialist will do a series of tests to check how far the cancer has progressed. Once this has been determined she or he will devise a treatment plan that centres on the complete removal of the cancer.

Anti-Ageing Skin Care

There are certain things that you can do to prevent your skin ageing too quickly. Of course, if you've got good genes, that's first prize. My mother was well into her eighties and had the skin of a 40-year-old woman. She always cared for her skin. I can remember watching her having facials from the time I was a little girl, but ultimately, I think that her genes determined the way her skin looked. Exercise is excellent for waking up your skin and helping it glow, but if you're walking always wear a sunscreen and a hat and see that your lips and all exposed areas of your body are protected.

If you are a swimmer, rinse your skin well after your swim and moisturise it. Don't smoke. You know all about the dangers of smoking by now but some people do not realise how appalling it is for your skin. Eat a healthy, balanced diet and don't drink too much. Keep yourself hydrated. If you are drinking enough water, it will be reflected in your skin tone. Protect your skin during the day with a moisturiser and a sunscreen or a good base containing a sunscreen. At night you must clean your skin well. At your age, you should be using treatments that not only moisturise but also exfoliate.

As you know to your cost and from the crowded shelves in your bathroom, there are thousands of skincare products in the marketplace that promise you a glowing skin, a finer skin, a youthful skin and a radiant skin. The problem is that these creams and potions may be beautifully packaged and look and feel wonderful but they may not work. Because the baby boomers are now ready to spend a lot of money on their appearance, new and exciting research is being done on skincare products to try to find the 'magic' anti-ageing formula.

The issue is whether one should buy prescription products that have been seen to work but are often costly and complicated to use, or trust the over-the-counter products which promise us so much. As you get older, the collagen, which is a fibrous tissue found throughout your body, and the elastin, which are the fibres that make the skin elastic, begin to age with wear and tear so that your skin looks less plump and supple. In addition, exposure to the sun, the build-up of dead skin cells on the surface of the skin, fine lines and wrinkles, and the thinning appearance of the skin make us look older.

Anti-ageing products play several roles in the rejuvenation of the skin: they exfoliate (slough off) the dead layers; they help build up the collagen and elastin; and they thicken the skin so that it looks firmer and more glowing. Below is a list of ingredients that appear time and again in anti-ageing creams. Read the labels of products carefully and buy those that contain the appropriate ingredients. And sometimes just pamper yourself with a wonderfully scented product that will be good for your soul, even if it doesn't do much for your skin.

Glycolic Acid is found in green fruit and young plants. It is also made from sugarcane. It is the most powerful of the *Alpha Hydroxy Acids*, or the fruit acids, and stimulates the surface of the skin to peel by a chemical action, which helps to reduce the build-up of dead skin cells. It is used as a skin peel, which means that it exfoliates the dead cells of the epidermis or surface layer of the skin. This means that when you use it, your skin looks younger and glowing. Another of its functions is to trigger the production of collagen, which makes your skin look plumper. If you see either of the above ingredients listed on your product you are on the right track.

Retinol or *retinoids* are derived from vitamin A. Because one of the main functions of vitamin A is to preserve the skin's elasticity and prevent excessive wrinkling and accelerated ageing, vitamin A derivatives are an ideal anti-ageing ingredient. If you see any of the following: *retinol, retinyl palmitate, retinyl linoleate,* or *retinyl acetate* on the label of a product you know that you are dealing with an anti-ageing product. It is thought that retinoids or retinol can correct the damage caused to the skin by the sun and strengthen the epidermis (the outer layer of the skin) by thickening it, which helps to prevent sun damage. Retinoids are natural exfoliators. *Retin A* is a stronger version of the retinoids and is used under a doctor's supervision rather than sold over the counter.

The following ingredients are often found in over-the-counter anti-ageing skincare products, but a great deal more scientific research, using well-designed trials, needs to be carried out to prove whether any of them are really effective in reversing the ageing process:

Vitamin E (α-*tocopherol*) may act as an antioxidant on the epidermis and help to repair damage by preventing the actions of free radicals that cause ageing, helping the skin to become smoother and refining fine lines and wrinkles. It also seems to have an effect on plumping out the skin.

Vitamin C (L-ascorbic acid) is another ingredient you will find in many over-the-counter skincare products. It helps lighten the skin, improves skin pigmentation and sun damage, and may also act as an antioxidant, which helps to prevent the damage caused by free radicals.

Coenzyme Q10 (ubiquinone) antioxidants, as I explained earlier, can help prevent skin damage and play a role in repairing the skin. Some researchers have reported that CoQ10 levels decrease in our skin as we age and believe that by adding this ingredient to our skincare regimen we can reverse some sun damage, smooth out some wrinkles and increase the collagen levels.

Soy isoflavones are also popular ingredients in the new spate of anti-ageing products directed at postmenopausal women. One of the reasons for this is that they are plant estrogens, as you saw in Chapter 5, which suggests that they might have a beneficial effect on the estrogen receptors in the skin and contribute to the reversal of age-related damage.

There are some very powerful new anti-ageing agents available called *cosmoceuticals*, some of which I describe below, but these should only be used by an expert dermatologist or plastic surgeon. It would be very unwise to buy them in over-the-counter products. If you find a 'miracle' anti-ageing cream that contains them, ask your dermatologist about it and only use it under strict supervision.

Kinerase, a growth hormone found in plants, is one of the newest, most powerful anti-ageing products. It is thought to reduce fine lines and wrinkles, smooth out the skin and diminish skin mottling and pigmentation. It can also be used very effectively in combination with *retinol palmitate* but should only be used under medical supervision.

Hydroquinone is a very powerful skin-lightening agent, or bleach. Like Kinerase, it should only be used under a doctor's supervision. It can cause extreme sensitivity and should be used with caution. It can be applied in combination with *glycolic acid* to refine and smooth an ageing, sun-damaged skin.

Plastic Surgery

Many postmenopausal women who feel that the available products do not work quickly or dramatically enough turn to plastic surgery to help them recover a much younger looking skin or face. Several procedures, which used to be extremely costly and difficult, have been refined and can be performed in an outpatient situation in the plastic surgeon's rooms. You should make extensive enquiries before you commit yourself to any of the following treatments and make sure that the practitioner is very well trained and well versed in these procedures.

Some women are very happy with the lines on their faces and, like Sue, who I quote at the beginning of this chapter, think they add interest and character. However, this is a very personal choice and the decision must be yours alone. Do not allow anyone to judge you, or label you frivolous. If it feels right to you, go ahead.

You can improve the texture of your skin by means of botox injections. Botox is a poison (*botulinum toxin*) that is injected in tiny amounts into the skin and helps to smooth out wrinkles and frown lines by temporarily paralysing the tiny facial muscles. It relaxes the muscles on each side of the wrinkle and flattens it out. The problem is that this procedure wears off in four or five months, so that you may need to make frequent visits to maintain the effect.

Some women want a lighter, smoother skin and want to refine the fine lines and wrinkles. For this, they would have a chemical peel, where a strong exfoliating product is applied to the skin to remove the damaged layer or layers and unsightly bumps and pigmentation. The strength of the peel depends on the extent of the damage. The time the skin takes to heal and stop looking sensitive depends on the strength of the peel. The peel also causes the skin to regenerate while it is healing, giving you a smoother, younger looking skin.

The same type of result may be obtained through laser treatments, where the imperfections of the skin are burnt off using a very fine, high intensity beam of light. Some laser and peel treatments are very mild or superficial and need to be repeated monthly for four to six months before changes can be seen. The recovery time is rapid, with some skin redness for only 24 hours.

Other treatments are more aggressive or deeper and result in more noticeable changes in skin texture and pigment. The recovery time is longer, more in the order of a few days to a week of skin redness or sensitivity. Deeper lines can be plumped out using injections of one of the many available 'fillers' like fat, collagen or *hyaluronic acid*.

Finally, you can investigate the possibility of a facelift, the only effective treatment for the excess hanging skin in the neck, jowl and cheek areas. The latest procedure in this type of surgery has gone beyond 'pull and tuck'. Surgeons now operate in such a way that they reposition the face and fill it out. If you don't want anything as drastic as a facelift, you can have surgery to remove the bags above or under your eyes.

And talking about eyes, many women really battle with dry, red, itchy, and blurred eyes when they reach menopause; the blurring is caused by the fact that the eye no longer has a smooth film over it. Apart from the fact that red, blurry eyes don't look great, these symptoms can make you feel very tired at the end of a day because when clear vision is compromised and you are struggling to see clearly, it can be exhausting.

Here's a tip: don't wait until your eyes are dry all the time. When you reach perimenopause start to use products like eye drops that have the same composition as natural tears to keep your eyes moist. You can use them several times a day (hourly or once every two hours) and they really help. There is also a tear gel that mimics the moisturising action of your tears, coating the surface of the eye and protecting it from the drying effects – the dose depends on what works for you.

At night you can try a special lubricating eye ointment to help your eyes stay moist. If your eyes are very dry don't have the air conditioner on in your car, drink a lot of water and use a humidifier at night if you have a heater or air conditioner on in your bedroom. There is a new product, *cyclosporine ophthalmic emulsion* (Restasis), which may be helpful in treating a severe dry eye problem.

If the drops, gels or ointments are not at all helpful, there is a procedure that may relieve the dryness. The ophthalmologist will insert punctual plugs into your eyes. The *punctin* is a tiny duct that drains tears from your eyes into the nose. It is situated in the lower part of your eye, near your nose. The plug is a mechanical blockage and helps whatever tears you have left in your eye to stay there and not drain out. You should get your eyes checked annually for age-related problems such as cataracts and glaucoma. You've probably already noticed that your eyesight has changed in middle age and a lot of headaches are caused by impaired vision.

Is your mind working properly?

Many women and their healthcare practitioners have been confused and often unnecessarily worried by research which seems to suggest that women who are not on long-term HT may be at risk for dementia and damaged cognitive functioning. This means that they may suffer from poor memory and lose certain intellectual skills. According to the experts, cognition includes all kinds of brain functions like memory, the ability to learn, facility with language and the way you solve problems.

One of our great fears is the thought that if we are careless and don't use HT we might be candidates for diminished cognitive ability and, horror of horrors, Alzheimer's disease. Our worry is further compounded by the fact that we now know that the risks of HT may outweigh the benefits. We become afraid that if we are prone to severe hot flushes we may be putting ourselves at risk. I think that this kind of anxiety and fear can be very damaging because it can drive women to make emotive decisions without really understanding the facts. In Chapter 6 I described the mechanism of a hot flush but I didn't explain that the brain regulates its own blood supply so that it is not affected by changes in core body temperature. So even if you feel that you're going to burst into flame during a hot flush, your brain is taking care of itself.

Much of the early research seemed to indicate that menopausal women would do better intellectually if they took estrogen, but after the WHI, which I discussed at length in Chapter 3, these ideas were turned upside down. Although the experts agree that estrogen may have a protective effect on the brain there is no adequate clinical proof that this information is valid.

The WHI found that contrary to previous beliefs, the memories of women who had gone through the perimenopausal transition were no worse than those of any other women, nor was there a decline in the speed with which they calculated problems, and, guess what, they actually improved slightly in these areas over time! Once again, the results of many of the previous studies were influenced by the fact that the women in the trials who had decided to take HT were usually better educated, younger and healthier, so it was highly likely that they were going to do well in cognitive tests. Factors other than lowered levels of estrogen, for instance depression, anxiety, sleep deprivation and lifestyle, can affect memory and cognitive performance As far as the terror of dementia is concerned, research shows that there is no real evidence that HT reduces the risk of dementia in older menopausal women, in fact, as the WHI showed, it may put them at greater risk.

Studies have shown that the risk of dementia is greater in older women who start HT later in life. There is no clinical trial evidence that hormone therapy at any age protects women against Alzheimer's disease. However, proponents of the timing hypothesis believe that more research is needed to establish whether the age at which women have HT, or if they start HT at onset of menopause, will reduce the risk of dementia.

Research has shown that sudden and dramatic falls in estrogen in younger women who have had an abrupt surgical menopause may affect brain function, so those women may want to have HT subject to the advice of their doctors. It is clear that when women are battling with hot flushes, distress and high levels of anxiety their cognitive ability may be affected. It is also thought that fluctuating levels of estrogen in naturally menopausal women produce those memory lapses so feared by menopausal women. But it has also been found that once a woman's hormones level out and stabilise in post- menopause, her memories are generally fine.

Generally, large observational studies on women with natural menopause show no strong evidence that there are any midlife cognitive changes during the transition from peri- to postmenopause. More research needs to be conducted to determine whether *some* mental abilities may be affected.

Very recent research looked into whether there was a difference between mental performance in pre-, peri- and post-menopausal women. The study tested whether there was a relationship between the amount of estrogen in the blood of these different women and their mental abilities. This research found that once the effects of getting older were taken into account, there was no difference between the three groups in relation to: *long-term memory*, which includes *episodic memory* (storage of facts and personal experiences that belong to particular places and times); *semantic memory* (facts, ideas, words, problem solving); *ease in using spoken or written language*; *visuospatial ability* (an ability to understand the way objects work together in a space like doing a jigsaw); or in *the ability to recognise faces*. In addition, there was no relationship between the amount of estrogen in the blood of each group of women and they way they performed in these tests. Two longitudinal studies (studies that follow subjects over a period of time, documenting changes) found that being menopausal did not relate to the women's cognitive decline.

It's important to ensure that you live healthily and control the amount of saturated fats in your diet so that you lower your risk of developing arteriosclerosis, which could cause the arteries in your brain to get clogged up with plaque, affecting the blood supply to the brain and causing cognitive damage. There is ongoing research investigating the protective and anti-inflammatory effect of estrogen on the brain, but in the meantime, it seems sensible to consider revising

253

the old adage and, in pursuit of 'healthy body, healthy mind', keep your bad cholesterol levels low. Monitor your blood pressure (see Chapter 7) and live healthily. Be careful what you eat (see Chapter 10) because you also need to keep your blood sugar levels stable, since both too much and too little glucose can affect brain function. Don't drink too much and exercise regularly. Physical fitness is essential for good brain health.

Don't get too hung up on everything you read – all the conflicting information or every scary newspaper article. If you have a family history of dementia or Alzheimer's disease, or any of the other risk factors that I have mentioned above, get expert help from a good neurologist or endocrinologist, see that you keep an open mind about all the available treatment options and never be afraid to ask questions and get answers that you understand. This will enable you to make careful, informed decisions about your cognitive functioning. Your doctor should be staying abreast of all the current research in this area, and there are robust, ongoing studies. There is work being done to develop a selective estrogen receptor modulator for the brain called a *neuroSERM*, which may shed some light on the role estrogen plays in the brain.

I am a believer in 'use it or lose it', so I think it's very important that middle-aged women don't just 'veg out' but exercise their brains as thoroughly as they do their bodies. If you don't have a career or an interesting job, find an intellectual pursuit. Join a book club that demands a written report on the books you have read. Learn a language, play bridge. Join a music appreciation group. Study something new. Go back to university and get a second or first degree. Start becoming involved in politics or world issues and stretch your mind by reading differently. Some midlife women develop a fascination with share portfolios and investments. Once you start using your brain, you'll be amazed at just how well it works.

Headaches and Migraines

While on the subject of the brain, I think this is a good time to look at headaches and migraine in peri- and postmenopause. There's no doubt if you think back to the headaches you suffered when you had PMS that fluctuating hormone levels can cause these.

Many perimenopausal women battle with headaches, even though some of them have had many headache-free years after their adolescent episodes, while others who never had a headache in their lives are suddenly experiencing some real shockers. Some women find their headaches get better in perimenopause, other long-time migraine sufferers battle as never before.

Usually women with migraines find that they have warning of an attack when they experience an aura. This means either lots of little flashing lights, or a funny zigzag light which cuts your vision in half, or a kind of sparkling at the side of your eye which pursues you when you turn your head. You can also get blurred vision, a funny taste in your mouth, slur your words, feel a tingling on your face and have numb fingertips. These are usually accompanied by a sinking heart as you prepare for what's in store.

Many women who have, in the past, had these warning signs before they plunge into their migraine with all its attendant symptoms, such as blinding pain, nausea and sensitivity to light, find suddenly in perimenopause that they just go straight into the migraine. Strangely though, some women whose aura was always followed by migraine just experience the aura, which continues for a short while and then disappears, leaving them without a headache. If you have always suffered from migraines, you won't be too concerned, but if you start to get migraines with an aura, or if you just get the aura, you should have yourself thoroughly checked by a neurologist. In fact, it might be a good idea not to take migraines or severe headaches of any kind for granted, have a neurological check-up and rule out any sinister possibilities, like a risk for stroke.

A very common type of perimenopausal headache seems to cause a pounding in the head accompanied by the sensation of a vice-like grip at the back of the head.

It is thought that the fluctuating levels of estrogen may be associated with bad migraines in perimenopausal women, but it's not the temporary high levels of estrogen that causes it but the sudden drop afterwards. The bad news is that if you were the kind of woman who got bad headaches during your period, you will probably find that your sensitivity to fluctuating hormone levels affects you quite badly now.

If you were a migraine sufferer you might have found that your headaches got worse immediately after your surgical menopause, which is probably the result of the rapid drop in your estrogen level. HT has sometimes helped balance the hormone levels of perimenopausal women with migraines. But be careful: if you were the kind of woman whose hormone fluctuations caused migraines, it would be better for you to take continuous combined rather than sequential HT (first the estrogen and then the progestin) and don't forget, as I explained in Chapter 4, the best method is through your skin, using a patch, cream or gel.

The good news is that once the hormones have stabilised after the perimenopausal stage most women stop having migraines or have far fewer episodes. However, a very large study showed that women who use HT were more likely to get migraines, and that the actual risk of getting a migraine was increased in these women whether they used ET or an EPT. The problem is that the study could not determine if using HT caused the headaches or if there is a tendency among menopausal women who suffer from migraines to use hormone therapy. So if you find you are suffering worse migraines since you have been on HT, it would probably be wise to stop until there is clearer evidence. All postmenopausal women who have battled with headaches and/or migraines (which are vascular events) should discuss all their options with their doctors; the best dose, type of hormone, and whether or not a transdermal hormone might be better. In general, migraine sufferers should be extremely cautious when deciding whether or not to take HT.

Vanessa laughed ruefully: 'Since I've become perimeno-pausal if I have more than one glass of wine, no matter what I do, even drinking several glasses of water before I

go to sleep, I wake with a dreadful, pounding headache.
I can't stand it. My husband and I are wine fundis and
get such pleasure from our wine collection, which we've
built up over the years. I'm sure it's connected to meno-
pause because my periods are irregular and I'm now in
my fifties, but I'd rather have hot flushes than this!'

As Vanessa's hormone levels changed, so has something in her body's chemistry that is telling her that her body can no longer tolerate more than one glass of wine at a time. It is highly likely that this problem will resolve itself once she is through the perimenopausal stage, but for the moment she just has to grin and bear it, carefully choosing and savouring the one glass she is able to drink. It's important to look out for other headache triggers in peri- and postmenopause: dieting excessively (especially the high protein, low carbohydrate diets), dehydration, tension in your back and neck muscles, stress, anxiety or depression, and certain foods which contain MSG or sulphur, or are highly processed.

Some women may find they have increased sinus headaches caused by hormonally related changes in their nasal membranes. A healthy diet, a proper exercise regimen, massages, anti-inflammatory medication, drinking six to eight glasses of water daily, dealing with your problems in a constructive way and learning to relax should help prevent bad headaches if you are prone to them.

And the correct medication, such as beta-blockers, antiepileptics, antidepressants, some calcium channel blockers, selected painkillers and anti-inflammatory medication, prescribed by a specialist physician or a neurologist, will help. Triptans are a group of medications used to treat migraine headaches. A migraine is a disorder involving nerves and blood vessels, thought to be caused by swelling of the blood vessels of the head due to on and off activation and inflammation of nerve cells in the brain. Triptans work by shrinking these swollen blood vessels and reducing the inflammation. They help relieve migraine pain and the associated symptoms of nausea and vomiting. Some supplements like magnesium have been found to be helpful, but don't give up too quickly if it doesn't seem to work immediately; it needs to be taken for at least three months for the benefits to be felt. Certain antioxidant supplements like Coenzyme Q10 may also be helpful, but there is not enough research yet to prove that they are truly effective.

Rebound headaches may cause huge problems for many peri- and postmenopausal women. The supplement fanatic Laurie, quoted in Chapter 5, was addicted to painkillers. Many of these drugs have a two-fold effect because they have a type of sedative in them which makes a woman feel good, and they also contain a painkiller. The problems arise when you take them for more than three days, because once you are hooked on them, if you don't take them they initiate a headache which will only get better when you treat it with the same medication.

You would be surprised how common this kind of headache is among middle-aged women. You need to see a headache specialist if you are getting these kind of headaches and wean yourself off the medication, although some specialists may suggest that you go 'cold turkey' and get some kind of anti-inflammatory medicine to help you deal with the pain. If you are really addicted to painkillers, you will find the withdrawal period very hard, but it's worth the anguish, and about five weeks after stopping these drugs, you should be either headache-free or much improved.

Depression

One of the main causes of lack of sexual desire in middle-aged women is depression. Many of the symptoms of perimenopause are mood-related and many of you will recognise them – mood swings, panic attacks, a lack of positive feeling or the absence of your usual cheerfulness, weepiness, anxiety, impatience, a short temper, grumpiness, lowered tolerance, unwarranted anger at what you feel to be invasions of your space, tension, jumpiness or restlessness, a sense of worthlessness and hopelessness. Depression is an umbrella term that can encompass all or some of those emotions.

A lot of trials have been dedicated to determining whether depression in peri- and postmenopausal women is related to estrogen levels. One interesting finding was that once women had gone through the perimenopausal years and become fully menopausal, levels of depression dropped, which means that the depression can be blamed on fluctuating levels of estrogen since women who have bad hot flushes and/or night sweats seem to become more depressed. This may also be related to the discomfort and lack of sleep caused by these symptoms, or by other issues that crop up at this stage of your life. Medical research has shown that menopausal women may suffer from bad hot flushes as a result of reduced serotonin levels, which are probably caused by lowered levels of estrogen. In Chapter 4 I discussed the use of various selective serotonin re-uptake inhibitors (SSRIs) – venlafaxine, fluoxetine, paroxetine, sertraline and citalopram – which appear to alleviate hot flushes.

It seems logical to use these same antidepressants to treat depression in perimenopausal women. Depression is a very debilitating illness, yet many women are ashamed that they feel depressed, subscribing to the old notion that it's 'all in their heads' and if they just 'pulled themselves together', they would feel better. This just isn't so, and even if many of the contributing factors are psychological, once you are not well it makes sense to get the appropriate medication so that you can cope better.

Some women try complementary medicines during this time, but there isn't enough evidence to show that these are safe and effective in the long run. I find it strange that people have no problem taking medication for diabetes or for bad headaches but baulk at antidepressants. This is a great pity, because as I wrote earlier, many depressed women find that when they are no longer in the perimenopausal stage they feel less depressed.

Many psychiatrists suggest medication for a short time – between six months and a year. If you're feeling depressed ask your doctor to refer you to a psychiatrist and have a proper assessment. If you decide to take an antidepressant, be warned that it might aggravate any libido problems you may have, but since depression dampens sexual desire in any case, it may be okay just to feel better, so that you can have pleasant sex. For some women antidepressants may have other side effects, such as weight gain or loss, but usually women are so relieved to feel better that these are not problematic.

There are other ways to deal with depression – a relatively easy solution is to exercise regularly. There is a plethora of literature showing that mood improves with a good workout or a brisk walk. Many women say that they notice that their mood worsens when they don't exercise and they definitely feel more depressed.

In my experience, many women become depressed during perimenopause for reasons other than fluctuating levels of estrogen. When they reach midlife women may be dealing with many losses. Although many find it fun to be alone with their partners when their children leave home, some find that the reason for their existence has been taken away and, more frightening, that they are no longer needed as their children make their way in the world. At the same time though, the demands of their children may have been replaced by the demands of elderly and infirm parents.

When the house is empty, women are forced to interact on a one-on-one basis with their partners for the first time in many years and the experience may not fill their souls. Some realise that their marriage is empty or a sham, or that in the intervening years they and their partner have grown apart and are no longer in love. Those women who have given up their identities and careers to look after their families may feel unfulfilled, as though they have wasted their lives. Their partners may still be busy and occupied, while they have a lot of empty time on their hands. There are women who are content with the status quo, but others find themselves unaccountably sad as they examine lost opportunities or missed chances. Some women who have never had children, and have been happy with the fact, suddenly feel bereft when menopause is inexorably upon them. Still others mourn their lost youth and beauty.

These feelings of loss may be aggravated by the fact that this is a time in many of our lives when we begin to lose those who have been closest to us – parents, spouses, partners and friends.

My sense is that menopause is a time to come to terms with these losses and the unresolved grief in our lives. Perhaps we have never had time before to stop and carefully examine our lives. Perhaps we are suddenly aware of the passage of time and the fact that it is running out. We are confronted with elderly parents who are signposts of our own mortality. Is it any surprise that so many middle-aged women suffer from depression?

Some kind of therapy may be a very good idea. There are different types of therapy out there and you should choose something that appeals to you personally. It is probably a good idea to work through these issues with a woman, preferably a middle-aged one. This is not because I don't believe there are good male therapists or young therapists available, but because I believe you may need someone who's been there. Menopause is a uniquely feminine and midlife experience. For those women who are suddenly struggling with their relationships, couples therapy may be a good idea. Although your marriage may be basically sound, certain issues need to be aired and dealt with. If you feel you can no longer stay in your relationship, you may need help in making the decision to change the situation.

If you can come to terms with your life in menopause, a new phase will open up to you, and there will be all kinds of extraordinary possibilities. Honouring your body and your psyche will help you to be more energised, interested and live better than ever before.

Empowerment points

- Be brave. If you are having a problem with sex, speak frankly and openly to your partner about it. There are ways to deal with it. Good sex in middle age is possible.

- There are excellent products to help dry vaginas. Find the one that suits you best.

- Regular exercise is a must: it increases sexual desire, helps you to sleep, protects against depression, cognitive decline and ill health, and makes you look and feel great.

- Choose your skincare products carefully. The fact that something smells and feels good is no guarantee that it will benefit your skin.

- Check out all very bad headaches. If you have an aura without a migraine or a migraine with an aura, check that nothing untoward is happening.

- Exercise your brain as you do your body.

- Get some professional help when you're negotiating the sometimes rocky emotional path of peri- and postmenopause.

Notes

_____

_____

_____

_____

_____

_____

_____

_____

_____

_____

_____

_____

_____

_____

_____

CONCLUSION

Speaking Loud and Clear: The Authentic Voice of Menopause

When I began to write this book I went to a talk given by Carol Gilligan, a well-known feminist psychologist who taught at Harvard for more than 30 years and is now a university professor at New York University and the author of several books, including the groundbreaking *In a Different Voice*.

The light that went on in my head stayed with me as I wrote but it is only now as I reach these concluding paragraphs that I truly understand the concept. The stories I have heard and the knowledge I have gained inspired me. I know now that menopause is not an end, but the beginning of a different and possibly a better time for women. It simply depends on how we live the menopausal years.

The very authentic voice of a famous woman in her eighties, who still works tirelessly for human rights, who looks wonderful and who still parties up a storm, echoes in my head: 'I'll flirt till the day I die. It might not get the results it used to but it makes me feel great!' Being menopausal didn't stop her, couldn't stop her. She took charge of her life and lived it all as well as possible; both the serious parts and the most light-hearted. If we choose, the final third of our lives will be extraordinary.

If we take responsibility for our health, if we understand what is happening to our bodies and if we determine what is best for us, the fear that menopause heralds the end of our lives and the myth that we will become estrogen deficient, dried-out, intellectually impaired, sad little old ladies, will be dispelled. We can take charge of ourselves as women and spend the rest of our lives living authentically with humour, vitality, wisdom and wit. Strong, powerful, interesting and sexy, we can go forward and live well in menopause.

A comprehensive list of symptoms of peri- and postmenopause

These symptoms, listed here in alphabetical order, are very individual. You may never experience any of them, you may experience some of them, and very, very rarely will any woman experience all of them. However, you may just not feel great or you may feel different but cannot specify why, and because you are not having hot flushes, for example, a friend may say: 'Oh you can't be having menopause.' Don't listen. Any of the symptoms below may be heralding your menopause. You may sail through menopause as you did through your menstrual periods, when you never experienced PMS, or your pregnancy, when you didn't have morning sickness. It all depends on your own body's chemistry. These are symptoms that may start now that you are in middle age, not symptoms that you have experienced for most of your adult life. When you read this list remember that about 76 per cent of women will probably have some kind of hot flush during menopause while only about 3 per cent will suffer bad headaches or migraines, but even if you aren't suffering from hot flushes, the headaches may be a sign that you are menopausal.

Be warned, however, that some of these symptoms may not be related to the climacteric (the transition period from being fertile to becoming fully menopausal) but may indicate a medical condition, so it is always wise to talk to your doctor when you start experiencing symptoms you haven't had before to rule out any more sinister causes. If you are middle-aged and have a constellation of the symptoms that usually indicate changing hormonal levels, they are probably related to perimenopause, but it is always sensible to make sure.

- Aching ankles, knees, wrists or shoulders
- Altered sleeping patterns
- Bleeding gums
- Bloating
- Breast swelling and tenderness
- Changes in urinary function (urinating more frequently, especially at night)
- Confusion
- Depression
- Difficulty in falling asleep
- Disturbed sleep
- Dizzy spells (people sometimes think they have an inner ear infection)
- Dry eyes
- Dry skin
- Erratic bleeding and spotting
- Feelings of worthlessness and hopelessness
- Forgetfulness
- Generalised anxiety and free-floating anxiety
- Greater urgency in the need to urinate
- Hairs suddenly appearing on your chin
- Headaches and migraines
- Heart palpitations
- Heavy menstrual periods
- Hot flushes (there are several types of hot flushes – see the description on page 116)
- Increased anger, impatience, short-temper, grumpiness
- Insomnia

- Irregular periods
- Itchiness around the vaginal area
- Joint pain
- Jumpiness and restlessness
- Leaking
- Less tolerance of things that irritate you
- Long silky facial hairs
- Loss of libido
- Low-grade fatigue
- Mood swings
- More frequent flatulence, wind pains and indigestion
- Negativity or absence of your usual cheerfulness
- Night sweats
- Painful intercourse
- Panic attacks
- Reluctance to be too close to someone
- Skin that is highly sensitive to human touch or fabrics
- Strange dreams and nightmares
- Sudden bouts of nausea or faintness
- Tension
- Thinning hair
- Unusually bad menstrual cramps
- Unusual skin sensations: prickly or tingling
- Unwarranted anger at what you feel to be an 'invasion' of your space
- Urinary infections
- Vaginal dryness
- Waking much earlier than usual
- Weepiness
- Weight gain, especially round the hips and thighs.

A quick course in empowerment during the peri- and postmenopausal years

- Choose your doctor or gynaecologist carefully. You can question your friends or healthcare practitioners if they have recommended him or her. When you call the practice, you can get a good idea of the doctor's attitude from his receptionist. If she acts like St Peter guarding the gates of heaven, that attitude stems directly from the boss. I know two sets of receptionists/practice administrators who are wonderful, sympathetic and respectful and they are exactly like the doctors for whom they work. The opposite applies to those who are curt, patronising and disrespectful of your time. You have been warned.

- Your doctor should address you respectfully and be prepared to spend time with you, listening carefully to your problems and asking questions. Beware the doctor who leaves you undressed for a serious amount of time in a small consulting room while she or he moves from patient to patient. She or he may be a superb clinician, but is often not paying enough attention. When your hairdresser does your hair, would you be comfortable with him or her moving between you and another client? You are consulting a doctor; you are not a cog in an assembly line.

- It is completely reasonable and sensible to ask your doctor to explain your symptoms and the results of your tests in a way that is clear and easy for you to understand. You should never feel rushed or stupid or that you are wasting his/her time. You have paid for the consultation and this is your time. If she or he does not respond in a manner that is acceptable to you, you must seriously question whether she or he is the correct practitioner for you.

- Never feel awkward about asking questions or asking for a point of information to be clarified.

- Don't accept it when your doctor tells you that she or he thinks you are too young to be perimenopausal or that you will get your menopause when you're 40. Doctors aren't psychic. Insist that you have your FSH and E2 levels tested if you think you may be perimenopausal. There is never any harm in being sure. Even if you aren't experiencing the symptoms of menopause you may want to have a record of your levels as a baseline comparison for the future.

- If you have had tests, the practice should phone you with the results as soon as they are available, and you should be able to discuss these results in detail with your doctor at a follow-up appointment. If the doctor has asked you to call for your results, it is your responsibility to call; don't wait.

- Because so many women in their fifth decade suffer from some kind of thyroid dysfunction, it is vital to eliminate this possibility when you experience what you and your doctor may assume are the symptoms of perimenopause. If your doctor does not recommend that your thyroid function be tested, ask for it.

- In midlife many women find that their lives have become exponentially more stressful for a wide variety of reasons: the empty nest syndrome, changing relationship patterns, self-doubt and angst over lifestyle choices, and a partner who may also be suffering from a midlife crisis. As a result of these stressors, you may be suffering from raised levels of cortisol. If you know that you are unduly stressed and have been so for any length of time, ask your doctor to prescribe a test to check your cortisol levels. Raised levels of cortisol can cause huge physiological and emotional problems. If you think that you have these symptoms they may not only be in your imagination.

- When you are having a check-up before starting HT, or when you return to your gynaecologist for your annual check-up, make a point of telling him or her if you are on any new medication or if you have had any illnesses or medical incidents during the year. For example, you can't expect your doctor to be psychic and intuit that a cardiologist has put you on a blood thinner or that since your last appointment you have been diagnosed with high blood pressure. It's not up to you to decide what is and isn't relevant about your medical history. Let the expert decide. If you don't impart the information you can't blame your doctor for making a bad decision.

- When your doctor quotes a bunch of statistics to show you how beneficial a hormone treatment is, don't be overwhelmed. Ask him or her to explain the statistics to you. Ask whether the risk is relative or absolute. Ask about the research; check out the sample numbers and find out whether the research is recent and whether it has been published in a prestigious journal such as the *New England Journal of Medicine*, *The Lancet*, and the *Journal of the American Medical Association*.

- Don't get carried away when searching the Internet. Recent research has shown that much of the information on the Internet may be incorrect and also dangerous, because the sites may belong to those whose commercial interests are paramount, or who may have developed crackpot theories which look sensible but have no substantial medical basis. Remember, just because it's on the Net doesn't mean that it's correct. So follow the same rules that you would when evaluating printed information. Are the authors identified and have they declared their commercial interests? Ask your doctor to recommend some good sites. She or he should be delighted to help you get the most useful information.

- If you're anxious about taking a particular medication, don't be afraid to question your practitioner or get a second opinion. You might not want to take a risk that your practitioner deems acceptable.

- Think for yourself and use your own judgement. The fact that your doctor's wife is on 0.625 mg of CEE doesn't mean that it's okay for you.

- When you decide to stop your HT you should probably wean yourself off it slowly. The way in which you do this depends on the type of HT you are taking. Discuss this with your doctor. I believe that it is better for your body to become gradually accustomed to having lower levels of estrogen. If you stop it abruptly you may experience the same sort of symptoms that come from fluctuating levels of estrogen in perimenopause.

- Always tell your healthcare practitioner what supplements you are taking. Many supplements have been shown to have side effects and others may react with medicines that you are taking, interfering with them or causing unwanted reactions. A good doctor today will have taken the trouble to make him or herself aware of the latest research on supplements and should be able to advise you. If your practitioner can't help you in this regard, find a certified dietician or a specialist physician who has this knowledge and spend some time discussing your lifestyle, especially your daily diet, with him or her. She or he will soon pick up areas where you may be lacking in vital supplements or be able to tell you that you are on the right track.

- Don't be gullible or naïve. Always ask yourself about the self-interest of the person who is trying to sell you supplements.

- Be sure to buy your supplements from someone who is really knowledgeable. A person who is selling supplements as part of a pyramid group just can't be as knowledgeable as an expert, and once again his or her advice may be biased by a profit motive.

- Eat a healthy, varied diet. You can get most of the vital nutritional supplements you need from a sensible, well-balanced meal plan.

- Have a baseline hormone test before you have your ovaries removed to check whether or not you are peri-menopausal. If you are already menopausal or have very low levels of estrogen and have not been battling with symptoms before surgery, you may or may not need a very low dose of estradiol. Many women find that their problems start after a surgical menopause because the dose of ET they are on is just too high.

- Always get a second, or even a third, opinion before you decide to have major surgery like a hysterectomy.

- Be aware of the risk of heart disease and take control of your life. All your particular risk factors, such as your lifestyle and family history, whether you smoke or are overweight, plus any others should be taken into consideration and carefully discussed with your doctor. If you're a smoker, stop smoking immediately.

- Women who are having heart attacks don't often complain of chest pain; they are more likely to report pain in their necks, the middle of their backs or their jaws. They often describe palpitations, a feeling of indigestion, shortness of breath and often nausea, which may be combined with vomiting.

- Until there is more evidence, HT should not be used to prevent cardiovascular disease when other studies show unambiguously that there are other drugs, like statins, which really work.

- Make a comprehensive list of questions before your consultation with a specialist, especially if you are dealing with surgery or a major illness. Take someone with you to take notes or use a tape recorder. It is impossible to assimilate all the information you will be given when you are in a highly emotional state. However it is sensible to prepare a list of questions in advance no matter what your problem is. When we find ourselves in a doctor's consulting room we may get flustered or anxious.

- Live as healthily as possible but don't ever blame yourself if you get cancer.

- Be sure to have an annual gynaecological examination. An annual mammogram is a must if you have specific, individual reasons, are older than 50, or are on HT. For peace of mind, if you are at high risk for breast cancer, arrange to have an ultrasound every six months in addition to your annual examination.

- Work in partnership with your oncologist to get the best out of your treatment; if something worries you or you don't understand some point of information, don't be afraid to ask over and over again until you are satisfied that you understand what's going on.

- Get good counselling once you are diagnosed with cancer. Having a safe place to let off steam, scream, weep and shout will help deal with those overwhelming feelings.

- Osteoporosis is a silent disease and only proper screening will show whether you are at risk for it.

- Living well is a good way to help protect yourself against osteoporosis: eat sensibly and exercise at least five times a week.

- Know your risk factors for osteoporosis. If you do, you can eliminate any risks that are in your control and protect yourself against those that aren't, like a family history, a particular medication or illness.

- Take adequate calcium and vitamin D: 1200-1500 mg of elemental calcium; 800 IU of vitamin D.

- There is no such thing as a painless way to lose weight.

- Stay away from fad diets. Lose weight on a sensible meal plan at a sensible rate: not more than two to four kilograms a month.

- Watch your calories and refuse second helpings. It doesn't matter what the diet is, once the portions and calories are restricted, women lose weight.

- If you know you're going to a dinner party or will be eating at a special restaurant, pace yourself during the day.

- Some women do better when they eat every couple of hours. So you may have breakfast at 8am, a snack at 10am, lunch at 1pm, a snack at 4pm, dinner at 7pm, with a snack at about 9pm. If the food you eat is sensible, your insulin levels will be balanced and you won't have unwarranted food cravings.

- Learn to know what true hunger feels like. Don't eat out of habit, boredom or for comfort, and don't wait until you're ravenous before you eat.

- Vary your diet. You'll be surprised at how many things you can eat and still lose weight.

- Find someone to monitor you. Research has shown that those women who had support when they were on a diet and then went on to a weight maintenance programme did much better than those who had to go it alone.

- Watch the amount of alcohol you consume.

- Don't fall into despair if you've pigged out. Get straight back to your meal plan and your exercise regimen. Take the emotion out of eating once and for all. When you eat well and exercise, you're being kind to and looking after yourself

- Treat yourself occasionally and do it guilt-free.

- Exercise for at least 30 minutes, five times a week. See that you have a varied exercise programme and always work up a sweat. Regular exercise is a must for middle-aged women; it increases sexual desire, helps to you to sleep, protects against depression, cognitive decline and ill health, and makes you look and feel great.

- Ensure that you drink enough, but not too much, water. Six to eight glasses a day will stop that hungry feeling you may get when you're dehydrated.

- You are not a 'bad girl' when your diet goes awry or you diverge from your meal plan. What you've done may not be great for your health but that's it. A middle-aged woman doesn't need to be bullied and bossed about her weight or judged on it. It's no one's business but your own. Do it for your health's sake and the rest will follow.

- Be brave. If you are having a problem with sex, speak frankly and openly to your partner about it.

- There are excellent products to help dry vaginas. Find the one that suits you best.

- Check out all very bad headaches. If you have an aura without a migraine, or a migraine with an aura, check out that nothing untoward is happening.

- Exercise your brain as you do your body.

- Get professional help when you're negotiating the sometimes rocky emotional path of peri- and postmenopause.

Glossary: medical terms guaranteed to confuse you when you discuss menopause

Absolute risk – the exact number of people at risk per a specific number

Adipose tissue – fat tissue

Adjuvant therapy – treatment that is given in addition to the primary treatment or therapy

Adrenal cascade – the order in which the hormones in the body are manufactured from pregnenolone

Adrenal gland – small gland situated on top of each kidney, which secretes certain sex steroid hormones and cortisol

Amenorrhoea – not having a period when you are still in your reproductive years

Amino acid – a chemical messenger in the body

Antioxidant – a supplement that slows down the rate at which something in the body decays or breaks down because of its interaction with oxygen

Aromatase inhibitors – drugs that block certain tissues, especially in menopausal women, from producing estrogen

Arteriosclerosis – hardening of the arteries

Benign – not life threatening or dangerous – not malignant

Beta-blocker – a medicine that helps to regulate the heart-beat by calming down specific body responses

Bio-available – able to be metabolised by the body

Biochemistry – the chemical interactions that take place in the body, from the cells to the major organs – the chemistry of life

Bioidentical – chemically exactly the same as the biological substance

Bisphosphonate – a medicine that controls the activity of the osteoclasts to limit the breaking down of bone

Bone mineral density – the amount of bone material that is packed into a certain volume of bone

Bone mineralisation – when bone tissue or material is broken down, releasing calcium and phosphate

Carbohydrates – compounds that are made up of carbon, hydrogen and oxygen, eg, sugars, starches, cellulose and gums

Cardiovascular disease – disease of heart, blood vessels

Cervix – the opening of the womb; the narrow end of the uterus that leads into the vagina

Chemotherapy – a chemical treatment in either pill or injection form that travels through the bloodstream killing the cancer cells in the body

Cholesterol – a fatty substance that is found throughout the body in cells, blood, tissues, brain, muscles, and liver. It is found in proteins like meat, chicken, fish and eggs and in dairy products. The liver produces cholesterol and synthesises it. It is essential for healthy living because it plays a vital role in cell repair and the storage and production of energy. All sex steroid hormones come from cholesterol

Cognitive – intellectual functioning. Cognition is the action of knowing and includes all kinds of brain functions like memory, the ability to learn, facility with language and the way people solve problems

Collagen – a fibrous tissue, found throughout the body

Colposcopy – a procedure whereby the cervix is examined with a high-powered magnifying lens and a light inserted into the vagina

Conjugated equine estrogens (CEE) – an estrogen called equinol is synthesised to become this type of estrogen

Core needle biopsy – a biopsy performed on a breast lump so that material can be collected

Corpus luteum – from the Latin meaning yellow body. When the follicle releases the egg by rupturing, it becomes this yellow body

Cortical bone – very hard bone on the outside of the bone which makes up the shaft of the bones

C-reactive protein (CRP) – a very specific protein that is produced by the liver only when the body is experiencing severe injury, infection or inflammation

DEXA scan – dual energy X-ray absorptiometry. The DEXA measures the amount of bone present in a specific area

Double-blind randomised controlled study – a study in which both the patients and the doctor are 'blinded' to the therapy being given

Ductal carcinoma in situ (DCIS) – a cancer in the breast duct that has not invaded the surrounding tissue

Ducts – tubes or canals. In this book the tubes or canals in the breasts

Elastin – fibres that make the skin elastic

Embolisation of fibroids – an advanced X-ray technique where the blood supply to the fibroid is cut off, so that it shrinks

Embolism – the blocking of a blood vessel by a plug

Endocrine system – the system of glands that controls all the body's hormones

Endocrinologist – a specialist who deals in the complex interaction of hormones

Endogenous estrogen – the estrogen found in the body

Endometrial ablation – the lining of the womb is burnt away

Endometrial hyperplasia – thickening of the lining of the womb

Endometriosis – endometriosis occurs when endometrial cells grow outside the uterus. The endometrial cells can be found in the ovaries, the fallopian tubes and the pelvic cavity

Endometrium/endometrius – lining of the womb

Endothelium – the layer of thin, flat cells that lines the inside surface of blood vessels. Endothelial cells line the entire circulatory system, from the heart to the smallest capillary

Enzyme – a protein that helps or causes certain chemical reactions in the body

Equinol – estrogen found in pregnant mares

Estrogenic or estrogenated – a state caused by estrogen

Exogenous estrogen – estrogen taken or applied to the body

Fallopian tubes – the two tubes leading from the ovaries to the uterus, down which the egg travels to the womb

Fibroid – benign growth of muscle and connective tissue in the walls of the uterus

Fine needle biopsy – a procedure during which the specialist uses an ultrasound and a very fine needle to take a sample of tissue and the cells

Fluctuating levels – changing levels

Fluid retention – when the body holds excess water

Follicle – a sac-like structure containing the egg

G-spot – the region situated in a woman's genital area, behind her pubic bone. This area surrounds the urethra. Tiny glands called Skene's glands are found here, in the upper wall of the vagina and the lower end of the urethra. The name G-spot is given to the area where the Skene's glands are found

Homocysteine – an amino acid, which can be toxic in high amounts and may be a risk factor in heart disease

Hormones – chemical substances that act as messengers throughout the body

Hydrogenated fats – vegetable oils that have been heated to a very high temperature, then bubbled through with hydrogen

Hypercalcemia – too much calcium

Hypertension – high blood pressure

Hyperthyroidism – an overactive thyroid

Hypocalcemia – too little calcium

Hypothalamus – part of the base of the brain to which the pituitary gland is attached. It regulates many important body functions, memory and emotions

Hypothyroidism – an underactive thyroid

Hysterectomy – surgical removal of the womb

Hysteroscopy – a procedure whereby an instrument is passed through the mouth of the womb to allow the inside of the womb to be viewed

Immune system – the series of organs and chemical reactions that the body uses to protect itself from disease. It also helps the body fight and control the spread of disease

Insulin resistance – although there is enough insulin available in the system, the cells it regulates do not respond to it

Involuted breast – a breast that has collapsed inward so the fatty tissue is not too dense

Isoflavone – a plant estrogen found in soy

Laparoscopy – a procedure whereby a surgeon inserts a small instrument (laparoscope) through the navel into the abdomen, looks at and then treats the patient

Laparotomy – A technique whereby the surgeon makes a cut in the abdomen and removes the fibroid

Libido –sexual desire

Lignans – plant estrogens

Lobes – sections – in this book, specifically sections of the breast

Lobules – smaller lobes

Malignant – life-threatening, virulent. The word refers to a growth which tends to spread and recur and so proves fatal

Mammogram – special X-ray of the breast

Melanoma – a type of skin cancer

Melatonin – a hormone secreted by a small gland in the brain called the pineal gland which is associated with sleep and biological rhythms

Menopause – the last day of a woman's last period

Menstrual cycle – the cyclical changes that occur in the lining of the womb in preparation for accepting a fertilised egg. If there is no fertilised egg the lining is shed, causing a bleed, which is called a period

Metabolic syndrome – a group of symptoms which can cause insulin resistance leading to glucose intolerance or type 2 diabetes. Today it is generally called Insulin Resistance Syndrome

Metabolises – breaks down or builds up

Mineral – a natural inorganic substance with a specific chemical make-up that is vital for healthy body function

Monounsaturated fat – found in avocado, olive oil, canola oil and peanut oil

MRI – magnetic resonance imaging. A specialised medical technique using magnetic resonance rather than X-rays to produce pictures of the inside of the body

Myomectomy – procedure during which a fibroid is surgically removed. It is frequently the chosen treatment for premenopausal women because it usually helps to preserve fertility

Myocardial infarction – heart attack

Neurotransmitter – chemical that allows the transmission of impulses along the nerves

Norepinephrine – a chemical involved with the sympathetic nervous system

Nutraceuticals – products taken from foods, which are said to have proven medical benefits, especially in the prevention of heart disease

Omega-3 and omega-6 fatty acids – vital fats, crucial for the efficient functioning and maintenance of every single cell in the body

Oophorectomy – removal of the ovaries

Osteocytes – cells in the bone that send out `messages' to the body that a specific area of bone needs to be remodelled

Osteoblast – special cells in the bone that build new bone tissue

Osteoclast – special cells in the bones that break down old bone tissue

Ovary – one of two structures in the female body, about the size of an almond, containing all the eggs of your reproductive life

Ovulation – the process whereby the egg is developed and released from the ovary

Ovum – an egg in your ovary

Pancreas – a long gland situated behind and below the stomach, which produces insulin and digestive juices

Perimenopause – the time before and after the actual moment of menopause, around menopause

Pessary – a type of tablet that is inserted into the vagina

Physiological – the normal function of living things

Phytoestrogens – estrogens that are found in plants

Pituitary gland – the most important gland in the endocrine system, situated at the base of the hypothalamus, which produces and controls the actions of many of the most important hormones in the body

Polyunsaturated fat – the fat found in vegetable oils, like corn and sunflower oil as well as fish oils, flaxseed oils, sesame and walnut oil

Postmenopause – after menopause

Precursor – a building block which causes a particular chemical reaction

Radiation – procedure during which the cancer is blasted with X-rays

Radical hysterectomy – surgery during which the womb, cervix and part of the upper area of the vagina, as well as the ovaries, are removed

Receptor – a minute place on the surface of a cell that bonds to one particular substance which then sends a message through the cell membrane

Relative risk – the percentage of people at risk per a given number

Remodelling – in this book, the process whereby bone is broken down and reformed

Resorption – the removal of old bone tissue by the osteoclasts

SERM – selective estrogen receptor modulator. These hormones have a beneficial estrogen effect in certain areas of the body and block unwanted estrogen effects in other parts of the body, so that the amount of active estrogen in the body is not increased

Serotonin – a brain chemical involved with mood, appetite and sleep

Sex-steroid hormones – special hormones that are involved with the growth and functioning of the reproductive organs. They are the hormones that affect male or female sexual characteristics

SSRI – selective serotonin re-uptake inhibitor; a drug that slows the action of the enzyme that destroys excess serotonin and helps a certain amount of serotonin to remain circulating throughout the body, making people feel better. Many antidepressants are SSRIs

Statins – drugs that act on a certain enzyme in the liver, causing a lowering of cholesterol in the blood

Statistics – a method of collecting, analysing and interpreting data

Synthesised – manufactured

Thromboembolic disease – blood clots

Total hysterectomy – surgery during which the uterus and part of the cervix or the entire cervix are removed

Trabecular bone – spongy and soft, it is found at the ends of long bones and in the spine

Transdermal – taken through the skin

Transvaginal ultrasound – an ultrasound performed via the vagina

Tumour – a swelling or enlargement of any part of the body

Type 2 diabetes – this occurs when the pancreas keeps making higher and higher amounts of insulin but eventually becomes exhausted and stops producing the appropriate insulin

Ultrasound – high frequency sound that produces an image

Urethra – a thin tube that carries urine from the bladder through the vagina and from there to the outside of the body

Urinary tract – all the organs that are involved in the production and expulsion of urine from the body

Uterus – womb

Vagina – the passage that leads from the womb to the outside of the body; the area where the penis usually enters the body during intercourse

Vasomotor symptoms – the symptoms caused by the effect of blood vessels when they constrict or dilate. Often used to describe symptoms like the hot flushes and night sweats that women suffer in menopause

Vitamin – organic substances that the human body needs in varying but usually small quantities in order to grow; they help break down and use (metabolise) the food we eat in the most efficient way, ensuring that we function healthily.

Bibliography and Resource List

This list of books, journal articles and websites is intended to help those of you who wish to read further and learn more about aspects of the subjects I have covered in the book. With that in mind I have divided the list into the chapters to which these publications and Internet sites relate.

Chapters 1, 2, 3 and 4

A service of the US National Library of Health and the National Institutes of Health (2004). Cortisol Level. Medline Plus Medical Encyclopaedia. Available online: http://www.uptodate.com.

AACE Menopause Guideline Revision Task Force (2006). 'American Association of Clinical Endocrinologists medical guidelines for clinical practice for the diagnosis and treatment of menopause'. *Endocrinological Practice* 12(3): 315-37.

ACOG Committee (2005). 'Compounded bioidentical hormones: Opinion No. 322'. *Obstetrics & Gynecology* 106: 1139-40.

Al-Azzawi, F and Buckler, HM (2003). 'For the United Kingdom Vaginal Ring Investigator Group. Comparison of a novel vaginal ring delivering estradiol acetate versus oral estradiol for relief of vasomotor menopausal symptoms'. *Climacteric* 6: 18-127.

Alster, T et al (2004). *The aging face: More than skin deep*. The Discovery Institute of Medical Education.

Angier, N (1999). *Woman: An Intimate Geography*. London: Virago.

Arana, A et al (2006). 'Hormone therapy and cerebrovascular events: a population-based nested control study'. *Menopause: The Journal of the North American Menopause Society* 13(5): 730-36.

Archer, DF et al (2007). 'Drosperinone, a progestin with added value for added hypertensive postmenopausal women'. *Menopause: The Journal of the North American Menopause Society* 14(3): 352-4.

Australian Government. National Health and Medical Research Council. Available online: http://www.nhmrc.gov.au/publications/pdf/hrtsumm.pdf.

Balasubramanyam, A (2004). *Disentangling the Threads of the Metabolic Syndrome*. Medscape Conference Coverage based on selected sessions at the ENDO: The Endocrine Society 86th Annual Meeting. Available online: http://www.medscape.com/viewarticle/494115.

Barclay, L and Lie, D (2004). 'Estrogen does not prevent chronic disease in postmenopausal women with hysterectomy'. Medscape Medical News. Available online: http://www.medscape.com/px/urlinfo.

Barclay, L (2004). 'NIH stops estrogen-alone arm of WHI: a newsmaker interview with Jacques Roussouw, MD'. Medscape Medical News. Available online: http://www.medscape.com/px/urlinfo.

Barton, D (2007). 'Clinical assessment and management of hot flashes and sexual function'. *American Society of Clinical Oncology*: 73-7.

Bell, RJ et al (2007). 'Endogenous androgen levels and cardiovascular risk profile in women across the adult life span'. *Menopause: The Journal of the North American Menopause Society* 14(4): 630-38.

Bentley, G and Muttukrishna, S (2007). 'Potential use of biomarkers for analyzing interpopulation and cross-cultural variability in reproductive aging'. *Menopause: The Journal of the North American Menopause Society* 14(4): 668-79.

Birnbaum, L (2002). 'The Case against Relative Risk'. Professionalism of Exercise Physiology 5(2). Available online: http://www.css.edu/users/tboone2/asep/relativeRISK

Buckler, H and Al-Azzawi, F (2003). 'The effect of a novel vaginal ring delivering estradiol acetate on the climacteric symptoms in postmenopausal women'. *British Journal of Obstetrics and Gynaecology* 110: 753-9.

Burger, H et al (2004). 'Practical recommendations for hormone replacement therapy in the peri and post menopause'. Climacteric 7: 1-7. Available online: http://www.imsociety.org/PDF/news_prac_rec.pdf.

Cameron, DR and Braunstein, GD (2004). 'Androgen replacement therapy in women'. *Fertility and Sterility* 82(2): 273-89.

Chatterton, R (2005). 'Characteristics of salivary profiles of oestradiol and progesterone in premenopausal women'. *The Journal of Endocrinology* 186(1): 77-84.

Chatterton, RT (2006). 'Validation of hormone testing'. *Proceedings from the Postgraduate Course presented prior to the 17th Annual Meeting of the North American Menopause Society.*

Cicinelli, E (2007) 'Bioidentical estradiol gel for hormone therapy in menopause'. *Expert Review of Obstetrics & Gynecology* 2(4): 423-430.

Coney, S (1994). *The Menopause Industry: How the medical establishment exploits women*. Almeda, CA: Hunter House.

Cooper, DS (2003). 'Hyperthyroidism'. *The Lancet* 362(9382): 459-68. Available online: http://www.thelancet.com.

Crowther, N (2004). 'The clinical relevance of fasting serum insulin levels in obese subjects'. *South African Medical Journal* 94(7): 519-20.

Cummings, SR (2006). 'LIFT study is discontinued'. *British Menopause Journal* 8(331): 667.

Davey, M (2005). 'Progestogen use in the menopause'. *SAMS Journal* 23(4).

De Villiers, T et al (2007). 'SAMS revised position statement on menopausal hormone therapy'. *SAMS News* 4(2): Issue 8.

Dennerstein, L et al (2007). 'A cross-cultural approach to understanding women's health experiences: a cross-cultural comparison of women aged 20 to 70 years'. *Menopause: The Journal of the North American Menopause Society* 14(4): 688-696.

Dennerstein, L et al (2007). 'Modeling women's health during the menopausal transition: a longitudinal analysis'. *Menopause: The Journal of the North American Menopause Society* 14(1): 53-62.

Drug Digest (2001). 'What are Tibolone Tablets?' Available online: http://www.drugdigest.org/DD?PrintablePages/Monograph/07765,8144%.html.

Ecker, J (2007). 'Evidence and opinion: closing the gap'. *Menopause: The Journal of the North American Menopause Society* 14(1): 3-4.

Ettinger, B (2006). 'When is it appropriate to prescribe postmenopausal hormone therapy?'. *Menopause: The Journal of the North American Menopause Society* 13(3): 404-10.

Ettinger, B et al (2004). 'Effects of ultra low dose transdermal estradiol on bone mineral density: a randomised clinical trial'. *Obstetrics and Gynecology* 104: 443-51.

General Nutrition. *Testing Testosterone.* Available online: http://www.bodyandfitness.com/Information/Menhealth/testosterone.htm

Germano, C and Cabot, W (1999). *The Osteoporosis Solution: New therapies for prevention and treatment.* New York: Kensington Books.

Gilson, GR and Zava, DT (2003). 'Picking up the pieces after the Women's Health Initiative Trial Part 1'. *International Journal of Pharmaceutical Compounding* 7(4).

Goldman, JA (2004). 'The Women's Health Initiative Review and Critique'. *Medscape Ob/Gyn and Women's Health* 6(3). Available online: http://www.medscape.com/px/urlinfo.

Goldstein, S (2005). 'The case for less-than-monthly progestogen in women on HT: Is transvaginal ultrasound the key?'. *Menopause: The Journal of the North American Menopause Society*12(1): 110-13.

Goldstein, SR and Ashner, L (1998). *Could it be ... Perimenopause?*. Boston, New York, Toronto, London: Little, Brown and Company.

Goldstein, SR and Ashner, L (1998). *The Estrogen Alternative: What every women needs to know about Hormone Replacement Therapy and SERMs, the new estrogen substitute*. New York: GP Putnam & Sons.

Gompel, A et al (2007). 'The EMAS update on clinical recommendations on postmenopausal hormone therapy'. *Maturitas* 56: 227-29.

Gruber, C et al (2002). 'Productions and actions of estrogens'. *New England Journal of Medicine* 346(6): 340-52.

Grundy, SM et al (2004). 'Definition of Metabolic Syndrome: Report of the National Lung and Blood Institute/American Heart Association Conference on Scientific Issues Related To Definition'. *Circulation* 109: 433-8.

Henrich, JB et al (2006). 'Limitations of follicle -stimulating hormone in assessing menopause status: findings from the National Health & Nutrition Examination Survey (NHANES 1999-2000)'. *Menopause: The Journal of the North American Menopause Society* 13(2): 171-77.

Herrington, DM (1999). 'The HERS trial results: paradigms lost? Heart and Estrogen/progestin Replacement Study'. *Annals of Internal Medicine* 131(6): 463-6.

Hormone Replacement Therapy The Agents (2002): 26-45. Available online: http://www.Harcourt-international.com/e-books pdf/449.pdf.

'Interview with Christiane Northrup MD, FACOG' (1998). *International Journal of Pharmaceutical Compounding* 2(1): 12-17.

Jacobs, G et al (2004). 'Cognitive Behavior Therapy Should Be First-Line Therapy for Sleep-Onset Insomnia'. *Archives of Internal Medicine* 164: 1888-96.

Jadad, AR and Gagliardi, A (1998). 'A Rating Health Information on the Internet: Navigating to Knowledge or to Babel?' *Journal of the American Medical Association* 279: 611-14.

Landau, C, Cyr, MG and Moulton, AW (1994). *The Complete Book of Menopause*. New York: Perigee.

Larsen, R; Kronenberg, HM; Melmed, S and Polonsky, KS (eds) (2003). *Williams Textbook of Endocrinology, 10th ed.* Philadelphia, PA: W B Saunders.

Long, C et al (2006). 'A randomized comparative study of the effects of oral and topical estrogen therapy on the vaginal vascularization and sexual function in hysterectomized postmenopausal women'. *Menopause: The Journal of the North American Menopause Society* 13(5): 737-43.

Love, SM and Lindsay, K (1997). *The Hormone Dilemma. Should you take HRT?* New York: Random House.

Lundstrom, E et al (2002). 'Effects of Tibolone and Continuous Combined Hormone Replacement Therapy on Mammographic Breast Density'. *American Journal of Obstetrics and Gynecology* 186(4): 717-22.

Manson, J et al (2006). 'Postmenopausal hormone therapy: new questions and the case for new clinical trials'. *Menopause: The Journal of the North American Menopause Society* 13(1): 139-47.

Martens, M (2007). 'Ecology and the health of the menopausal vagina'. *Menopause Management* 16(4): 30-6.

McGaugh, JL. Panel: 'The Science of Memory and Emotion. How Emotions Strengthen Memory'. Project on the Decade of the Brain, Library of Congress.1990-2000. Available online: http://www.loc.gov/loc/brain/emotion/Mcgaugh.html.

Menon, U et al (2007). 'Decline in use of hormone therapy amongst postmenopausal women in the United Kingdom'. *Menopause: The Journal of the North American Menopause Society* 14(3): 462-67.

Mills, D. 'Because you're trying to get off HRT, here's the approach we recommend'. Available online: http://www.womentowomen.com/chooseoffhrt.asp.

Morris, C E (1996). *Psychology: an introduction.* 9th ed. New Jersey: Prentice Hall.

Murray, J (1998). 'Natural Progesterone: What Role in Women's Healthcare?' Project Aware. Part 1. September 1998. Available online: http://www.project-aware.org/Resource/articlearchives/Progesterone_Murray1.shtml.

Nachtigall, L (2004). 'The Forum: Hormone Therapy'. *OB/GYN Special Edition* (Spring).

Nachtigall, LE (2006). 'Bioidentical versus non-bioidentical hormones'. *Proceedings from the Postgraduate Course presented prior to the 17th Annual Meeting of the North American Menopause Society.*

Nappi, RE et al (2001). 'Course of Primary Headaches During Hormone Replacement Therapy'. *Maturitas* 38(2).

National Women's Health Network: 'A Voice for Women, a Network for Change'. Available online: http://www.nwhn.org/about/index.php.

Nauton, M et al (2006). 'Estradiol gel: a review of the pharmacology, pharmokinetics, efficacy and safety in menopausal women'. *Menopause: The Journal of the North American Menopause Society* 13(3): 517-27.

North American Menopause Society Hormone Therapy Advisory Panel (2003). 'Estrogen and Progestogen use in peri- and postmenopausal women: September 2003 position statement of the North American Menopause Society'. *Menopause: the Journal of The North American Menopause Society* 10(6): 497-506.

Northrup, C (2001). *The Wisdom of Menopause*. London: Piatkus.

Northrup, C (2004). 'Women to Women'. Available online: http://www.womentowomen.com/howitworks.asp.

Notelovitz, M and Tonneson, D (1993). *Menopause and Midlife Health*. New York: T Martin's Press.

Patching van der Sluijs, C et al (2007). 'Women's health during mid-life survey: the use of complementary and alternative medicine by symptomatic women transitioning through menopause in Sydney'. *Menopause: The Journal of the North American Menopause Society* 14(3): 397-403.

Peled, Y et al (2007). 'Levonorgestrel-releasing intrauterine system as an adjunct to estrogen for the treatment of menopausal symptoms-a review'. *Menopause: The Journal of the North American Menopause Society* 14(3): 550-54.

Pick, M (2004). 'Perspective on the Risks of HRT'. *Women to Women*. Available online: http://www.womentowomen.com/LIB-perspectiveonrisks.asp.

Position Statement (2006). 'Bioidentical hormones'. *The Endocrine Society*.

Position Statement (2007). 'Estrogen and progestogen use in peri- and postmenopausal women: March 2007. Position statement of the North American Menopause Society'. *Menopause: The Journal of the North American Menopause Society* 14(2): 168-82.

Position Statement (2007). 'The role of local vaginal estrogen for treatment of vaginal atrophy in postmenopausal women: 2007 position statement of the North American Menopause Society'. *Menopause: The Journal of the North American Menopause Society* 14(3): 357-69.

Position Statement. 'Recommendations for estrogen and progestogen use in peri- and post menopausal women: October 2004 position statement of the North American Menopause Society'. *Menopause: the Journal of the North American Menopause Society* (11)6: 589-600.

Power, ML et al (2007). 'Evolving practice and attitudes toward hormone therapy of obstetrician-gynecologists'. *Menopause: The Journal of the North American Menopause Society* 14(1): 20-28.

Preston, R et al (2007). ' Randomized, placebo-controlled trial of the effects of drosperinone-estradiol on blood pressure and potassium balance in hypertensive postmenopausal women receiving hydrochlorothiazide'. *Menopause: The Journal of the North American Menopause Society* 14(3): 408-14.

Pritchard, K (2004). 'Debating the issues: Should we bury Tamoxifen? Should we disclose positive data early?' Medscape Ob/Gyn and Women's Health. Available online: http://www.medscape.com/viewarticle/47405?.

ProjectAware (2002). Association of Women for the Advancement of Research and Education. *About Progesterone*. Available online: http://www.project-aware.org/Managing/Hrt/progesterone.shtml.

Redmond, G (1995). *The Good News About Women's Hormones: Complete information and proven solutions for the most common hormonal problems*. New York: Warner Books Inc.

Rigby, A et al (2007). 'Women's awareness and knowledge of hormone therapy post-Women's Health Initiative'. *Menopause: The Journal of the North American Menopause Society* 14(5): 853-58.

Roberts, CGP and Laderson PW (2004). 'Hypothyroidism'. *The Lancet* 363: 793-803. Available online: http://www.thelancet.com.

Rolnick, SJ et al (2007). 'Provider management of menopause after the findings of the Women's Health Initiative'. *Menopause: The Journal of the North American Menopause Society* 14(3): 441-49.

SAMS News 1(1), September 2004.

Santoro, N et al (2007). 'Helping midlife women predict the onset of the final menses: SWAN, the Study of Women's Health Across the Nation'. *Menopause: The Journal of the North American Menopause Society* 14(3): 415-24.

Sarkar, NN (2003). 'Low-dose intravaginal estradiol delivery using a Silastic vaginal ring for estrogen replacement therapy in postmenopausal women: a review'. *European Journal of Contraception and Reproductive Health Care* 8(4): 217-24.

Shakir, Y et al (2004). 'Combined hormone therapy in postmenopausal women with features of metabolic syndrome. Results from a population-based study of Swedish women: Women's Health in the Lund Area study'. *Menopause: the Journal of the North American Menopause Society* 11(5): 549-55.

Shifren, JL et al (2006). 'Testosterone patch for the treatment of hypoactive sexual desire disorder in naturally menopausal women: results from the INTIMATE NM1 study'. *Menopause: The Journal of the North American Menopause Society* 13(5): 770-79.

Simon, JA et al (2006). 'A clinical review and discussion of the efficacy and safety of a new transdermal form of hormone therapy'. *Women's Health Update.*

Simon, JA et al (2006). 'Understanding the controversy; hormone testing and bioidentical hormones'. *Proceedings from the Post-*

graduate Course presented prior to the 17th Annual Meeting of the North American Menopause Society.

Slater, CC et al (2001). 'Markedly Elevated Levels of Estrone Sulfate After Long-term Oral, but Not Transdermal, Administration of Estradiol in Postmenopausal Women'. *Menopause: the Journal of the North American Menopause Society* 8(3): 200-3.

Somers, S (2002). *The Sexy Years*. New York: Crown, Random House.

Speroff, L (2003). 'Efficacy and tolerability of a novel estradiol vaginal ring for relief of menopausal symptoms'. *Obstetrics and Gynecology* 102(4): 823-34.

Speroff, L et al (2006). 'Efficacy of a new oral estradiol acetate formulation for relief of menopausal symptoms'. *Menopause: The Journal of the North American Menopause Society* 13(3): 442-50.

Sturdee, DW et al (2004). 'The acceptability of a small intrauterine progestogen-releasing system for continuous combined hormone therapy in early postmenopausal women'. *Climacteric* 7: 404-11.

Templeton, Allan (ed) (1998). *Evidence Based Fertility Treatment*. London: RCOG Press.

United States Department of Health and Human Services. *Women's Health Initiative: WHI Background and Overview*. Available online: http://www.nhlbi.nih.gov/whi/background.htm.

Utian, W (2004). 'Development and clinical application of guidelines, consensus opinions, and position statements. The need for clinical judgement beyond the evidence'. *Menopause: the Journal of the North American Menopause Society* 11(6): 583-4.

Vogel, JJ (2006). 'Selecting bioidentical hormone therapy'. *Proceedings from the Postgraduate Course presented prior to the 17th Annual Meeting of the North American Menopause Society.*

Vongpatanasin, W (2003). 'Differential effects of oral versus transdermal estrogen replacement therapy on C-reactive protein in postmenopausal women'. *Journal of American Cardiology* 41: 1358-63.

Waknine, Y (2004). 'Testosterone patch can improve sexual function in women'. *Medscape Medical News*. Medscape NAMS 15th Annual Meeting: Abstracts S-3 and S-11. Presented 8

October 2004. Available online: http://www.medscape.com/px/urlinfo.

Weisberg, E et al (2005). 'Endometrial and vaginal effects of low-dose estradiol delivered by vaginal ring or vaginal tablet'. *Climacteric* 8(1): 83-92.

Wilson, R (1966). *Feminine Forever*. New York: Evans & Company.

Woods, NF et al (2006). 'Increased urinary cortisol levels during the menopausal transition'. *Menopause: The Journal of the North American Menopause Society* 13(2): 212-21.

Wylie-Rosett, J (2005). 'Menopause, micronutrients and hormone therapy'. *The American Journal of Clinical Nutrition* 81(s5): 1223s-31s.

Ziel, HK and Finkle WD (1975). 'Increased risk of endometrial carcinoma among users of conjugated estrogens'. *New England Journal of Medicine* 293(23): 1167-70.

Available Online

http://www.healthscout.com/ency/68/352/main.html

http://www.nlm.gov/medlineplus/ency/article/003456.htm

http://www.drugsdigest.com/MMX/Estrone.html

http://www.brainyencyclopedia.com/encyclopedia/e/en/endothelium.html

http://www.quackwatch.com

http://www.mayoclinic.com

http://www.cushings-help.com/definitions.htm

http://www.brainyencyclopedia.com/encyclopedia/a/at/atherosclerosis.html

http://my.athernet/~nrsprng/stpindex.html

http://www.cancer.org

http://www.healthywomen.org/content.cfm?L1=3&L2=52

Chapter 5

Allen, LV et al (2000). *A Healthcare Professional's Guide to Evaluating Dietary Supplements, The American Dietetic Association and American Pharmaceutical Association Special Report. From the Joint Working Group on Dietary Supplements*. Available online: http://www.pharmacist.com/pdf/dietary_supplements. pdf.

Amato, P and Christophe, S (2002). 'Estrogenic activity of herbs commonly used as remedies for menopausal symptoms'. *Menopause: the Journal of the North American Menopause Society* 9(2): 145-50.

Atkinson, C et al (2000). 'The effects of isoflavone phytoestrogens on bone; preliminary results from a large randomized, controlled trial'. Endocrine Society, 82nd Annual Meeting, Toronto, Canada, June 21-4.

Bejelakovic, G et al. (2007). 'Mortality in randomized trials of anti-oxidant supplements for primary and secondary prevention: systematic review and meta-analysis'. *Menopause: The Journal of the American Medical Association*. 297(8): 842-57.

Berkow, R and Beers, M (1999). *The Merck Manual of Diagnosis and Therapy* 17th ed. USA: Merck & Co.

Bisseker, C (2002). 'Homeopathic and legal'. *Financial Mail*. Available online: http://secure.financialmail.co.za/indexfront. html.

Bodinet, C and Freudenstein, J (2004). 'Influence of marketed herbal menopause preparations on MCF-7 cell prolifieration'. *Menopause: the Journal of the North American Menopause Society* 11(3): 281-9.

Booth, NL et al (2006). 'Clinical studies of red clover (Trifolium pratense) dietary supplements in menopause: a literature review'. *Menopause: The Journal of the North American Menopause Society* 13(2): 251-64.

Boothby, LA et al (2004). 'Bioidentical Hormone Therapy: A Review'. *Menopause: the Journal of the North American Menopause Society* 11(3): 356-67.

Brett, K et al (2007). 'Complementary and alternative medicine use among midlife women for reasons including menopause in the United States: 2002'. *Menopause: The Journal of the North American Menopause Society* 14(2): 300-7.

Bruyere, O et al (2004). 'Glucosamine sulfate reduces osteoarthritis progression in postmenopausal women with knee osteoarthritis: evidence from two 3-year studies'. *Menopause: the Journal of the North American Menopause Society* 11(2): 138-43.

Chen, Y et al (2004). 'Beneficial effects of soy isoflavones on bone mineral content was modified by years since menopause, body weight and calcium intake: a double-blind randomised, controlled trial'. *Menopause: the Journal of the North American Menopause Society* 11(3): 246-54, 290-8.

Chertow, B (2004). 'Advances in Diabetes for the Millennium: Vitamins and Oxidant Stress in Diabetes and its Complications'. *Medscape CME Activity*. Available online: http://www.medscape.com/viewarticle/490306.

Coghlan, A (2004). 'Special Report: A health fad that's hard to swallow'. *New Scientist*. Available online: http://www.newscientist.com/article.ns?id=dn4853.

Coghlan, A (2004). 'Special Report: Big errors in herbal remedy labels revealed'. *New Scientist*. Available online: http://www.newscientist.com/article.ns?id=dn4665.

Cohen, M H (2003). 'Complementary and integrative medical therapies, the FDA, and the NIH: definitions and regulation'. *Dermatologic Therapy* 16(2): 77.

Cunnae, S et al (1993). 'High alpha-linolenic acid flaxseed (Linum usitatissimum): some nutritional properties in humans'. *British Journal of Nutrition* 69(2): 443-53.

D'Anna, R et al (2007). 'Effects of the phytoestrogen genestein on hot flashes, endometrium and vaginal epithelium in postmenopausal women: a 1-year randomized, double-blind placebo-controlled study'. *Menopause: The Journal of the North American Menopause Society* 14(4): 648-55.

Daost, J et al (2006). 'Prevalence of natural health product use in healthy postmenopausal women'. *Menopause: The Journal of the North American Menopause Society* 13(2): 241-50.

Gallagher, JC et al (2004). 'The Effect of soy protein isolate on bone metabolism'. *Menopause: the Journal of the North American Menopause Society* 11(3): 290-8.

Geller, SE and Studee, L (2007). 'Botanical and dietary supplements for mood and anxiety in menopausal women'. *Menopause: The Journal of the North American Menopause Society* 14(3): 541-49.

Gold, E et al (2007). 'Cross-sectional analysis of specific complementary and alternative medicine (CAM) use by racial/ethnic group and menopausal status: the Study of Women's Health across the nation (SWAN)'. *Menopause: The Journal of the North American Menopause Society* 14(4): 612-23.

Griffin, MD et al (2006). 'Effects of altering the ratio of dietary n-6 to n-3 fatty acids on insulin sensitivity, lipoprotein size, and postpranadial lipemia in men and postmenopausal women aged 45-70: the OPTLIP Study'. *American Journal of Clinical Nutrition* 84(6):1290-8.

Haan, MN (2003). 'Can vitamin supplements prevent cognitive decline and dementia in old age?' *American Journal of Clinical Nutrition* 77(4): 762-3.

Hasler, CM (2000). *Functional Foods: Their Role in Disease Prevention and Health Promotion*. A publication of the Institute of Food Technologists Expert Panel on Food Safety and Nutrition. Available online: http://www.nutriwatch.org/04Foods/ff.html.

Hercberg, S et al (2004). 'The SU.VI.MAX Study: a randomized, placebo-controlled trial of the health effects of antioxidant vitamins and minerals'. *Archives of Internal Medicine* 164(21): 2335-42.

Hodgson, JM et al (2004). 'Supplementation with isoflavonoid phytoestrogens does not alter serum lipid concentrations: a randomized controlled trial in humans'. *Fertility and Sterility* (1): 145-8.

Hodis, H and Mack, W (2007). 'Postmenopausal hormone therapy in clinical perspective'. *Menopause: The Journal of the North American Menopause Society* 14(5): 944-57.

Huntley, A and Ernst, E A (2003). 'Systematic review of herbal medicinal products for the treatment of menopausal symptoms'. *Menopause: the Journal of the North American Menopause Society* 10: 465-76.

Kaszkin-Bettag, M et al (2007). 'The special extract Err 731 of the roots of Rheum Rhaponticum decreases anxiety and improves health state and general well-being in perimenopausal women'. *Menopause: The Journal of the North American Menopause Society* 14(2): 270-83.

Kohrt, W and Gonzansky, W (2006). 'Anti-aging strategies: science or hype'. *Menopause Management* 15(3): 12-18.

Ma, J et al (2006). 'US women desire greater professional guidance on hormone and alternative therapies for menopausal symptom management'. *Menopause: The Journal of the North American Menopause Society* 13(3): 506-516.

Mangialetti, N and Raso, J (1999). 'Should We Thank God for Julian Whitaker?' *American Council on Science and Health*. Available online: http://www.acsh.org/healthissues/newsID.901/healthissue_detail.asp.

Maxwell, J and Mehlman, JD (2000). 'Nutraceuticals: Do They Spell the End of FDA Regulation of Drugs?' The Doctor will see you now. Available online: http://www.thedoctorwillseeyounow.com/articles/bios/bioethics.shtml.

McAlindon, TE et al (2000). 'Glucosamine and chondroitin for treatment of osteoarthritis: a systematic quality assessment and meta-analysis'. *Journal of the American Medical Association* 283(11): 1469-75.

Meisler, JG (2003). 'Towards Optimal Health: The experts discuss the use of botanicals by women'. *Journal of Women's Health* 12(9): 847-52.

Meltzer, HM et al (2004). 'Are vitamin and minerals supplements required for good health?' *Journal of the Norwegian Medical Association* 124(12): 1646-9.

Olshansky, SJ et al (2002). 'Position Statement on Aging'. *Scientific American Magazine and the Journal of Gerontology* 57(8): B292-7. Available online: http://www.biomed.gerontology.org.

Safi, AM et al (2003). 'Role of Nutriceutical Agents in Cardiovascular Diseases: An Update-Part 1'. *Cardiovascular Reviews*

& *Reports* 24(7): 381-5, 391. Available online: http://www.medscape.com/viewarticle/460060.

Scambia, G and Gallo, G (2006). 'The role of phyto chemicals in menopause: a new actor on the scene of alternative treatment options'. *Menopause: The Journal of the North American Menopause Society* 13(5): 724-6.

Scott, GN and Elmer, GW (2002). 'Update on Natural Product-Drug Interactions'. *American Journal Health System Pharmacy* 59(4): 339-47. Available online: http://www.ajhp.org/cgi/content/abstract/59/4/339.

Singh, RB et al (2003). 'Effect of coenzyme Q10 on risk of atherosclerosis in patients with recent myocardial infarction'. *Molecular Cell Biochemistry* 246(1-2): 75-82.

Solomen, P et al (2002). 'Ginkgo for Memory Enhancement: A Randomized Controlled Trial'. *Journal of the American Medical Association* 288: 835-40.

Stuenkel, CA (2007). 'Isoflavones and cardiovascular risk in post-menopausal women: no free lunch'. *Menopause: The Journal of the North American Menopause Society* 14(4): 606-608.

Taylor, DA (2004). 'Botanical Supplements: Weeding Out the Health Risks'. *Environmental Health Perspective* 12(13): A750-A753. Available online: http://www.medscape.com/viewpublication/1084_index.

Tice, JA et al (2003). 'Phytoestrogen supplements for the treatment of hot flashes: the Isoflavone Clover Extract (ICE) Study: a randomized controlled trial'. *Journal of the American Medical Association* 290(2): 207-14.

Turunen, M et al (2004). 'Metabolism and function of coenzyme Q'. *Biochimica et Biophysica Acta* 1660(1-2): 171-99.

Unfer, V et al (2004). 'Endometrial effects of long-term treatment with phytoestrogens: a randomized, double-blind, placebo-controlled study'. *Fertility and Sterility* 82(1): 145-8.

Walter, P (2001). 'Towards ensuring the safety of vitamins and minerals'. *Toxicology Letters* 120(1-3): 83-7.

Weil, A (2000). *Eating Well for Optimum Health.* London: Little, Brown and Company.

Wilburn, A J et al (2004). 'The Natural Treatment of Hypertension'. *Journal of Clinical Hypertension* 6(5): 242-8.

Wu, J et al (2007). 'Possible role of equol status in the effects of isoflavone on bone and fat mass in postmenopausal Japanese women: a double-blind, randomized controlled trial'. *Menopause: The Journal of the North American Menopause Society* 14(5): 866-74.

Wuttke, W et al (2006). 'Effects of Black Cohosh (Cimcifuga Racemosa) on bone turnover, vaginal mucosa, and various blood parameters in postmenopausal women: a double-blind placebo-controlled, and conjugated estrogens-controlled study'. *Menopause: The Journal of the North American Menopause Society* 13(2):185-96

Available Online

http://www.healthatoz.com/healthatoz/Atoz/dc/cen/cam/altdicnew.html

http://ods.od.nih.gov/

http://www.dietandbody.com/article1143.html

http://www.dietandbody.com/article1145.html

http://www.quackwatch.org/index.html

http://innerself.com/

http://www.cfsan.fda.gov/~dms/supplmnt.html

http://nccam.nih.gov/health/supplements.htm

http://www.drugdigest.org/DD/Home/AllAboutDrugs/0,4081,,00.html

http://www.biochem.northwestern.edu/holmgren/Glossary/Definitions/Def-V/vitamin.html

http://www.nlm.nih.gov/medlineplus/ency/article/002399.htm

http://www.healthcentral.com/mhc/top/000339.cfm

http://www.nlm.nih.gov/medlineplus

http://health.allrefer.com/alternative-medicine/dietary-supp-4.html

http://http://www.food.gov.uk/healthiereating/vitaminsminerals

http://www.urbanext.uiuc.edu/thriftyliving/index.html

http://www.food.gov.uk/multimedia/pdfs/vitmin2003.pdf

http://dietary-supplements.info.nih.gov/factsheets/dietary-supplements.asp

http://ww.oasisfoods.com/wild_life/health_guides/nutrition_glossary_n.html

http://nccam.nih.gov/health/

http://www.bodyandfitness.com/Information/Health/Research/minerals.htm

http://www.diagnose-me.com/glossary/G668.html

Chapter 6

Aiello, EJ et al (2004). 'Effect of a yearlong, moderate-intensity exercise intervention on the occurrence and severity of menopausal symptoms in postmenopausal women'. *Menopause: the Journal of the North American Menopause Society* 11(4): 369-71.

Balfour, R P (1999). 'Laparoscopic assisted vaginal hysterectomy, 190 cases: complications and training'. *Journal of Obstetrics and Gynaecology* 19(2): 164-6.

Bordeleau, L et al (2007). 'Therapeutic options for the management of hot flashes in breast cancer survivors: an evidence-based review'. *Clinical Therapeutics* 29(2): 230-41.

Carmody, J et al (2006). 'A pilot study of mindfulness-based stress reduction for hot flashes'. *Menopause: The Journal of the North American Menopause Society* 13(5): 760-69.

Carpenter, JS et al (2004). 'Hot flashes, core body temperature and metabolic parameters in breast cancer survivors'. *Menopause: the Journal of the North American Menopause Society* 11(4): 375-81.

Crisafulli, A et al (2004). 'Effects of genistein on hot flushes in early postmenopausal women: a randomised, double-blind EPT and placebo controlled study'. *Menopause: the Journal of the North American Menopause Society* 11(4): 400-4.

Debernardo, RL, MD (2005). Fibroid Tumours. Department of Obstetrics & Gynecology, Massachusetts General Hospital, Boston, MA. Review provided by VeriMed Healthcare Network. Available online: https://ssl.adam.com/content.aspx?productId=10&pid=10&gid=000529&site=morehead2.adam.com&login=MORE6662.

Elkind-Hisch, K (2004). 'Cooling off hot flashes: uncoupling of the circadian pattern of core body temperature and hot flash frequency in breast cancer survivors'. *Menopause: the Journal of the North American Menopause Society* 11(4): 369-71.

Evans, ML et al (2005). 'Management of postmenopausal hot flushes with venlafaxine hydrochloride: a randomized, controlled trial'. *Journal of Obstetrics and Gynaecology* 105(1): 161-6.

Freedman, RR (2001). 'Physiology of hot flashes'. *American Journal of Human Biology* 13(4): 453-64.

Freedman, RR et al (1995). 'Core body temperature and circadian rhythm of hot flashes in menopausal women'. *Journal of Clinical Endocrinology and Metabolism* 80(8): 2354-8.

Garreau, JR et al (2006). 'Side effects of aromatase inhibitors versus tamoxifen: the patients' perspective'. *American Journal of Surgery* 192(4): 496-8.

Gordon, P et al (2006). 'Sertraline to treat hot flashes: a randomized controlled, double-blind, crossover trial in a general population'. *Menopause: The Journal of the North American Menopause Society* 13(4): 568-75.

Gould, SA et al (1999). 'Emergency obstetric hysterectomy an increasing incidence'. *Journal of Obstetrics and Gynaecology* 19(6): 580-3.

Guttuso, T et al (2003). 'Gabapentin's effects on hot flashes in postmenopausal women: a randomized controlled trial'. *Obstetrics and Gynaecology* 101: 337-45.

Haney, AF and Wilde, RA (2007). 'Options for hormone therapy in women who have had a hysterectomy'. *Menopause: The Journal of the North American Menopause Society* 14(3): 592-97.

Kerwin, J et al (2007). 'The variable response of women with menopausal hot flashes when treated with sertraline'. *Menopause:*

The Journal of the North American Menopause Society 14(5): 841-5.

Lorraine, A et al (2002). 'Hot Flashes: The Old and the New, What Is Really True?' *Mayo Clinic Proceedings* 77: 1207-18. Mayo Foundation for Medical Education and Research.

Miller, ER et al (2004). 'Meta-analysis: High dose vitamin E supplementation may increase all-cause mortality'. *Annuals of Internal Medicine* 142(1): 37-46

Nelson, HD et al (2005). 'Management of menopause related symptoms: Agency of Healthcare Research and Quality'. Evidence Report/Technology assessment 120.

Nelson, HD et al. (2006). 'Non-hormonal therapies for menopausal hot flashes: systematic review and meta-analysis'. *JAMA* 295(17): 2057-71.

North American Menopause Society (2003). *Menonote*: 32.

Obermeyer, C et al (2004). 'Therapeutic decisions for menopause: results of the DAMES project in central Massachusetts'. *Menopause: the Journal of the North American Menopause Society* 11(4): 456-65.

Pinkerton, JV and Pastore, LM (2007). 'Perspective on menopausal vasomotor symptoms, CAM and SWAN'. *Menopause: The Journal of the North American Menopause Society* 14(4): 601-5.

Reddy, SY et al (2006). 'Gabapentin, estrogen, and placebo for treating hot flushes: a randomized controlled trial'. *Obstetrics and Gynecology* 108(1): 41-8.

Sicat, BL and Brokaw, DK (2004). 'Non-hormonal Alternatives for the Treatment of Hot Flashes'. *Pharmacotherapy* 24(1): 79-93.

Stearns, V et al (2003). 'Controlled Release in the Treatment of Menopausal Hot Flashes, A Randomized Controlled Trial'. *Journal of the American Medical Association* 289: 2827-34.

Tait, D et al (2002). 'Research and Pathophysiology and Treatment of Hot Flashes'. Mayo Clinic Proceedings 77: 1207-18. *Mayo Foundation for Medical Education and Research*. Available online: http://www.mayoclinicproceedings.com/inside.asp?AID=219&UID.

The HOPE and HOPE-TOO Trial Investigators (2005). 'Effects of long-term vitamin E supplementation on cardiovascular events and cancer: A randomized trial'. *Journal of the American Medical Association* 293(11): 1338-1347.

Thurston, R et al (2007). 'SSRIs for menopausal hot flashes: a promise yet to be delivered'. *Menopause: The Journal of the North American Menopause Society* 14(5): 820-2.

'Treatment of menopause-associated vasomotor symptoms; position statement of the North American Menopause Society'. *Menopause: the Journal of the North American Menopause Society* 11(1): 11-33.

Whiteman, MK et al (2003). 'Smoking, body mass and hot flashes in midlife women'. *Obstetrics and Gynaecology* 101: 264-72.

Wilde, RA (2007). 'Introduction to special issue on surgical menopause'. *Menopause: The Journal of the North American Menopause Society* 14(3): 556-61.

Available Online

http://www.chclibrary.org/micromed/004820.htm

http://sharedjourney.com/define/endometriosis.html

http://www.dyspareunia.org/html/uterine_prolapse.htm

http://www.nlm.nih.gov/medlineplus/ency/article/000914.htm

Chapter 7

'AHA Guidelines. Evidence Based Guidelines for cardiovascular disease prevention in women'. (2004). *Circulation* 109: 672-93.

American Heart Association (2003). *Heart disease and stroke statistics*.

Astma, F et al (2006). 'Postmenopausal status and early menopause independent risk factors for cardiovascular disease: a meta-analysis'. *Menopause: The Journal of the North American Menopause Society* 13 (2): 256-79.

Barclay, L (2004). 'Many Type 2 Diabetics Should Take Statins'. *Medscape Medical News*. Available online: http://www.medscape.com/viewarticle/474226_print.

Barnes, J et al (2005). 'Effects of two continuous hormone therapy regimens on C-reactive protein and homocysteine'. *Menopause: the Journal of the North American Menopause Society* 12(1): 92-8.

Barrett-Connor, E (2007). 'Hormones and Heart Disease in Women: The Timing Hypothesis'. *American Journal of Epidemiology* 166(5): 506-10.

Berg, G et al (2004). 'Lipid and lipoprotein profile in menopausal transition: effects of hormone, age and fat distribution'. *Hormone & Metabolic Research* 36: 215-220.

Caboral, M (2004). 'Women: The Target of the New American Heart Association Guidelines in Cardiovascular Prevention'. *Topics in Advanced Nursing Journal* 4(3). Available online: http://www.medscape.com/viewarticle/487462.

Canonico, M et al (2007). 'Hormone Therapy and Venous Thromboembolism Among Postmenopausal Women: Impact of the Route of Estrogen Administration and Progestogens'. *Circulation*. 115: 840-845.

Carels, R et al (2004). 'Reducing Cardiovascular Risk factors in Postmenopausal Women through a Lifestyle Intervention'. *Journal of Women's Health* 13(4): 412-26.

Chataigneau, T et al (2004). 'Chronic treatment with progesterone but not medroxyprogesterone acetate restores the endothelial control of vascular tone in the mesenteric artery of ovariectomized rats'. *Menopause: the Journal of the North American Menopause Society* 11(3): 255-63.

Cholesterol definition and glossary of related terms for cholesterol. com © Pfizer Inc.

Clearfield, M (2004). 'Coronary Heart Disease Risk Reduction in Postmenopausal Women: the Role of Statin Therapy and Hormone Replacement Therapy'. *Preventative Cardiology* 7(3): 131-6.

Healy, K and Mosca, L (2004). 'New Strategies to Prevent and Treat Coronary Heart disease in Women'. *Menopause Management* 13(4).

Herrington, DM et al (1999). 'Completed and Ongoing Trials of Women and Heart Disease: PEPI and HERS'. *48th Annual Scientific Session American College of Cardiology*. Available online: http://www.medscape.com/viewarticle/439518.

Hsia, J et al (2007). 'Calcium/vitamin D supplementation and cardiovascular events'. *Circulation* 115(7): 846-54.

January 09 2004 HQ00269. 'Aspirin: From pain relief to preventive medicine'. *Mayo Foundation for Medical Education and Research*. Available online: http://www.mayoclinic.com/invoke. cfm?id=HQ00269.

Khor, LL et al (2004). 'Sex- and age-related differences in the prognostic value of C-reactive protein in patients with angiographic coronary artery disease'. *American Journal of Medicine* 117(9): 657-64.

Kopernik, G et al (2004). 'Tools for making the correct decisions regarding hormone therapy. Part II, Organ response and clinical applications'. *Fertility and Sterility* 81(6).

Kullo, IJ and Ballantyne, CM (2005). 'Conditional risk factors for atherosclerosis'. *Mayo Clinic Proceedings* 80(2): 219-30. Available online: http://www.mayoclinicproceedings.com/ inside.asp?AID=681&UID=.

Lammers, C (2003). 'Novel Risk Factors Are Now Being Used to Identify New Culprits in Heart Disease'. Available on line: http://www.mayoclinic.org/news2003-rst/1885.html.

Lobo, R (2007). 'Surgical Menopause and cardiovascular risks'. *Menopause: The Journal of the North American Menopause Society* 14 (3): 562-66.

Martins, D et al (2007). 'Prevalence of cardiovascular risk factors and the serum levels of 25-hydroxyvitamin D in the United States: data from the Third National Health and Nutrition Examination Survey'. *Archives of Internal Medicine* 167 (11): 1159-65.

Meinert, C L et al (2000). 'Gender representation in trials'. *Controlled Clinical Trials* 21(5): 462-75.

Mohandas, B and Jawahar, LM (2007). 'Lessons from hormone replacement therapy trials for primary prevention of cardiovascular disease'. *Current Opinion in Cardiology* 22: 434-42.

Naftolin, F et al (2004). 'The Women's Health Initiative could not have detected cardioprotective effects of starting hormone therapy during the menopausal transition'. *Fertility and Sterility* 81(6): 1498-501.

Nainggolan, L (2007). 'Oral Contraceptives Increase Risk of Plaques'. *Medscape Medical News*.

Nandur, R et al (2004). 'Cardiovascular Actions of Selective Estrogen Receptor Modulators and Phytoestrogens'. *Preventative Cardiology* 7(2): 73-9.

Pettee, KK (2007). 'The relationship between physical activity and lipoprotein subclasses in postmenopausal women: the influence of hormone therapy'. *Menopause: The Journal of the North American Menopause Society* 14(1): 115-22.

Polotsky, AJ and Santoro, N (2007). 'Menopause and cardiovascular disease: Endogenous reproductive hormone exposure affects risk factors'. *Menopause Management* 16(2): 21-26.

Rietzschel, E (2007). American Heart Association 2007 Scientific Sessions: Abstracts 3537 and 3614. Presented November 6.

Sanada, M et al (2004). 'Substitution of transdermal estradiol during oral estrogen-progestin therapy in postmenopausal women: effects on hypertriglyceridemia'. *Menopause: the Journal of the North American Menopause Society* 11(3): 331-36.

Scarabin, P et al (2003). 'Differential association of oral and transdermal oestrogen-replacement therapy with venous thromboembolism risk'. *The Lancet* 362(9382): 428-32.

Simoncini, T et al (2005). 'Activation of nitric oxide synthesis in human endothelial cells by red clover extracts'. *Menopause: the Journal of the North American Menopause Society* 12(1): 69-77.

'The British Guidelines-Plus Race, Alcohol, Exercise and More'. (2004). *Medscape Cardiology* 8(1): 1-8. Available online: http://www.medscape.com/viewarticle/473321.

The Merck Manual Second Home Edition. 'Melanoma' in Chapter 216 'Skin cancer'. USA: Merck & Co Inc. Available online: http://www.merck.com/mmhe/sec08/ch113/ch113d.html.

The National Institute of Health and the Expert Group on Vitamins and Minerals [EVM] Report (2003). Published by the Food Standards Agency.

The Writing Group for the PEPI Trial (1995). 'Effects of estrogen or estrogen/progestin regimens on heart disease risk factors in postmenopausal women. The Postmenopausal Estrogen/Progestin Interventions (PEPI) Trial'. *Journal of the American Medical Association* 273(3):199-208. Erratum in: *Journal of the American Medical Association* (1995) 274(21): 1676.

Update of US National Cholesterol Education Program (NCEP) Adult Treatment Panel (ATP) III Guidelines: 'An Expert Interview with Christie M Ballantyne, MD' (2004). *Medscape Cardiology* 8(1). Available online: http://www.medscape.com/viewarticle/491820.

Welty, F (2004). 'Preventing clinically evident coronary heart disease in the postmenopausal woman'. *Menopause: the Journal of the North American Menopause Society* 11(4): 484-94.

Wilde, RA (2007). 'Endogenous androgens and cardiovascular risk'. *Menopause: The Journal of the North American Menopause Society* 14(4): 609-10.

Yin, WH et al (2004). 'Independent Prognostic Value of Elevated High-Sensitivity C-Reactive Protein in Chronic Heart Failure'. *American Heart Journal* 147(5): 931-8. Available online: http://www.medscape.com/viewarticle/477549.

Zouridakis, E et al (2004). 'Markers of inflammation and rapid coronary artery disease progression in patients with stable angina pectoris'. *Circulation* 110(13): 1747-53.

Available Online

http://www.answers.com/phytochemicals&r=67

http://www.answers.com/homocysteine&r=67

http://www.lifeclinic.com/focus/blood/whatisit.asp

http://www.healthcentral.com

http://www.fda.gov/fdac/features/2003/503_aspirin.html

http://www.mayoclinic.com/invoke.cfm?id=HQ00269

http://quitsmoking.about.com/od/tobaccostatistics/a/heartdis-eases.htm

http://www.healthcentral.com/mhc/top/000171.cfm

http://www.hyperdictionary.com/medical/cholesterol

http://www.answers.com/cholesterol&r=67

http://www.forcholessterol.com/cwp/appmanager/for_cholessterolDesktop?_nfpb=true&_pageLabel=FC_glossary

http://www.altvetmed.com/face/8304-cholesterol-and-ldl.html

http://www.uihealthcare.com/reports/cardiovascular/011203cholesterol.html

http://www.neurologychannel.com/stroke/

http://www.cancer.org

http://www.wordreference.com/definition/fibrinogen

http://www.answers.com/cardiovascular+disease&r=67

http://en.wikipedia.org/wiki/Circulatory_system

http://www.clevelandclinicmeded.com/diseasemanagement/cardiology/vthromboembolism/vthrombembolism.htm

http://www.medicinenet.com/script/main/hp.asp

http://www.ahrq.gov/clinic/tp/menopstp.htm

Chapter 8

American Cancer Society (2005). *Overview: Breast Cancer. What causes breast cancer?*

Arnould, L et al (2006). Trastuzumab for the adjuvant treatment of early-stage HER2-positive breast cancer'. *National Institute for Health and Clinical Excellence* (NICE).

Arnould, L et al (2006). 'Trastuzumab-based treatment of HER2-positive breast cancer: an antibody dependent cellular cytotoxicity mechanism?'. *The British Journal of Cancer* 94(2): 259-267.

Azar, B (1999). 'Probing links between stress, cancer'. APA *Monitor online* 30(6). Available online: http://www.intensivenutrition.com/stress.pdf.

Barclay, L and Vega, C (2004). 'MRI more sensitive than mammography in women at high risk of breast cancer'. *Medscape Medical News*. Available online: http://www.medscape.com/viewarticle/484354.

Baum, M (2004). 'Current. Status of Aromatase Inhibitors in the Management of Breast Cancer and Critique of the NCIC MA-17 Trial'. *Cancer Control* 11(4): 217-21. Available online: http://www.moffitt.usf.edu/pubs/ccj/v11n4/pdf/217.pdf.

Bond, B et al (2002). 'Women like me: reflections on health and hormones from women treated for breast cancer'. *Journal of Psychosocial Oncology* 20(3): 39-57.

Bulun, S et al (1999). 'Aromatase in Aging Women'. *Seminars in Reproductive Medicine* 17(4): 349-58.

Cho, E et al (2003). 'Premenopausal Fat Intake and Risk of Breast Cancer'. *Journal of the National Cancer Institute* 95: 1079-85.

Clemons, M and Verma, S (2003). 'Aromatase Inhibitors in the Treatment of Early Breast Cancer: Highlights of the 26th Annual San Antonio Breast Cancer Symposium'. *Medscape Hematology-Oncology* 6(2). Available online: http://www.medscape.com/viewarticle/467141.

De Lignières, B (2002). 'Effects of progestogens on the postmenopausal breast'. *Climacteric* 5: 229- 35.

De Lignières, B et al (2002). 'Combined hormone replacement therapy and risk of breast cancer in a French cohort study of 3175 women'. *Climacteric* 5: 332-40.

Douchi, T (2007). 'Difference in segmental lean and fat mass components between pre- and postmenopausal women'. *Menopause: The Journal of the North American Menopause Society* 14(5): 875-878.

Evans, EM et al (2007). 'Effects of soy protein isolate and moderate exercise on bone turnover and bone mineral density in postmenopausal women'. *Menopause: The Journal of the North American Menopause Society* 14(3) 481-88.

Fabian, CJ et al (2004). 'Breast Cancer Chemoprevention Phase I Evaluation of Biomarker Modulation by Arzoxifene, a Third Generation Selective Estrogen Receptor Modulator'. *Clinical Cancer Research* 10: 5403-5417.

Gainford, MC et al (2005). 'A practical guide to the management of menopausal symptoms in breast cancer patients'. *Support Care Cancer*. 13(8): 573-8.

Gertig, G et al (2006) 'Hormone therapy and breast cancer: what factors modify the association?'. *Menopause: The Journal of the North American Menopause Society* 13(2): 178-84.

Harms, SE et al (2006). 'ACR Practice Guideline for the performance of Magnetic Resonance Imaging (MRI) of the breast'. *ACR Practice Guideline* (Res. 35).

Howell, A et al (2004).'Comparison of fulvestrant versus tamoxifen for the treatment of advanced breast cancer in postmenopausal women previously untreated with endocrine therapy: A multinational, double-blind, randomized trial'. *The Journal of Clinical Oncology* 22(9): 1605-13.

Ingle, JN (2006). 'Evaluation of fulvestrant in women with advanced breast cancer and progression on prior aromatase inhibitor therapy: a phase II trial of the North Central Cancer Treatment Group'. *The Journal of Clinical Oncology* 24(7): 1052-56.

Jarvis, W (2004). 'How Quackery Harms Cancer Patients'. Quackwatch Home Page www.quackwatch.com.

Johnston, SRD (2006). 'New Approaches to Preventing Resistance to Aromatase Inhibitors'. *Medscape Hematology-Oncology* 9(1).

Komm, BS et al (2005). 'Bazedoxifene Acetate: A Selective Estrogen Receptor Modulator with Improved Selectivity'. *Endocrinology* 146(9): 3999-4008.

Kubow, S et al (2000). 'Lipid peroxidation is associated with the inhibitory action of all trans- retinoic acid on mammary cell transformation'. *Anticancer Research* 20: 843-48.

Lewis-Wambi, JS and Jordan, VC (2005). 'Treatment of postmenopausal breast cancer with Selective Estrogen receptor Modulators (SERMs)'. *Breast Disease* 24: 93-105.

Lurie, G et al (2007). 'Association of estrogen and progestin potency of oral contraceptives with ovarian carcinoma risk'. *Obstetrics and Gynaecology* 109(3): 597-607.

McLemore, MR (2006). 'Gardasil: introducing the new human papilloma virus vaccine'. *Clinical Journal of Oncology Nursing* 10(5): 559-60.

Menon, U et al (2005). 'Prospective Study Using the Risk of Ovarian Cancer Algorithm to Screen for Ovarian Cancer'. *Journal of Clinical Oncology* 23(31): 7919-26.

Merck Manual Second Home Edition 'Chapter 216: Paget's Disease Skin Cancer'. USA: Merck & Co Inc. Available online: http://www.merck.com/mmhe/sec08/ch113/ch113d.html.

Moreno, V et al. (2002). 'Effect of oral contraceptives on risk of cervical cancer in women with human papillomavirus infection: the IARC multicentric case-control study'. *The Lancet* 359: 1085-92.

Munoz, N et al. (2002). 'Role of parity and human papillomavirus in cervical cancer: the IARC multicentric case-control study'. *The Lancet* 359(9312): 1093-1101.

Musa, MA et al (2007). 'Medicinal chemistry and emerging strategies applied to the development of selective estrogen receptor modulators (SERMs)'. *Current Medicinal Chemistry* 14(11): 1249-61.

Naieralski, J (1998). 'Alcohol and the Risk of Breast Cancer'. *Program on Breast Cancer and Environmental Risk Factors Cornell University (BCERF)*. Available online: http://envirocancer.cornell.edu/factsheet/diet/fs13.alcohol.cfm.

Nandur, R et al (2004). 'Cardiovascular Actions of Selective Estrogen Receptor Modulators and Phytoestrogens'. *Preventative Cardiology* (92): 73-9.

Nolan, T et al (2004). 'HRT and SERMS: New Guidelines for Patient Management-Part 1'. *Medscape Ob/Gyn & Women's Health*. Available online: http://www.medscape.com/viewarticle/448832_25.

Olsen, O and Gøtzsche, PC (2001). 'Screening for breast cancer with mammography'. *The Cochrane Database of Systematic Reviews* 4 (CD001877). DOI: 10.1002/14651858.CD001877.

Perez, E et al. (2005). 'Women with Early Stage, HER2-Positive Breast Cancer'. *American Society of Clinical Oncology Annual Meeting*: 419-424.

Pritchard, K (2004). 'Impact of the Women's Health Initiative (WHI) on the Practising Oncologist: Putting the WHI results into Perspective'. 2004 ASCO Annual Meeting. Available online: http://www.asco.org/ac/1,1003,12-002673-00_18-0026-00_19-00543-00_29-00E,00.asp.

Rojas, M et al (2005). 'Follow-up strategies for women treated for early breast cancer'. *Cochrane Database Systems Review* (1): CD001768.

Scott Lind, D (2004). 'Breast Complaints ACS Surgery'. *WebMD* 5: 1-16. Available online: www.acssurgery.com:6200/wnis/acs_0604a.htm-66k.

Smith, RA et al (2004). 'The randomized trials of breast cancer screening: what have we learned?' *Radiologic Clinics of North America* 42(5): 793-806.

Sporn, MB (2004). 'Commentary re CJ Fabian et al, Breast Cancer Chemoprevention Phase I Evaluation of Biomarker Modulation by Arzoxifene, a Third Generation Selective Estrogen Receptor Modulator'. *Clinical Cancer Research* 10(16): 5403-17.

Strasser-Weippl, K and Goss, PE (2005). 'Advances in Adjuvant Hormonal Therapy for Postmenopausal Women'. *Journal of Clinical Oncology* 10: 1751-59.

Tang, T (2003). 'Questions about the CA-125 Test'. *John Hopkins Pathology*. Available online: http://pathology2.jhu.edu/ovca/OvarianCancer_VSearchResult.cfm?RequestTimeout=120.

The ESHRE Capri Workshop Group (2005). 'Non-contraceptive health benefits of combined oral contraception'. *Human Reproduction Update* 11(5): 513-25.

The Five Steps of a Breast Self Exam (2004). Available online: http://www.breastcancer.org/dia-detec-exam-idx.html.

The Oncology Channel. 'Endometrial cancer'. healthcommunities.com, 8 Feb 2005.

Van Veen, WA and Knottnerus, JA (2002). 'The evidence to support mammography screening'. *Netherlands Journal of Medicine (Amsterdam)* 60(5): 200-6.

Vogel, VG (2006). 'Managing breast cancer risk in postmenopausal women'. *Menopause Management* 16(s1): 19-21.

Widdice, LE and Kahn JA (2006). 'Using the new HPV vaccines in clinical practices'. *Cleveland Clinical Journal of Medicine* 73(10): 929-35.

Winer, EP (2005). 'American Society of Clinical Oncology Technology Assessment on the Use of Aromatase Inhibitors as Adjuvant Therapy for Postmenopausal Women With Hormone Receptor-Positive Breast Cancer: Status Report 2004'. *American Society of Clinical Oncology* 23(3): 619-29.

Yu, B et al (2007). 'Structural modulation of reactivity/activity in design of improved benzothiophene selective estrogen receptor modulators: induction of chemopreventive mechanisms'. *Molecular Cancer Therapeutics* 6(9): 2418-28.

Zebecchi, L et al (2003). 'Comprehensive menopausal assessment: an approach to managing vasomotor and urogenital symptoms in breast cancer survivors'. *Oncology Nursing Forum* 30(3): 393-405.

Zielinski, SL (2005). 'Hormone replacement therapy for breast cancer survivors: an unanswered question?'. *Journal of the National Cancer Institute* 97: 955.

Available Online

http://www.infoforyourhealth.com/Cancer/ovarian%20cancer.htm

http://www.oncologychannel.com/ovariancancer/

http://dictionary.laborlawtalk.com/

http://www.answers.com/ovarian+cyst&r=67

http://www.girlzone.com?FEMedia?RareBreastCancer.html

http://www.medicinenet.com/ovarian_cysts/index.htm

http://www.cochrane.org

http://www.medicinenet.com/endometriosis/page4.htm

http://www.drsuzman.com/procedureset.htm

http://www.positivehealth.com/permit/Articles/Nutrition/
byrnes64.htm

http://envirocancer.cornell.edu/factsheet/diet/fs13.alcohol.cfm

http://www.cancer.org

http://www.medicinenet.com/ovaraian-cancer/article.htm

http://www.answers.com/ovarian%20cancer

http://www.mayoclinic.com/health/breast-cancer/AN00495

http://www.cancerbackup.org.uk/Cancertype/Breast/Causes-
diagnosis/HER2testing

http://www.cancer.org/docroot/CRI/content/CRI

Chapter 9

Adochi, JD and Cosman, F. (2007). 'Osteoporosis: A disease across the skeleton'. *Menopause Management* 16 (1): 22-24.

Aftab M, et al (2003). 'Effects of Growth Hormone Replacement on Parathyroid Hormone Sensitivity and Bone Mineral Metabolism'. *The Journal of Clinical Endocrinology & Metabolism* 88(6): 2860-68.

Akesson, K et al (1997). 'Rationale for active vitamin D analog therapy in senile osteoporosis'. *Calcified Tissue International* 60: 100-5.

Al-Ghazal et al (2000). 'The psychological impact of immediate rather than delayed breast reconstruction'. *European Journal of Surgical Oncology* 26(1): 17-19.

Balasubramanyam, A (2005). 'Osteoporosis: New Insights and Novel Treatments'. *Medscape* ENDO 2005.

Barclay, L (2004). 'Exercise Program Improves Osteoporosis'. *Medscape Ob/Gyn & Women's Health*. Available online: http://www.medscape.com/viewarticle/478726.

Barclay, L (2004). 'Long-term use of alendronate continues to protect against osteoporosis'. *Medscape Medical News*. Available online: http://www.medscape.com/viewarticle/471934.

Birge, S (2007). 'Non-vertebral 'osteoporotic' fractures: a brain disease or bone disease'. *Menopause: The Journal of the North American Menopause Society* 14(1): 1-2.

Bischoff-Ferrari, H (2007). 'How to select the doses of vitamin D in the management of osteoporosis'. *Osteoporosis International* 18(4): 401-407.

Bischoff-Ferrari, HA et al (2006). 'Effect of calcium supplementation on fracture risk: a double-blind randomized controlled trial'. *Journal of Bone & Mineral Research* 21(sl1): s1-s530.

Bischoff-Ferrari, HA et al (2006). 'Estimation of optimal serum concentrations of 25-hydroxyvitamin D for multiple health outcomes'. *American Journal of Clinical Nutrition* 84: 18-28.

Biskobing, D M et al (2002). 'Novel Therapeutic Options for Osteoporosis'. *Current Opinion in Rheumatology* 14(4): 447-52.

Bjarnason, NH and Christiansen, C (2000). 'The influence of thinness and smoking on bone loss and response to hormone replacement therapy in early postmenopausal women'. *Journal of Clinical Endocrinology and Metabolism* 85: 590-6.

Black, D (2004). 'Which regions of spine and hip should be used to assess osteoporosis and/or risk of fracture? Ask the experts about osteoporosis'. *Medscape Ob/Gyn & Women's Health*.

Bliuc, D et al (2004). 'Barriers to effective management of osteoporosis in moderate and minimal trauma fractures: a prospective study'. *Osteoporosis International*.

Boonen, S et al (2007). 'Need for Additional Calcium to Reduce the Risk of Hip Fracture with Vitamin D Supplementation: Evidence from a Comparative Meta-analysis of Randomized Controlled Trials'. *Journal of Clinical Endocrinology & Metabolism* 92: 1415-1423.

Brooke-Wavell, K (1997). 'Brisk walking reduces calcaneal bone loss in post-menopausal women'. *Clinical Science* 92(1): 75-80.

Brown, S (1996). *Better Bones, Better Body: Beyond estrogen and calcium: a comprehensive self-help program for preventing, halting and overcoming osteoporosis*. New Canaan, CT: Keats Publishing Inc.

Centers for Disease Control and Prevention (CDC) (2004). 'Awareness of family health history as a risk factor for disease, United States 2004'. *Morbidity & Mortality Weekly* Report 53(44): 1044-47.

Clegg D, et al (2006). 'Glucosamine, chondroitin sulfate and the two in combination for painful knee osteoarthritis'. *New England Journal of Medicine* 354(8): 795-808.

Coetzee, M and Kruger (2004). 'Osteoprotegerin-Receptor Activator of Nuclear Factor [kappa] B Lignan Ratio: A new approach to Osteoporosis Treatment?' *Southern Medical Journal* 97(5): 506-11.

Colon-Emeric, CS et al (2004). 'The HORIZON Recurrent Fracture Trial: design of a clinical trial in the prevention of subsequent fractures after low trauma hip fracture repair'. *Current Medical Research Opinions* (6): 903-10.

Compston, JE (2001). 'Sex steroids and bone'. *Physiological Reviews* 81: 419-47.

Cornuz, J et al (1999). 'Smoking, smoking cessation, and risk of hip fracture in women'. *American Journal of Medicine* 106: 311-4.

Cortet et al (2004). 'Does quantitative ultrasound of bone reflect more bone mineral density than bone microarchitecture?' *Calcified Tissue International* 74(1): 60-7.

Cosman, F (2003). 'Selective estrogen-receptor modulators'. *Clinics in Geriatric Medicine* 19(2): 371-9.

Cosman, F (2007). 'Secondary causes of postmenopausal osteoporosis'. *Menopause Management* 16(1): 22-24.

Cox, D et al (2004). 'Effect of raloxifene on the incidence of elevated low-density lipoprotein (LDL) and Achievement of LDL target goals in postmenopausal women'. *Current Medical Research & Opinion* 20(7): 1049-55.

Crandall, C (2002). 'Combination treatment of osteoporosis: a clinical review'. *Journal of Women's Health and Gender Based Medicine* 11(3): 211-24.

Cranney, A et al (2006). 'Parathyroid hormone for the treatment of osteoporosis: a systematic review'. *Canadian Medical Association Journal* 175 (1):52-9.

Crans, GG et al (2004). 'Association of severe vertebral fractures with reduced quality of life: reduction in the incidence of severe vertebral fractures by teriparatide'. *Arthritis & Rheumatism* 50(12): 4028-34.

Definition of Osteoporosis. www.bonehealthforlife.org (2004).

Dennison, E (2003). 'Growth hormone predicts bone density in elderly women'. *Bone* 32(4): 434-40.

Doggrell, SA (2003). 'Present and future pharmacotherapy for osteoporosis'. *Drugs Today* 39(8): 633-57.

Emkey, R (2004). 'Alendronate and Risedronate for the Treatment of Postmenopausal Osteoporosis: Clinical Profiles of the Once-Weekly and Once-Daily Dosing Formations'. *Medscape General Medicine* 6(3), Available online: http://www.medscape.com/viewarticle/480498_print.

Farley, D (1997). 'Bone Builders: Support Your Bones with Healthy Habits'. *U.S. Food and Drug Administration* FDA Consumer September-October.

Fielding, RA (1995). 'The role of progressive resistance training and nutrition in the preservation of lean body mass in the elderly'. *Journal of American College Nutrition* 14(6): 587-94.

Follin, SL and Hansen, LB (2003). 'Current Approaches to the Prevention and Treatment of Postmenopausal Osteoporosis'. *American Journal Health System Pharmacy* 60(9): 883-901.

Gallagher, JC (2007). 'Effect of early menopause on bone mineral density and fractures'. *Menopause: The Journal of the North American Menopause Society.* 14(3): 567-71.

Germano, C and Cabot, M (1999). *The Osteoporosis Solution: New Therapies for Prevention and Treatment.* New York: Kensington Books.

Geusens, P and Boonen, S (2002). 'Osteoporosis and the Growth Hormone-Insulin-Like Growth Factor Axis'. *Hormone Research* 58.

Gold, DT, Lee, LS and Tresolini, CP (eds) (2001). *Working with patients to prevent, treat and manage osteoporosis: a curriculum guide for the health professions*. 3rd ed. Durham: Center for the Study of Aging and Human Development, Duke University.

Harris, ST et al (1999). 'Effects of risedronate treatment on vertebral and nonvertebral fractures in women with postmenopausal osteoporosis: a randomized controlled trial. Vertebral Efficacy with Risedronate Therapy (VERT) Study Group.' *Journal of the American Medical Association* 282: 1344-52.

Hartard, M et al (1996). 'Systematic strength training as a model of therapeutic intervention: a controlled trial in postmenopausal women with osteopenia'. *American Journal of Physical Medicine & Rehabilitation* 75(1): 21-8.

Health Encyclopedia. 'Hip Fracture'. Available online: http://www.healthscout.com/ency/68/110/main.html.

Heaney, RP (2003). 'Long-latency deficiency disease: insights from calcium and Vitamin D'. *American Journal of Clinical Nutrition* 78(5): 912-19.

Hill, AP (2007) 'Hormone therapy and oral health'. *Menopause: The Journal of the North American Menopause Society*. 16(3): 16-40.

Hodsman, A et al (2003). 'Efficacy and Safety of Human Parathyroid Hormone (1-84) in Increasing Bone Mineral Density in Postmenopausal Osteoporosis'. *The Journal of Clinical Endocrinology & Metabolism* 88(11): 5212-20.

Hoidrup, S et al (2000). 'Tobacco smoking and risk of hip fracture in men and women'. *International Journal of Epidemiology* 29: 253-9.

Holden, M (2005). 'PILATES: the best kept secret in back rehabilitation'. Available online: http://www.medic8.com/health-guide/articles/pilates.html.

'Interpretation of DEXA measures'. www.bonehealthforlife.org.

Ives, JC and Sosnoff, J (2000). 'Beyond the Mind-Body Exercise Hype'. *The Physician And Sports Medicine* 28(3).

Kanis, J et al (2005). 'Assessment of Fracture Risk'. *Osteoporosis International* 16: 581-9.

Kasukawa, Y et al (2004). 'The anabolic effects of GH/IGF system on bone'. Current *Pharmaceutical Design* 10(21): 2577-92.

Katz, W and Sherman, C (1998). 'Exercise for Osteoporosis'. Series Editor: Nicholas A DiNubile. *The Physician And Sports Medicine* 26(2).

Katz, WA and Sherman, C (1998). 'Osteoporosis'. Series Editor: Nicholas A DiNubile. *The Physician And Sports Medicine* 26(2).

Kelley, GA et al (2001). 'Resistance training and bone mineral density in women: a meta-analysis of controlled trials'. *American Journal of Physical and Medical Rehabilitation* 80(1): 65-77.

Krall, EA and Dawson-Hughes, B (1994). 'Walking is related to bone density and rates of bone loss'. *American Journal of Medicine* 96(1): 20-6.

Kremer, C et al (2000). 'Patient satisfaction with outpatient hysteroscopy versus day case hysteroscopy: randomised controlled trial'. *BMJ* 320: 279-282.

Lang T, et al (2004). 'Cortical and trabecular bone mineral loss from the spine and hip in long- duration spaceflight'. *Journal of Bone & Mineral Research* 19(6): 1006-12.

Laszlo, D (2003). 'Teriparatide Reduces Fracture-Related Back Pain Over Long Term'. *Medscape Medical News*. ©2003 Medscape.

Lemaire, V et al (2004). 'Modeling the interactions between osteoblast and osteoclast activities in bone remodeling'. *Journal of Theoretical Biology* 229(3): 293-309.

Lian, J, Gorski, J and Ott, S (2004). *American Society for Bone Mineral Research. Bone Curriculum; Bone Structure and Function*.

Lindsay, R et al (1997). 'Randomised controlled study of effect of parathyroid hormone on vertebral-bone mass and fracture incidence among postmenopausal women on oestrogen with osteoporosis'. *The Lancet* 350(9077): 550-5.

Lindsay, R et al (2004). 'Sustained vertebral fracture risk reduction after withdrawal of Teriparatide in postmenopausal women with osteoporosis'. *Archives of Internal Medicine* 164(18): 2024-30

Lindsay, R et al. (2002). 'Effect of lower doses of conjugated equine estrogens with and without medroxyprosgeterone acetate in early postmenopausal women'. *Menopause: The Journal of the American Medicine Association* 287: 2667-668.

Liu-Ambrose, T et al (2004). 'Resistance and agility training reduce fall risk in women aged 75 to 85 with low bone mass: a 6-month randomised controlled trial'. *J Am Geriatr Soc* 52(5): 657-65.

Maricic, M et al (2002). 'Early effects of raloxifene on clinical vertebral fractures at 12 months in postmenopausal women with osteoporosis'. *Archives of Internal Medicine* 162(10): 1140- 43.

McClung, M et al (2006). 'Prevention of bone loss in postmenopausal women treated with lasofoxifene compared with raloxifene'. *Menopause: The Journal of the North American Menopause Society* 13(3): 377-86

McLean, RR et al (2004). 'High Homocysteine Levels linked to Fracture Risk in two reports'. *New England Journal of Medicine* 350: 2042-49. First to Know, North American Menopause Society Released June 2004.

McTiernan, A et al (2004). 'Effect of exercise on serum estrogens in postmenopausal women: A 12-month randomized clinical trial'. *Cancer Research* 64: 2923-28.

Meunier, PJ et al (2004). 'The effects of strontium ranelate on the risk of vertebral fracture in women with postmenopausal osteoporosis'. *New England Journal of Medicine* 350(5): 459-68.

Miller, L et al (2004). 'Bone Mineral Density in Postmenopausal Women: Does Exercise Training Make a Difference?' *The Physician And Sports Medicine* 32(2).

NIH Consensus Development Panel on Optimal Calcium Intake (1994). *Journal of the American Medical Association* 272.

Orenstein, B (2004). 'Lost in Space: Bone Mass'. *Radiology Today* 5(6): 10.

Peck, P (2004). 'Ultra-low dose estradiol patch stops bone turnover, increases bone density'. *Medscape Medical News*. Available online: http://www.medscape.com/viewarticle/475033.

Pouilles, JM et al (1995). 'Effect of menopause on femoral and vertebral bone loss'. *Journal of Bone and Mineral Metabolism* 10: 1534-6.

Rapuri, PB et al (2000). 'Smoking and bone metabolism in elderly women'. *Bone* 27: 429-36.

Reginster, JY et al (2004). 'Strontium ranelate: a new paradigm in the treatment of osteoporosis'. *Expert Opinion on Investigational Drugs* 13(7): 857-64.

Reginster, JY et al (2005). 'Strontium ranelate reduces the risk of non-vertebral fractures in postmenopausal women with osteoporosis: TROPOS study'. *Journal of Clinical Endocrinology & Metabolism* 90(5): 2816-22.

Richman, S et al (2006). 'Low dose estrogen therapy for prevention of osteoporosis: working our way back to monotherapy'. *Menopause: The Journal of the North American Menopause Society.* 13(1): 148-55

Riera-Espinoza, G et al (2004). 'Changes in bone turnover during Tibolone treatment'. *Maturitas* 47(2): 83-90.

Ringa, V (2004). 'Alternatives to hormone replacement therapy for menopause: an epidemiological evaluation'. *Journal de Gynecologie, Obstetrique et Biologie de la Reproduction (Paris)* 33(3): 195-209.

Rowland, JH et al (2000). 'Role of breast reconstructive surgery in physical and emotional outcomes among breast cancer survivors'. *Journal of National Cancer Institute* Sept 6 92(17): 1422-29. Erratum in: *Journal of National Cancer Institute* 2001 93(1): 68.

Rymer, J et al (2002). 'Ten years of treatment with tibolone 2.5mg daily: effects on bone loss in postmenopausal women'. *Climacteric* 5(4): 390-8.

Sambrook, PN (2004). Skeletal benefits with alendronate twice those of raloxifene. *Journal of Internal Medicine* 255: 503-11.

Sartori, L et al (2003). 'Injectable bisphosphonates in the treatment of postmenopausal osteoporosis'. *Aging-Clinical & Experimental Research* 15(4): 271-83.

Sawicki, A et al (2004). 'Strontium ranelate reduces the risk of vertebral fractures in postmenopausal women'. *Calcified Tissue International* 74 (s84):153.

Scott-Lind, D et al (2004). 'Breast Procedures'. *ACS Surgery: Principles and Practice* (5): 1-16. Available online: http://www.acssurgery.com/sample/ACS0305.pdf.

Seeman, E et al (2006). 'Strontium Ranelate reduces the risk of vertebral and non-vertebral fractures in women eighty years or older'. *Journal of Bone & Mineral Research* 21(7): 1113-20.

Seeman, E, (2007). 'Is change in bone mineral density a sensitive and specific surrogate of anti fracture efficacy?'. *Bone* 41: 308-317.

Shangold, M and Sherman, C (1998). 'Exercise and Menopause: A Time for Positive Changes'. Series Editor: Nicholas A DiNubile. *The Physician And Sports Medicine* 26(12).

Slipman, C et al (2004). 'Osteoporosis (secondary)'. *eMedicine*. Available online: http://www.emedicine.com/pmr/topic95.htm.

Swegle, JM and Kelly, MV (2004). 'Tibolone: a unique version of Hormone Replacement Therapy'. *Annals of Pharmacotherapy* 38(5): 874-81.

Tekeoglu, I et al (2005). 'Comparison of cyclic and continuous calcitonin regimens in the treatment of postmenopausal osteoporosis'. *Rheumatology International* 211-224.

The Board of Trustees of the North American Menopause Society (2006). 'Management of osteoporosis in postmenopausal women: position statement of the North American Menopause Society'. *Menopause: The Journal of the North American Menopause Society.* 13(3): 340-67.

Ward, KD and Klesges, RC (2001). 'A meta-analysis of the effects of cigarette smoking on bone mineral density'. *Calcified Tissue International* 68(5): 259-70.

Wilkins, EG et al (2000). 'Prospective analysis of psychosocial outcomes in breast reconstruction: one-year postoperative results from the Michigan Breast Reconstruction Outcome Study'. *Plastic Reconstructive Surgery* 106(5): 1014-25; discussion 1026-7.

Ylikorkala, O and Metsa-Heikkila, M (2002). 'Hormone Replacement Therapy in Women with a History of Breast Cancer'. *Gynecological Endocrinology* 16(6): 469-78.

Yu, Z et al (2004). 'Two to three years of Hormone Replacement Therapy in healthy women have long term preventative effects on bone mass and osteoporotic fractures: the PERF study'. *Bone* 34(4): 728-35.

Available Online

http://www.nlm.nih.gov/medlineplus/osteoporosis.html

http://www.phoenix5.org/glossary/bisphosphonates.html

http://arbl.cvmbs.colostate.edu/hbooks/pathphys/endocrine/thyroid/calcitonin.html

http://arbl.cvmbs.colostate.edu/hbooks/pathphys/endocrine/thyroid/pth.html

http://www.e-ds.com/healthinfo_view/i_00000007B9./e-MedspatientEducationCalciumImbalance

http://www.britannica.com/eb/article?tocId=9033466

http://www.meb.uni-bonn.de/cancer.gov/CDR0000062903.html

http://members.optushome.com.au/physio/glossa_m.html

http://www.4collegewomen.org/fact-sheets/osteoporosis.html

http://www.hersource.com/osteo/c1/smoking.cfm

http://www.ozestuaries.org/indicators/Def_decomposition.html

http://www.hyperdictionary.com/medical/cytokines

http://www.emedicine.com/pmr/topic95.htm

http://www.medicinenet.com/calcitonin/article.htm

http://www.infoaging.org/d-osteo-4-cause.html

http://www.medscape.com/viewarticle/510285

http://www.fore.org/patients/bmd_testing.html

http://www.earlymenopause.com/calcium.htm

http://www.opendoorclinic.org/hivglossary.htm

Chapter 10

Arterburn, LM et al. (2006). 'Distribution, inter conversion, and dose response of n-3 fatty acids in humans'. *American Journal of Clinical Nutrition* 83 (suppl):1467S-76S.

Aude, YW et al (2004). 'The national cholesterol education program diet vs a diet lower in carbohydrates and higher in protein and monounsaturated fat: a randomized trial'. *Archives of Internal Medicine* 164(19): 2141-6.

Avenell, A et al (2004). 'What are the long-term benefits of weight reducing diets in adults? A systematic review of randomized controlled trials'. *Journal of Human Nutrition and Dietetics* 17(4): 317-35.

Bantle, J P (2004). 'Weight Management and Type 2 Diabetes'. *Medscape Diabetes & Endocrinology* 6(1). Available online: http://www.medscape.com/viewarticle/473049.

Barclay, L (2004). 'Obesity increases risk of false-positive mammograms'. *Medscape General Medicine*. Available online: http://www.medscape.com/viewarticle/479111?src=mp.

Barclay, L (2004). 'Relationship of Obesity and Fitness Level to Cardiovascular Risk and Diabetes'. *Medscape Medical News*. Available online: http://www.medscape.com/viewarticle/488814_print.

Blackburn, G (2004). 'Making scientific sense of different dietary approaches, Part 2: Evaluating the Diets'. *Medscape Diabetes & Endocrinology* 6(1).

Bravata, DM (2003). 'Efficacy and safety of low-carbohydrate diets'. *Journal of the American Medical Association* 289(14).

Bray, G (2000). 'Physiology and Consequences of Obesity'. *MedscapeOb/Gyn & Women's Health*. Available online: http://www.medscape.com/viewprogram/707.

Brehm, BJ (2003). 'A randomized trial comparing a very low carbohydrate diet and a calorie- restricted low fat diet on body weight and cardiovascular risk factors in healthy women'. *Journal of Clinical Endocrinology & Metabolism* 88(4): 1617-23.

Canadian Diabetes Association. *Type 2 diabetes: Things you should know.*

Carnethon, MR et al (2004). 'Risk factors for the metabolic syndrome: the Coronary Artery Risk Development in Young Adults (CARDIA) study, 1985-2001'. *Diabetes Care* 27(11): 2707- 15.

Carroll, S and Dudfield, M (2004). 'What is the relationship between exercise and metabolic abnormalities? A review of the metabolic syndrome'. *Sports Medicine* 34(6): 371-418.

Centres for Disease Control. Department of health and human services Body Mass Index (BMI): 'BMI for Adults: Body Mass Index Formula for Adults'.

Crowther, NJ (2004). 'The clinical relevance of fasting serum insulin levels in obese subjects'. *South African Medical Journal* 94(7).

D'eon, T and Braun, B (2002). 'The roles of estrogen and progesterone in regulating carbohydrate and fat utilization at rest and during exercise'. *Journal of Women's Health & Gender Based Medicine* 11(3): 225-37.

Douchi, T et al (2007). 'Difference in segmental lean and fat mass components between pre- and postmenopausal women'. *Menopause: The Journal of the North American Menopause Society* 14(5): 875-8.

Engler, MB et al (2004). 'Flavonoid-rich dark chocolate improves endothelial function and increases plasma epicatechin concentrations in healthy adults'. *Journal of the American College of Nutrition* 23(3): 197-204.

Foster, GD et al (2003). 'A randomized trial of a low-carbohydrate diet for obesity'. *New England Journal of Medicine* 348(21): 2082-90.

Fox, M (2004). 'Low-carb fad seen as unhealthy and a rip-off'. *Reuters Health Information*.

Fung, TT et al (2004). 'Prospective study of major dietary patterns and stroke risk in women'. *Stroke* 35(9): 2014-19.

Gambacciani, M et al (1999). 'Climacteric modifications in body weight and fat tissue distribution'. *Climacteric* 2(1): 37-44.

Gambacciani, M et al (2001). 'Prospective evaluation of body weight and body fat distribution in early postmenopausal women with and without hormonal replacement therapy'. *Maturitas* 39(2): 125-32.

Grundy, S et al (2004). 'Definition of Metabolic Syndrome: Report of the National Heart, Lung and Blood Institute/American Heart Association Conference on Scientific Issues Related to Definition'. *Circulation* 109: 433-38.

Hagey, AR and Warren, MP (2006). 'Exercise and menopause: positive effects'. *Menopause Management* 15(3):19-25.

Harvard Health Publications. 'Answering your questions on trans fats'.

He, K (2004). 'Fish consumption and incidence of stroke: a meta-analysis of cohort studies'. *Stroke* 35(7): 1538-42.

HealthCentral.com (2001). 'What are the exercise basics?' Available online: http://healthcentral.com/fitorfat/408/42759.html.

Homehealth.uk 'What is a healthy balanced diet?' Available online: http://www.homehealth-uk.com.

Insulin resistance and pre-diabetes. NIH Publication No. 04-4893 May 2004.

Kerr, M (2004). 'Incidence of Metabolic Syndrome Low When Weight is Stable'. *Medscape Medical News, Medscape General Medicine.* Available online: http://www.medscape.com/viewarticle/493446.

Knowles, W et al (2002). 'Reduction in the Incidence of Type 2 Diabetes with Lifestyle Intervention or Metformin'. *New England Journal of Medicine* 346(6): 393-403.

László, B (2003). 'Central and peripheral fat mass have contrasting effect on the progression of aortic calcification in postmenopausal women'. *European Heart Journal* 24(16): 1531-37.

Lemoine, S et al (2007). 'Effect of weight reduction on quality of life and eating behaviors in obese women'. *Menopause: The Journal of the North American Menopause Society* 14(3): 432-40.

Lewis, JE (2006). 'A randomized controlled trial of the effect of dietary soy and flaxseed muffins on quality of life and hot flashes during menopause'. *Menopause: The Journal of the North American Menopause Society* 13(4): 631-42.

Lichtenstein, A et al (2006). 'Diet and Lifestyle recommendations revision 2006: A scientific statement from the American Heart Association Nutrition Committee'. *Circulation* 114: 82-96.

Lovejoy, J C (1998). 'The influence of sex hormones on obesity across the female life span'. *Journal of Women's Health* 7(10): 1247-56.

Marco, M et al (2006). 'Menopause, insulin resistance and risk factors for cardiovascular disease'. *Menopause: The Journal of the North American Menopause Society*13(5): 809-19.

Mayoclinic.com (2004). 'Low-carbohydrate diets: Are they safe and effective?'

McAuley, KA (2005). 'Comparison of high-fat and high-protein diets with a high-carbohydrate diet in insulin-resistant obese women'. *Diabetologia* 48(1): 8-16.

Meckling, KA et al (2004). 'Comparison of a low-fat diet to a low-carbohydrate diet on weight loss, body composition, and risk factors for diabetes and cardiovascular disease in free- living, overweight men and women'. *Journal of Clinical Endocrinology & Metabolism* 89(6): 2717-23.

MedicineNet.com 1996-2005. 'Low Carb-state of mind'. ©MedicineNet, Inc.

Milewicz, A et al (2001). 'Menopausal obesity: myth or fact?' *Climacteric* 4(4): 273-83.

Moller, S E (1992). 'Serotonin, carbohydrates, and atypical depression'. *Pharmacology & Toxicology* 71(1): 61-71.

Morgan, T et al (2004). 'Acute effects of nicotine on serum glucose insulin growth hormone and cortisol in healthy smokers'. *Metabolism* 53(5): 578-82.

Mursu, J (2004). 'Dark chocolate consumption increases HDL cholesterol concentration and chocolate fatty acids may inhibit lipid peroxidation in healthy humans'. *Free Radical Biology and Medicine* 37(9): 1351-59.

Norman, R et al (1999). 'Oestrogen and progestogen hormone replacement therapy for perimenopausal and post-menopausal women: weight and body fat distribution'. *The Cochrane Database of Systematic Reviews* 3(CD001018). DOI: 10.1002/14651858.CD001018.

'Partnership for essential nutrition'. Available online: http://www.Essentialnutrition.org/lowcarb.php.

Peck, P (2004). 'Both Uphill, Downhill Exercise Help Lipid and Glucose Metabolism'. *Medscape General Medicine*. Available online: http://www.medscape.com/viewarticle/493323.

Pittas, AG (2003). 'Nutrition interventions for prevention of type 2 diabetes and the metabolic syndrome'. *Nutrition in Clinical Care* 6(2): 79-88.

Rao, G (2001). 'Insulin resistance syndrome'. *American Family Physician* 63(6): 1159-63, 1165-6.

Raynor, HA et al (2004). 'Relationship between changes in food group variety, dietary intake, and weight during obesity treatment'. *International Journal of Obesity & Related Metabolic Disorder* 28(6): 813-20.

Rolls, BJ et al (2004). 'What can intervention studies tell us about the relationship between fruit and vegetable consumption and weight management?' *Nutrition Abstracts & Reviews* 62(1): 1-17.

Salodorf, MacNeil J (2004). 'High and Low carb Diets Produce Similar Results'. *Medscape General Medicine*. Available online: http://www.medscape.com/viewarticle/494078.

Salodorf, MacNeil J (2004). 'Water-Rich Diet More Effective than Low-Fat Regimen for Weight Loss'. Medscape General Medicine. Available online: http://www.medscape.com/viewarticle/494144?src=mp.

Salodorf, MJ (2004). 'Weight Loss Maintenance Program Keeps Pounds Off'. *Medscape General Medicine*. Available online: http://www.medscape.com/viewarticle/494143?src=mp.

Shipp, T (2005). 'Does ultrasound have a role in the evaluation of postmenopausal bleeding and among postmenopausal women with endometrial cancer?' *Menopause: the Journal of the North American Menopause Society* 12(1): 8-11.

Simkin-Silverman, LR et al (2003). 'Lifestyle intervention can prevent weight gain during menopause: results from a 5-year randomized clinical trial'. *Annals of Behavioral Medicine* 26(3): 212-20.

Song, Y et al (2004). 'A Prospective Study of Red Meat Consumption and Type 2 Diabetes'. *Diabetes Care* 27(9): 2108-15.

Sorenson, MB (2002). 'Changes in body composition at menopause age, lifestyle or hormone deficiency?' *Journal of the British Menopause Society* 8(4): 137-40.

South, J. 'L-Tryptophan, nature's answer to Prozac'. *Off-shore Pharmacy*. Available online: http://www.smart-drugs.com/JamesSouth-tryptophan.htm.

Staropoli, CA et al (1998). 'Predictors of menopausal hot flashes'. *Journal of Women's Health* 711: 1149-55.

Stern, L et al (2004). 'The effects of low-carbohydrate versus conventional weight loss diets in severely obese adults: one-year follow-up of a randomized trial'. *Annals of Internal Medicine* 10: 778-85.

St-Onge, MP and Heymsfield, SB (2004). 'Reducing CVD Risk Through Appropriate Weight Management'. *Medscape General Medicine*. Available online: http://www.medscape.com/viewprogram/3118.

Sutton-Tyrell, K (2004). 'Healthy Life Style Diet and Exercise Slow Atherosclerosis in Menopausal Women'. *Journal of the American College of Cardiology* 44: 579-87.

Tanko, LB and Christiansen, C (2004). 'An update on the antiestrogenic effect of smoking: a literature review with implications for researchers and practitioners'. *Menopause: the Journal of the North American Menopause Society* 11(1): 104-9.

Thompson, D et al (2004). 'Relationship between Accumulated Walking and Body Composition'. *Medicine & Science in Sports & Exercise* 36(5): 911-14.

Till, A. *The GI Factor*. ©Anne Till & Associates.

Utian, W et al (2004). 'Body mass index does not influence response to treatment, nor does body weight change with lower doses of conjugated estrogens and medroxyprogesterone acetate in early post menopausal women'. *Menopause: the Journal of the North American Menopause Society* 11(3): 306-14.

Volek, JS et al (2004). 'Comparison of energy-restricted very low-carbohydrate and low-fat diets on weight loss and body composition in overweight men and women'. *Nutrition & Metabolism* (London) 1: 13.

Wasnich, R (2004). 'Changes in bone density and turn over after alendronate or estrogen withdrawal'. *Menopause: the Journal of the North American Menopause Society* 11(6): 622-30.

Wholegrains for healthful eating recipe. (2005). Edited by NCND staff, technical review by the Nutrition Education for the Public Dietetic Practice Group. American Dietetic Association (ADA).

Wing, R (2004). 'NAASO Annual Scientific Meeting: Abstract 96-OR'. Presented 17 November.

Wing, R et al (1991). 'Weight gain at the time of menopause'. *Archives of Internal Medicine* 151: 97-102.

Wurtman, RJ and Wurtman, JJ (1996). 'Brain Serotonin, Carbohydrate-craving, obesity and depression'. *Advances in Experimental Medicine & Biology* 398: 35-41.

Yancy, WS et al (2004). 'Low-carbohydrate, ketogenic diet versus a low-fat diet to treat obesity and hyperlipidemia: a randomized, controlled trial'. *Annals of Internal Medicine* 140(10): 769-77.

Available Online

http://www.cdc.gov/nccdphp/dnpa/bmi/bmi-adult-formula.htm

http://www.mindbodyhealth.com/lowfatdietmyth.htm

http://www.answers.com/topic/carbohydrate

http://www.healthyeatingclub.com/info/articles/body-shape/lowcarbevidence.htm

http://syndromex.stanford.edu/InsulinResistance.htm

http://www.caloriecontrol.org/metricconversion.html

http://www.schering.de/scripts/en/20_busareas/gyn_andro/index.php

http://www.answers.com/topic/metabolism

Chapter 11

A Skin Care Directory. Skin Care & Beauty Glossary ©2002~2003. www.ASkinCareDirectory.com.

Alster, T et al (2004). 'The aging face: more than skin deep'. The Discovery Institute of Medical Education.

Alvarez, G and Ayas, N (2004). 'The impact of daily sleep duration on health: a review of the literature'. *Progress in Cardiovascular Nursing* 19(2): 56-9.

American Heritage® Dictionary of the English Language, Fourth Edition (2004). 'G-Spot'. Houghton Mifflin Company. Available online: http://www.answers.com/topic/g-spot.

Anastasia, L and Misakian, MD (2003). 'Postmenopausal Hormone Therapy and Migraine Headache'. *Journal of Women's Health* 12(10): 1027-36.

Anderson, M et al (2004). 'Are vaginal symptoms ever normal? A review of the literature'. *Medscape General Medicine* 6(4). Available online: http://www.medscape.com/viewarticle/490226.

Asbury, E et al (2006). 'The importance of continued exercise participation in quality of life and psychological well-being in previously inactive postmenopausal women: a pilot study'. *Menopause: The Journal of the North American Menopause Society* 13 (4):561-67.

Aysegul, E et al (2007). 'Efficacy of citalopram on climacteric symptoms'. Menopause: *The Journal of the North American Menopause Society* 14(2): 223-9.

Azcoitia I, et al (2003). 'Are gonadal steroid hormones involved in disorders of brain aging?' *Aging Cell* 2(1): 31-7.

Bagger, Y et al (2005). 'Early Postmenopausal Hormone Therapy May Prevent Cognitive Impairment Later in Life'. *Menopause: the Journal of the North American Menopause Society* 12(1): 12-17.

Barlow, D (2006). 'What do we think about cognition and menopause?'. *Menopause: The Journal of the North American Menopause Society* 13 (1):4-5.

Barnhart, KT et al (1999). 'Related Quality of Life'. *Journal of Clinical Endocrinology & Metabolism* 84(11): 3896-902.

Basson, R (2007). 'Recent conceptualization of women's sexual response'. *Menopause Management* 16(3): 16-27.

Begany, T (2003). 'Is diabetes a risk for cognitive impairment?' *Neuropsychiatry Reviews* 4(5).

Benca, RM (2005). 'Diagnosis and treatment of chronic insomnia: a review'. *Psychiatr Serv* 56(3): 332-43.

Berga, S et al (2007). 'Does estrogen use support cognition in post-menopausal women?'. *Menopause: The Journal of the North American Menopause Society* 14(2): 163-5.

Berkow, R and Beers, M (1999). 'Melanoma'. *The Merck Manual of Diagnosis and Therapy 17th ed*. USA: Merck & Co.

Berman, L et al (2003). 'Seeking help for sexual function complaints: what gynecologists need to know about the female patient's experience'. *Fertility & Sterility* 79(3): 572-6.

Beyene, Y et al (2007). 'I take the good with the bad, and I moisturize'. *Menopause: The Journal of the North American Menopause Society* 14(4): 734-41.

Boccardi, M et al (2006). 'Effects of hormone therapy on brain morphology of healthy postmenopausal women: a Voxel-based morphometry study'. *Menopause: The Journal of the North American Menopause Society* 13(4): 584-91.

Bommadevara, M and Zhu, L (2002). 'Temperature difference between the body core and arterial blood supplied to the brain during hyperthermia or hypothermia in humans'. *Biomechanics and Modeling in Mechanobiology* 1(2): 137-49.

Brandes, JL (2006) 'The influence of estrogen on migraine'. *Journal of the American Medicine Association* 295(15): 1824-30.

Braunstein, GD et al (2005). 'Safety and efficacy of a testosterone patch for the treatment of hypoactive sexual disorder in surgically menopausal women: a randomized placebo controlled trial'. *Archives of Internal Medicine*. 165:1582-89.

Briden, ME (2004). 'Alpha-hydroxyacid chemical peeling agents: case studies and rationale for safe and effective use'. *Cutis* 73 (2 Suppl): 18-24.

Brinton, RD (2004). 'Requirements of a brain selective estrogen: advances and remaining challenges for developing a Neuro-SERM'. *Journal of Alzheimer's Disease* 6 (6 Suppl): S27-35.

Buster, J et al (2005). 'Testosterone patch for low sexual desire in surgically menopausal women: a randomized trial'. *Obstetrics and Gynecology*.105: 944-52.

Cameron, D and Braunstein, G (2005). 'Androgen replacement therapy in women'. *Fertility and Sterility* 8(2): 273-89.

Carruthers, J et al (2004). Consensus recommendations on the use of botulinum toxin type A in facial aesthetics. *Plastic & Reconstructive Surgery* 114 (6 Suppl): 1S-22S.

Cheng, MH et al (2007). 'Does menopausal transition affect quality of life? A longitudinal study of middle-aged women in Kinmen?'. *Menopause: The Journal of the North American Menopause Society* 14(5): 885-90.

Chiu, A and Kimball, AB (2003). 'Topical Vitamins, Minerals and Botanical Ingredients as Modulators of Environmental and Chronological Skin Damage'. *British Journal of Sports Medicine* 149(4): 681-91.

Cohen, LS et al. (2002). 'Prevalence and predictors of premenstrual dysphoric disorder (PMDD) in older premenopausal women. The Harvard Study of Moods and Cycles'. *Journal of Affective Disorders* 70(2): 125-32.

Craig, M et al (2005). 'The Women's Health Initiative Memory Study: findings and implications for treatment'. *The Lancet Neurology* 4(3).

Criego, A B et al (2005). 'Brain glucose concentrations in patients with type 1 diabetes and hypoglycemia unawareness'. *Journal of Neuroscience Research* 79(1-2): 42-7.

Davison, SL and Davis, SR (2003). 'Androgens in women'. *Journal of Steroid Biochemistry & Molecular Biology* 85(2-5): 363-6.

Davison, SL et al (2005). 'Androgen levels in adult females: changes with age, menopause and oophorectomy'. *Clinical Endocrinology and Metabolism* 90(7): 3847-53.

Dennerstein, L (2004). 'A population-based study of depressed mood in middle-aged, Australian-born women'. *Menopause:*

the *Journal of the North American Menopause Society* 11(5): 563-8.

Dennerstein, L (2004). 'Mood and Menopause'. Conference Coverage, based on selected sessions at the 2nd World Congress on Women's Mental Health, Washington, DC March 17-20. *Medscape General Medicine*. Available online: http://www.medscape.com/viewarticle/473294.

Dickerson, L M et al (2003). 'Premenstrual syndrome'. *American Family Physician* 67(8): 1743-52.

Dimeo, F et al (2001). 'Benefits From Aerobic Exercise in Patients With Major Depression: A Pilot Study'. *British Journal of Sports Medicine* 35(2): 114-7.

Dimitrova, KR et al (2002). 'Estrogen and homocysteine'. *Cardiovascular Research* 53(3): 577-88.

Dormire, SL (2003). 'What we know about managing menopausal hot flashes: navigating without a compass'. *JOGN Nursing: Journal of Obstetric, Gynecologic & Neonatal Nursing* 2(4): 455-64.

Dragisic, KG and Milad, MP (2004). 'Sexual functioning and patient expectations of sexual functioning after hysterectomy'. *American Journal of Obstetrics & Gynecology* 190(5): 1416-18.

'Dyspareunia in women' (2002). The American Heritage® *Stedman's Medical Dictionary*.

Edmonds, M et al (2004). 'Exercise therapy for chronic fatigue syndrome'. *Cochrane Database of Systematic Reviews* (3): CD003200.

El-Toukhy, TA et al (2004). 'The effect of different types of hysterectomy on urinary and sexual functions: a prospective study'. *Journal of Obstetrics & Gynaecology* 24(4): 420-5.

Evans, MK et al (2005). 'Management of postmenopausal hot flashes with venalaxifine hydrochloride: a randomized controlled trial'. *Obstetrics & Gynecology* 105(1): 2059-63.

Farrell, S A & Kieser, K (2000). 'Sexuality after hysterectomy'. *Obstetrics & Gynecology* 95(6 Part 2): 1045-51.

Fettes, I (1999). 'Migraine in the Menopause'. *Neurology* 53(4), Supplement 1.

Freedman, R and Roehrs, T (2007). 'Sleep disturbances in menopause'. Menopause: *The Journal of the North American Menopause Society* 14(5):826-9

Freeman, EW (2004). 'Hormones and menopausal status as predictors of depression in women in transition to menopause'. *Archives of General Psychiatry* 61(1): 62-70.

Fuchs, KO et al (2003). 'The effects of an estrogen and glycolic acid cream on the facial skin of postmenopausal women: a randomized histologic study'. *Cutis* 71(6): 481-8.

Fugate, WN (2004). 'Prostate cancer: A Family Affair'. *Menopause Management* 13(3): 12-13.

Fuh, JL et al (2006). 'A longitudinal study of cognition change during menopausal transition in a rural community'. *Maturitas* 53(4): 447-53.

Garcia, C (2003). 'The influence of specific noradrenergic and serotonergic lesions on the expression of hippocampal brain-derived neurotrophic factor transcripts following voluntary physical activity'. *Neuroscience* 119(3): 721-32.

Gladstone, HB (2000). 'Efficacy of Hydroquinone Cream (USP 4%) Used Alone or in Combination with Salicylic Acid Peels in Improving Photodamage on the Neck and Upper Chest'. *Dermatologic Surgery* 26(4): 333.

Gracis, C et al (2004). 'Predictors of decreased libido in women during the late reproductive years'. *Menopause: the Journal of the North American Menopause Society* 11(2): 144-150.

Graesslin, O et al (2002). 'Local investigation concerning psychic and sexual functioning a short time after hysterectomy'. *Gynecology Obstetrique & Fertilité* 30(6): 474-82.

Greene, RA and Dixon, W (2002). 'The role of reproductive hormones in maintaining cognition'. *Obstetrics & Gynecology* 29(3).

Hansen, CJ et al (2001). 'Exercise Duration and Mood State: How Much is Enough to Feel Better?' *Gynecology Obstetrique & Fertilité* 20(4): 267-75.

Harlow, BL et al (2003). 'Depression and its influence on reproductive endocrine and menstrual cycle markers associated with perimenopause: the Harvard Study of Moods and Cycles'. *Archives of General Psychiatry* 60(1): 29-36.

Henderson, V (2004). 'Only a Matter of Time? Hormone Therapy and Cognition'. *Menopause: the Journal of the North American Menopause Society* 12(1): 1-3.

Henderson, VW and Sherwin, BB (2007). 'Surgical versus natural menopause: cognitive issues.' *Menopause: The Journal of the North American Menopause Society* 14(7): 572-579.

Henderson, VW (2006) 'Estrogen-containing hormone therapy and Alzheimer's disease risk: understanding discrepant inferences from observational and experimental research'. *Neuroscience* 138(3): 1031-9.

Herlitz, A et al (2007). 'Endogenous estrogen is not associated with cognitive performance before, during or after menopause'. *Menopause: The Journal of the North American Menopause Society* 14(3): 425-31.

Hewer, W et al (2003). 'Short-term effects of improved glycemic control on cognitive function in patients with type 2 diabetes'. *Gerontology* 49(2): 86-92.

Humphries, K and Gill, S (2003). 'Risks and benefits of hormone replacement therapy: The evidence speaks'. *Canadian Medical Association Journal* 168(8).

Hung, M (2003). 'Low dose DHEA increases androgen, estrogen levels in menopause'. *Medscape General Medicine*. Available online: http://www.medscape.com/viewarticle/465827.

Huppert, FA and Van Niekerk, JK (2003). 'Dehydroepiandrosterone (DHEA) supplementation for cognitive function'. *Cochrane Review Abstract*.

'Hysterectomy and your sexual response'. The Women's Sexual Health Foundation.

International Longevity Center USA (2001). 'Scientists advise older people how to maintain mental capacities'.

Ishunina, TA and Swaab, DF (2007) 'Alterations in the human brain in menopause' *Maturitas* 57(1)20-2

Joffee, H et al (2006). 'Estrogen therapy selectively enhances prefrontal cognitive processes: a randomized, double-blind placebo-controlled study with functional magnetic resonance imaging in perimenopausal and recently postmenopausal women'. *Menopause: The Journal of the North American Menopause Society* 13(3): 411-22.

Jones, JM (1999). 'Transformed Migraine'. *Clinician Reviews* 9(11): 67-9, 72-4, 77-80, 83.

Juska, J (2003). *A Round-heeled Woman: My Late-Life Adventures in Sex and Romance*. London: Chatto & Windus.

Kalantaridou, SN et al (2004). 'Reproductive functions of corticotropin-releasing hormone. Research and potential clinical utility of antalarmins (CRH receptor type 1 antagonists)'. *American Journal of Reproductive Immunology* 51(4): 269-74.

Kang, J et al (2004). 'Postmenopausal hormone therapy and risk of cognitive decline in community-dwelling women'. *Neurology* 63(1).

Katz, A (2002). 'Sexuality after hysterectomy'. *JOGN Nursing: Journal of Obstetric, Gynecologic & Neonatal Nursing* 31(3): 256-62.

Kennan, RP et al (2005). 'Human cerebral blood flow and metabolism in acute insulin-induced hypoglycemia'. *Journal of Cerebral Blood Flow & Metabolism* 25(4): 527-34.

Kerwin, J et al (2007). 'The variable response of women with menopausal hot flashes when treated with sertraline'. *Menopause: The Journal of the North American Menopause Society*. 14(5): 841-45.

Kim, DH et al (2003). 'Alteration of sexual function after classic intrafascial supracervical hysterectomy and total hysterectomy'. *Journal of the American Association of Gynecologic Laparoscopists* 10(1): 60-4.

Kinetin. Monograph. Natural Medicines Comprehensive Database, 10 March 2005. Available online: http://www.NaturalDatabase.com.

Kingsberg, S (2006). 'Prevalence of hypoactive sexual desire disorder in postmenopausal women: results from the WISHeS Trial'. *Menopause: The Journal of the North American Menopause Society* 13(1): 10-11.

Kingsberg, SA (2004). 'Helping Couples Cope with Prostate Cancer: The Role of the Gynaecologist'. *Menopause Management* 3: 14-17.

Knechtle, B (2004). 'Influence of physical activity on mental well-being and psychiatric disorders'. Schweizerische Rundschau Fuer Medizin *Praxis* 93(35): 1403-11.

Kockler, D and McCarthy, M (2004). 'Antidepressants as a Treatment for Hot Flashes in Women'. *American Journal of Health-System Pharmacy* 61(3): 287-92.

Kok, H et al (2006). 'Cognitive function across the life course and the menopausal transition'. *Menopause: The Journal of the North American Menopause Society* 13(1): 19-27.

Komisaruk, BR and Whipple, B (1998). 'Love as sensory stimulation: physiological consequences of its deprivation and expression'. *Psychoneuroendocrinology* 23(8): 927-44.

Krystal, AD (2004). 'Gonadal Hormone-Related Insomnia in Women'. *Medscape Primary Care* 6(1). Available online: http://www.medscape.com/viewarticle/478995.

Landy, S (2004). 'Migraine throughout the life cycle: treatment through the ages'. *Neurology* 62(5).

LeBlanc, E (2004). 'Hormone Therapy with oestrogen or oestrogen plus progesterone decreases cognitive function in older postmenopausal women'. *Evidence-based Healthcare and Public Health* 8(6).

LeBlanc, E et al (2007). 'Hot flashes and estrogen therapy do not influence cognition in early menopausal women'. *Menopause: The Journal of the North American Menopause Society* 14(2): 191-202.

Leiblum, S et al (1983). 'Vaginal Atrophy in the postmenopausal woman: the importance of sexual activity and hormones'. *Journal of the American Medical Association* 249(2): 195-8.

Leiblum, S et al (2006). 'Hypoactive sexual desire disorder in post-menopausal women: US results from the Women's International Study of Health and Sexuality (WISHeS)'. *Menopause: The Journal of the North American Menopause Society* 13(1): 46-56.

Loprinzi, CL (2006). 'New anti-depressants inhibit hot flashes', *Menopause: The Journal of the American Medicine Association* 13(4): 546-48.

Lukacs, JL et al (2004). 'Midlife Women's response to a Hospital Sleep Challenge: Age and Menopause Effects on Sleep Architecture'. *Journal of Women's Health* 13(3): 333-40.

MacLennan, A et al (2006). 'Hormone therapy, timing of intervention, and cognition in women older than 60 years: the REMEMBER pilot study'. *Menopause: The Journal of the North American Menopause Society* 13(1): 28-36.

Malouf Obermeyer, C and Sievert, L (2007). 'Cross-cultural comparisons: midlife aging and menopause'. *Menopause: The Journal of the North American Menopause Society* 14(4): 663-67.

Marks, SJ et al (2002). 'Estrogen replacement therapy for cognitive benefits: viable treatment or forgettable senior moment?' *Heart Disease & Stroke* 4(1): 26-32.

Martin, VT and Behbehani, M (2006). 'Ovarian hormones and migraine headaches: understanding mechanisms and pathogenesis-Part 2'. *Headache* 46(3): 365-86

Mazza, E et al (1999). 'Dehydroepiandroserone Sulfate levels in women. Relationships with age, body mass index and insulin levels'. *Journal of Endocrinological Investigation* 22(9): 681-7.

Medscape Conference Coverage, based on selected sessions at the International Society for Sexual Impotence research 11th World Congress (ISSIR) Female Sexual Dysfunction. *Medscape General Medicine*. Available online: http://www.medscape.com/viewprogram/3515.

Meyer, PM et al (2003). 'A population-based longitudinal study of cognitive functioning in the menopausal transition'. *Neurology* 61(6).

Meyer, PM et al (2003). 'A population-based longitudinal study of cognitive function in the menopausal transition'. *Neurology* 61(66): 801-6

Mitchell, JL et al (2003). 'Postmenopaual hormone therapy and its associations with cognitive impairment'. *Archives of Internal Medicine* 163(20): 2485-90.

Monheit, GD (2004). 'Chemical peels'. *Skin Therapy Letter* 9(2): 6-11. Available online: www.skintherapyletter.com.

Morales, AJ et al (1998). 'The effect of six months treatment with a 100 mg daily dose of dehydroepiandrosterone (DHEA) on circulating sex steroids, body composition and muscle strength in age-advanced men and women'. *Clinical Endocrinology (Oxford)* 49(4): 421-32.

Morley, JE and Kaiser, FE (2003). 'Female sexuality'. *Medical Clinics of North America* 87(5): 1077-90.

Morrison, MF et al (2004). 'Lack of efficacy of estradiol for depression in postmenopausal women: a randomized controlled trial'. *Biology & Psychiatry* 55: 406-12.

Muller, EE (2001). 'Steroids, cognitive processes and aging'. *Recenti Progressi in Medicina* 92(5): 362-72.

Nappi, RE (2006). 'Different effects of Tibolone and low dose EPT in the management of postmenopausal women with primary headaches'. *Menopause: The Journal of the North American Menopause Society* 13(5): 818-25.

National Cancer Institute. U.S. National Institutes of Health. 'Skin Cancer'. Available online: http://www.cancer.gov.

Nilsson, LG et al (2004) 'A prospective cohort study on memory, health and aging'. *Aging Neuropsychology & Cognition* 11(3): 134-48.

Nordberg, A (2003). 'Toward an early diagnosis and treatment of Alzheimer's disease'. *International Psychogeriatrics* 15(3): 223-37.

Owens, JF et al (2002). 'Cognitive function effects of suppressing ovarian hormones in young women'. *Menopause: the Journal of the North American Menopause Society* 9(4): 221-3.

Pine, A (2006). 'The healing properties of exercise'. *Menopause: The Journal of the North American Menopause Society* 13(4): 544-45

Pray, WS (2001). 'Self-Treatment for Minor Eye Conditions'. *US Pharmacist* 26(12).

Regenstein, QR et al (2004). 'Self reported sleep in postmenopausal women'. *Menopause: the Journal of the North American Menopause Society* 11(2): 198-207.

Regestein, QR (2006). 'Hot flashes and sleep'. *Menopause: The Journal of the North American Menopause Society* 13 (4): 549-52.

Resnick, SM and Maki, PM (2001). 'Effects of hormone replacement therapy on cognitive and brain aging'. *Annals of the New York Academy of Sciences* 949: 203-14.

Rhodes, JC et al (1999). 'Hysterectomy and sexual functioning'. *Journal of the American Medical Association* 282(20): 1934-41.

Roussis, NP et al (2004). 'Sexual response in the patient after hysterectomy: total abdominal versus supracervical versus vaginal procedure'. *American Journal of Obstetrics & Gynecology* 90(5): 1427-8.

Sall, K et al (2000). 'Two multicenter, randomized Studies of the efficacy and safety of cylosporine ophthalmic emulsion in moderate to severe dry eye disease'. *Opthalmology* 107(4): 631-39.

Sanel, P (2006). 'Testosterone therapy for postmenopausal decline in sexual desire: implications for a new study'. *Menopause: The Journal of the North American Menopause Society* 328-30.

Schorr, M (2004). 'Coenzyme Q 10 may ward off migraine attacks'. *Medscape Ob/Gyn & Women's Health*. Available online: http://www.medscape.com/viewarticle/474831?src=mp.

Schumacher, M et al (2003). 'Steroid hormones and neurosteroids in normal and pathological aging of the nervous system'. *Progress in Neurobiology (Oxford)* 71(1): 3-29.

Schwarz, S (2007) 'Menopause and determinants of quality of life in women at midlife and beyond: the Study of Health in Pomerania (SHIP)'. *Menopause: The Journal of the North American Menopause Society* 14(1): 123-34.

Shifren, JL and Avis, NE (2007). 'Surgical menopause: effects on psychological well-being and sexuality'. *Menopause: The Journal of the North American Menopause Society* 14(3): 586-91.

Shumaker, SA et al (2004). 'Conjugated Equine Estrogens and Incidence of Probable Dementia and Mild Cognitive Impairment in Postmenopausal Women: Women's Health Initiative Memory Study'. *Journal of the American Medical Association* 291(24): 2947-8.

Shumaker, SA et al (2004). Hormone therapy does not prevent cognitive decline or dementia in older women: WHIMS data. *NAMS First to Know.* PART B.

Stearns, V and Hayes, DF (2002). 'Cooling off hot flashes'. *Journal of Clinical Oncology* 20: 1436-8.

Suckling, J et al (2004). 'Local oestrogen for vaginal atrophy in postmenopausal women'. (Cochrane Review) in: *The Cochrane Library* 3. Chichester: John Wiley & Sons, Ltd.

Suzuki, T et al (2004). 'Mechanisms involved in apoptosis of human macrophages induced by lipopolysaccharide from Actinobacillus actinomycetemcomitans in the presence of cycloheximide'. *Infection & Immunity* 72(4): 1856-65.

Thurston, R et al (2006). 'Physical activity and risk of vasomotor symptoms in women with and without a history of depression: results from the Harvard Study of Moods and Cycles'. *Menopause: The Journal of the North American Menopause Society* 13(4): 553-60.

Toran-Allerand, CD (2004) 'Estrogen and the brain: Beyond ER-alpha and ER-beta'. *Experimental Gerontology* 1052: 136-44.

Tuohy, W. 'Sexual Healing in Life's Autumn'. *The Age.* Available online: http://www.theage.com.au.

Utian, W (2005). 'Problems with Desire and Arousal in Surgically Menopausal Women: Advances in Assessment, Diagnosis and Treatment'. *Menopause Management* 14(1): 10-22.

Vartanian, AJ and Dayan, SH (2005). 'Complications of botulinum toxin. A use in facial rejuvenation'. *Facial Plastic Surgery Clinics of North America Journal* 13(1): 1-10.

Vegeto, E et al (2004). Regulation of the lipopolysaccharide signal transduction pathway by 17β-estradiol in macrophage cells. *Journal of Steroid Biochemistry & Molecular Biology* 91(1- 2): 59-66.

Vermeer, S et al (2003). 'Silent brain infarcts and the risk of dementia and cognitive decline'. *New England Journal of Medicine* 348: 1215-22.

Weill-Engerer, S et al (2002). 'Neurosteroid quantification in human brain regions: comparison between Alzheimer's and nondemented patients'. *Journal of Clinical Endocrinology & Metabolism* 87(11): 5138-43.

Weill-Engerer, S et al (2003). 'In vitro metabolism of dehydroepi-androsterone (DHEA) to 7alpha-hydroxy-DHEA and Delta5-androstene-3β, 17β-diol in specific regions of the aging brain from Alzheimer's and non-demented patients'. *Brain Research* 969(1-2): 117-25.

Wolf, OT (2003). 'Cognitive functions and sex steroids'. *Annales d'Endocrinologie (Paris)* 64(2): 158-61.

Yazbeck, C (2004). 'Sexual function following hysterectomy'. *Gynecology Obstetrique & Fertilité* 32(1): 49-54.

Zee, P (2004). 'Expert Column: Insomnia and Menopause'. *Medscape Ob/Gyn & Women's Health.* Available online: http://www.medscape.com/viewarticle/484767.

Zobbe, V et al (2004). 'Sexuality after total vs. subtotal hysterectomy'. *Acta Obstetricia et Gynecologica Scandinavica* 83(2): 191-6.

Available Online

http://www.cdc.gov/nccdphp/drh/Africa_pdf/Chap_10.pdf

http://www.answers.com/polymer&r=67

http://www.citihealth.com/forsha/neova_.htm

http://en.mimi.hu/beauty/glycolic_acid.html

And Finally ...

Thank you to all my extraordinary friends for their help and encouragement during this odyssey. My particular gratitude to Celia (screaming 'No, no, no! Five more chapters!'), who made the supreme sacrifice, cheerfully lending me her husband, Mervyn Jacobson, for endless hours, and who helped me clarify the diagrams by drawing them so well, and to Bev, who with constant kindness distracted me, soothed me and put me back on track with many illicit cups of coffee. For their unique contribution, thank you too to Marina, Paula, Naomi, Helena, Marilyn, Kathy and Michelle.

Thanks to all the women whose stories are the hooks on which each chapter is hung. Their names have been changed and some of the anecdotes are composites, but the stories are all true and vivid examples of how women battle to come to terms with menopause.

This book and the first edition owe their existence to the faith of Alison Lowry, the chief executive of Penguin Books South Africa, who appreciated the need for it and gave me invaluable advice; to Pam Thornley, senior editor, who with kindness and warmth nursed me through the birth pangs and who is responsible for the indices; and to Jane Ranger for co-ordinating the first edition. Claire Heckrath's vision and sense of style helped to create the beautiful new cover for the second edition.

The editor of the first edition, Pat Tucker, helped me clarify my thoughts and ideas and applied her obsession with detail and consistency to a manuscript which required meticulous attention, given the complex nature of the subject. In a remarkably short time, with great humour and tolerance, especially given my predilection for clichés, she contributed to making this the book I had imagined it could be.

The task of revising and updating this edition has been made infinitely easier by the enthusiasm and meticulous attention of my editor, Gemma Harries. With good humour, patience and her much-appreciated talent for returning my constant calls and e-mails promptly, she laid my angst to rest, working speedily and thoroughly to ensure that this process was not only stress-free but fun.

Thank you to Caroline Molema for helping my life to run smoothly.

My daughters Sophie and Elizabeth have strengthened me with their ongoing love and pride in my achievements; menopause is not in their ambit and certain passages in this book have elicited shrieks of laughter, but they are my most vocal fans. My husband Nicholas has encouraged me in every turn my career has taken. He had absolute faith in me and in this book and without his nagging and his belief in me it might never have been written. He read every word and became my most valued critic. He also supported and calmed me when it all seemed too difficult.

Index

of hot flushes 122; regimens 77, 78-9; research findings 36-7; side effects 33-4; systemic ET/EPT 78; when indicated 56-7

Hormones: 16-26, 279; bioidentical 63-6; control of levels of production 19; fluctuation during perimenopause 10-12; imbalance in perimenopause 26

Hot flushes: 4, 50, 74, 114-25; after surgically induced menopause 116, 130; HT in management of 122; in relation to core body temperature 117; in relation to lifestyle 119-20; in relation to smoking and exercise 120-1; prevalence of 119

Human epidermal growth factor 165

Human papilloma virus (HPV) 179

Hydroquinone 248

Hypercalcemia 192, 279

Hypertension: 146-7; ACE inhibitors 146; beta blockers 147; systolic and diastolic pressure 146

Hyperthyroidism 24, 279

Hypocalcemia 192, 279

Hypothalamus: 7, 279; role in hormone secretion 17

Hypothyroidism 24, 279

Hysterectomy: 125-34, 172, 239-40, 279, 282; reasons for 129-30; surgical methods 128; total hysterectomy 127-8, 283; Wertheim's hysterectomy 180

Hysteroscopy 126, 280

Insomnia during menopause 241-2

Insulin 25-56, 212-3

Insulin-like growth factor 1 (IGF1) 69

Insulin resistance syndrome 26, 212-5. *See also* Metabolic syndrome

Intellectual functioning in menopause 251-4. *See also* Memory loss in menopause

International Menopause Society (IMS) 50, 139

Intrauterine device 180

Iron 95

Journal of the American Medical Association 44, 136, 270

Kinerase 248

Lancet, The 44, 270

Laparoscope 128, 132, 280

Laparoscopy 126, 128, 132, 133, 280

Laparotomy 132, 280

LDL 136, 144, 145

Letrozole 172, 173, 174

Libido, decreased: 67-8; caused by depression 258

Lifestyle: & mind 52, 54; & type 2 diabetes 214; & weight 209, 211, 219

Lignans, 280. *See also* Plant estrogens.

Linoleic acid. *See* Omega-6 fatty acids.

Linolenic acid. *See* Omega-3 fatty acids.

Linseed 106

Lipoproteins: 144, 148; lipoprotein(a) 148

Low density lipoproteins. *See* LDL.

Luteinising hormone 7, 173

Luteinising hormone-releasing hormone analogue 173

Lymphatic system 152

Lymph nodes 152, 155

Lymph vessels 152